THE VENTRICULAR SEPTUM OF THE HEART

BOERHAAVE SERIES
FOR POSTGRADUATE
MEDICAL EDUCATION
Vol. 21

PROCEEDINGS OF BOERHAAVE COURSES
ORGANIZED BY
THE FACULTY OF MEDICINE, UNIVERSITY OF LEIDEN,
THE NETHERLANDS

THE VENTRICULAR SEPTUM OF THE HEART

edited by

ARNOLD C.G. WENINK
Department of Anatomy and Embryology, University of Leiden

ARENTJE OPPENHEIMER-DEKKER
Department of Anatomy and Embryology, University of Leiden

ANDRÉ J. MOULAERT
Wilhelmina Children's Hospital, University of Utrecht

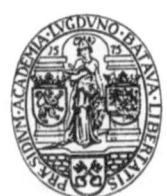

1981

LEIDEN UNIVERSITY PRESS

THE HAGUE / BOSTON / LONDON

Distributors:

for the United States and Canada

Kluwer Boston, Inc.
190 Old Derby Street
Hingham, MA 02043
USA

for all other countries

Kluwer Academic Publishers Group
Distribution Center
P.O. Box 322
3300 AH Dordrecht
The Netherlands

Library of Congress Cataloging in Publication Data   CIP

Main entry under title:

The ventricular septum of the heart.

(Boerhaave series for postgraduate medical education; v. 21)
Includes index.
1. Ventricular septal defects.   2. Heart septum.   I. Wenink, Arnold C.G.   II. Oppenheimer-Dekker, Arentje   III. Moulaert, André J.   IV. series.
RC685.V46V46   616.1'2   81-13727   ACCR2

ISBN-13:978-94-009-8626-8   e-ISBN-13:978-94-009-8624-4
DOI: 10.1007/978-94-009-8624-4

PREFACE

There continue to be disagreements concerning the embryology of the ventricular septum and the nomenclature of its various parts, as well as on its phylogenetic derivation. It must be obvious that until such time as these uncertainties have been resolved it will not be possible to understand the pathogenesis of ventricular septal defects and other anomalies involving the ventricular septum.

In an effort to clarify some of these difficulties a number of individuals, including anatomists, embryologists, pathologists, cardiologists, and surgeons, all acknowledged experts in their respective fields of endeavor, were invited to present their views and concepts in sessions devoted to the ventricular septum. In this "Boerhaave Course", detailed descriptions of the normal anatomy, embryology, and phylogeny of the septum were followed by papers on ventricular septal defects, atrioventricular defects, straddling valves, and various forms of univentricular heart. Major contributions were made through clinical accounts of these anomalies.

This course again clearly demonstrated the value of and the need for a multidisciplinary approach to the recognition, understanding, diagnosis, and management of congenital cardiac disease. While obviously it could not be expected that all of the problems and uncertainties concerning the normal and abnormal ventricular septum would be resolved, the lively and frank discussions among all participants of the course undoubtedly contributed to a better understanding of the still existing difficulties. All of the contributors to this monograph should be congratulated for a job superbly well done.

LODEWIJK H.S. VAN MIEROP
Gainesville, Florida

CONTENTS

CONTRIBUTORS

Anderson, Robert H. Cardiothoracic Institute, Brompton Hospital, London, U.K.

Becker, Anton E. Department of Pathology, Wilhelmina Gasthuis, Amsterdam, The Netherlands

Bruins, Caroline L.D.C. Department of Pediatric Cardiology, University Hospital, Leiden, The Netherlands

Draulans-Noë, H.A. Yvonne. Department of Pediatric Cardiology, University Hospital, Leiden, The Netherlands

Dumoulin, H. Department of Pediatric Cardiology, University Hospital Gasthuisberg, Leuven, Belgium

Duncan, Walter. Cardiology Department, The Hospital for Sick Children, Toronto, Ontario, Canada

Freedom, Robert. Cardiology Department, The Hospital for Sick Children, Toronto, Ontario, Canada

Gittenberger-de Groot, Adriana C. Department of Anatomy, University of Leiden, Leiden, The Netherlands

Hall, D. Department of Pediatric Cardiology, Deutsches Herzzentrum, München, F.R.G.

Harder, Joyce. Cardiology Department, The Hospital for Sick Children, Toronto, Ontario, Canada

Harinck, Eric. Department of Pediatric Cardiology, Wilhelmina Children's Hospital, University of Utrecht, Utrecht, The Netherlands

Ho, Siew Yen. Cardiothoracic Institute, Brompton Hospital, London, U.K.

Kutsche, Lynn M. Department of Pediatrics (Cardiology), University of Florida College of Medicine, Gainesville, Florida, U.S.A.

Ligtvoet-Gussenhoven, Elma. Thorax Center, Erasmus University, Rotterdam, The Netherlands

Middelhoff, Charles J.F.M. Department of Pathology, Wilhelmina Gasthuis, Amsterdam, The Netherlands

Moulaert, André J. Department of Pediatric Cardiology, Wilhelmina Children's Hospital, University of Utrecht, Utrecht, The Netherlands

Oppenheimer-Dekker, Arentje. Department of Anatomy, University of Leiden, Leiden, The Netherlands

Rowe, Richard. Cardiology Department, The Hospital for Sick Children, Toronto, Ontario, Canada

Sahn, David J. Department of Pediatrics, University of Arizona Health Sciences Center, Tucson, Arizona, U.S.A.

Sauer, Ursula. Department of Pediatric Cardiology, Deutsches Herzzentrum, München, F.R.G.

Van der Hauwaert, Luc G. Department of Pediatric Cardiology, University Hospital Gasthuisberg, Leuven, Belgium

Van Mierop, Lodewijk H.S. Department of Pediatrics (Cardiology), University of Florida College of Medicine, Gainesville, Florida, U.S.A.

Van Mill, Gertjan J. Department of Pediatric Cardiology, Wilhelmina Children's Hospital, University of Utrecht, Utrecht, The Netherlands

Voogd, Paul J. Department of Cardiology, University Hospital, Leiden, The Netherlands

Wenink, Arnold C.G. Department of Anatomy, University of Leiden, Leiden, The Netherlands

INTRODUCTION

In recent years, the study of the normal heart and of hearts with congenital malformations has led to more detailed knowledge of the anatomy, while new studies on development have provided more understanding of many anomalies. At the same time, refinement of existing diagnostic techniques and development of new methods have given pediatric cardiology the facility of gaining more detailed information from the living patient.

In the light of these advances, it was felt valuable to gather workers from different disciplines around a single topic and make as close a correlation among the different kinds of information as possible. The topic chosen was the ventricular septum, the development and the structure of which were discussed in the setting of normal and malformed hearts. The discussions took place at the Boerhaave Course on "The Ventricular Septum", held in Leiden, 12–13 June 1980. Most of the contributions to the course are included in the present volume.

An important feature of this book is the approach to congenital malformations of the septum, which may well be illustrated with the ventricular septal defect. Although the site and size of a defect are important features, it is still more valuable to know how the ventricular septum itself is built up in the case of a defect and how this buildup has to be correlated with the normal anatomy of the septum. This is a profitable approach since it has appeared that the septum is composed of several embryologically distinct constituents and that each of these constituents may grow out differently in malformed hearts. These facts seem to be in favor of complete and direct understanding among those who are working in different fields of investigation. But since no discussions on terms and definitions appear to have been final, every chance of misunderstanding has remained.

In this volume, we have chosen not to prescribe one set of terms all too rigorously. It should be appreciated that not every morphological detail is equally well distinguishable in the pathological specimen and in the living patient. Thus, the ventricular septum is known to have inlet and outlet (or infundibular) components, while a third component occupies the space between them. The boundaries between these components, however, have still to be defined. In the normal heart, the infundibular (or outlet) septum merges imperceptibly with the anterior (or bulboventricular or trabecular) septum. If for this latter component the term "trabecular septum" were chosen, then this term should not be taken in the most descriptive sense. First of all, the inlet septum also shows trabeculations while, secondly, the anterior septal component is not trabeculated to its full extent. Any meaningful distinction between infundibular and trabecular septal components should be applicable to both congenitally malformed and normal hearts. In the so-called "infundibular malalignment defect" it may be seen that the infundibular septum is a relatively small component, whereas the anterior (trabecular) septum is much larger and has both trabeculated and smooth portions. We have no specific term to indicate the boundary between these two portions but, evidently, this boundary should not be mistaken for the (invisible) boundary between the trabecular and infundibular septa of the normal heart.

On the other hand, most of the present contributors agree that the posterior boundary of the anterior (trabecular) septum is formed by the trabecula septomarginalis, the inlet septum being that component that borders upon the trabecula septomarginalis and that holds the tension apparatus of the septal leaflet of the tricuspid valve. But in the living patient, it may be difficult to identify the trabecula septomarginalis with certainty and identification of the complete tension apparatus seems to be impossible.

If one wants to stress the developmental background of the anterior (trabecular) septum, this component may be called the "bulboventricular septum". However, this term might cause confusion because, until now, there has been no general agreement as to the exact contribution of the embryonic bulbus to the adult left and right ventricles, nor is it generally understood that the term "embryonic ventricle" stands widely apart from the terms "right and left ventricles" as applicable to the normal adult heart. An additional problem is that the term "bulbus" is not universally used in the same sense by embryologists, and that different terms are currently used for the same structure.

We believe that our first aim in the near future should be a general agreement on nomenclature of the embryonic, the normal adult, and the congenitally malformed heart. In the present book, we have aimed at full comparability of the different terms used, without imposing one nomenclature upon the contributors.

In spite of the above problems, or perhaps rather on the basis of them, all contributors to this book have to be credited with their invaluable efforts to create a book which we hope will prove its value.

ARNOLD C.G. WENINK
ARENTJE OPPENHEIMER-DEKKER
ANDRÉ J. MOULAERT

1. MYOCARDIAL ARCHITECTURE OF THE VENTRICULAR SEPTUM

ARENTJE OPPENHEIMER-DEKKER

In textbooks on the anatomy of the heart, the morphological features of the ventricular septum are traditionally incorporated in the descriptions of the right and left ventricles. This is not surprising, for, although it is true that embryologically the ventricular septum has its own developmental background, the mature septum is a partition wall common to both chambers. In stating this, it is important to stipulate the fact that this quality of belonging to both chambers is not applicable over the whole extent of the septum. This, in turn, is related to the general buildup of the ventricles which, therefore, should be drawn into the picture. In the apical and the inflow (inlet) portions of the septum, the common character is clearly recognizable despite the differences in septal surface and even the demarcation of the borderlines with the free walls of the ventricles is not difficult. In the subarterial (outflow) regions, however, these points are less obvious due to a certain extent of divergence of the outflow tracts which makes the anatomical relationships more complicated both with regard to the exact demarcation of the portion which is really common to both left and right ventricular outflow tracts and to the precise localization of the transition into the free walls of the ventricles.

In defining the components of the mature ventricular septum macroscopically and without having dissected the septum, it is, in the nature of things, necessary to distinguish between the left ventricular aspect and the right ventricular aspect of the septum. It is not without significance that the descriptions of the septal components and characteristics differ largely depending upon whether the right or the left side is in the picture. Each chamber has its own markings influencing the morphology of its septal surface and a good knowledge of the various landmarks is important in enabling the investigator to differentiate between the various types of congenital cardiac anomalies in which the ventricular septum, or part thereof, is involved in the malformation.

As seen from the left ventricular side, the septal surface looks rather straight, regularly built, rather smooth without protrusions, especially in its anterior basilar portion, and it does not possess direct attachments to the papillary muscles of the mitral valve (Fig. 1a). Anterior to the membranous septum (which is found at the site of the junctional zone between the non-coronary and the right coronary semilunar cusps of the aortic valve) is the

A.C.G. Wenink et al. (eds.) The Ventricular Septum of the Heart, *1–8. All rights reserved.*
Copyright ©1981 by Martinus Nijhoff Publishers, The Hague/Boston/London.

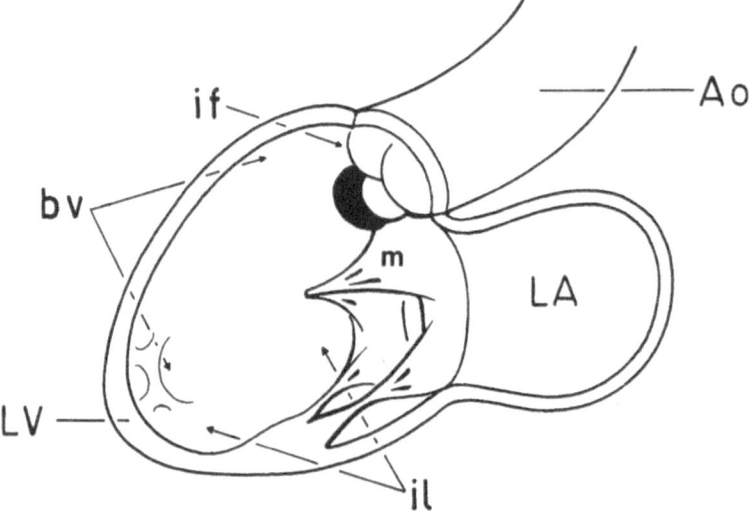

Fig. 1a. (Cf. Figure 1 of Chapter 6.) Schematic drawing of left aspect of ventricular septum and adjacent structures: Ao, aorta; LA, left atrium; LV, left ventricle; bv, bulboventricular septum; if, infundibular septum; il, inlet septum; m, mitral valve. The anterolateral papillary muscle is not in the drawing, because its insertion is less close to the septum than that of the posteromedial papillary muscle. The membranous septum is indicated in black.

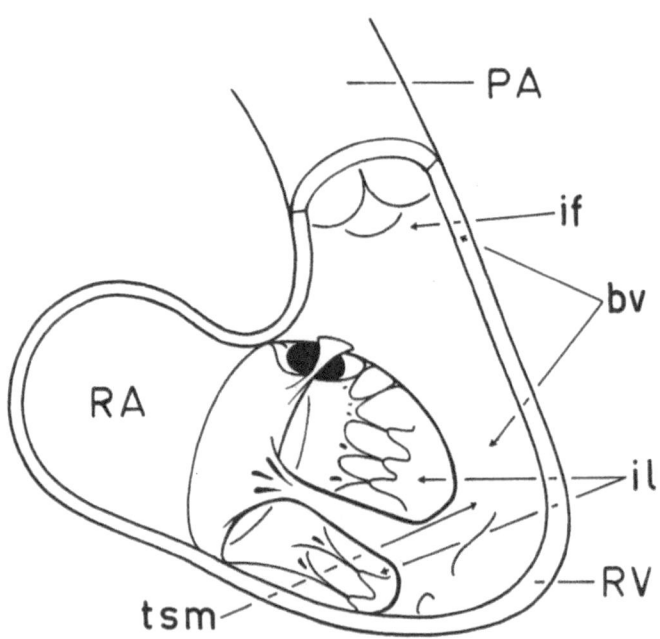

Fig. 1b. Schematic drawing of right aspect of ventricular septum and adjacent structures: PA, pulmonary artery; RA, right atrium; RV, right ventricle; tsm, trabecula septomarginalis. Further abbreviations as in Figure 1a. The membranous septum is indicated in black. Note the close relationship of the tricuspid valvular apparatus with the inlet septum.

location of the infundibular and the bulboventricular (anterior) parts of the ventricular septum. The infundibular septum is that septal component which separates the aortic and pulmonic orifices. This is but a small portion of the ventricular septum, because the arterial orifices, i.e., the valve rings, contact each other only in the region of the commissure between the right and left coronary aortic semilunar cusps, on the one hand, and in the area between the posterior and left anterior pulmonic semilunar cusps, on the other hand. The bulboventricular septum is the oblong anterior component of the septum, also comprising the apical region, with its basilar tip extending till in front of the infundibular septum. The left ventricular surface of this tip is usually very small. It often has a slight sinistroventral curvature and it does not really border on any aortic semilunar cusp. The latter features are related to the developmental processes in the anterior and basilar portions of the bulboventricular fold as described by Wenink in Chapter 3 of this book.

The borderlines between the infundibular and the bulboventricular septal components cannot be indicated in normal left ventricles. Neither is it possible to recognize the borderline between the bulboventricular component and the inlet septum, which is the posteroinferior part of the ventricular

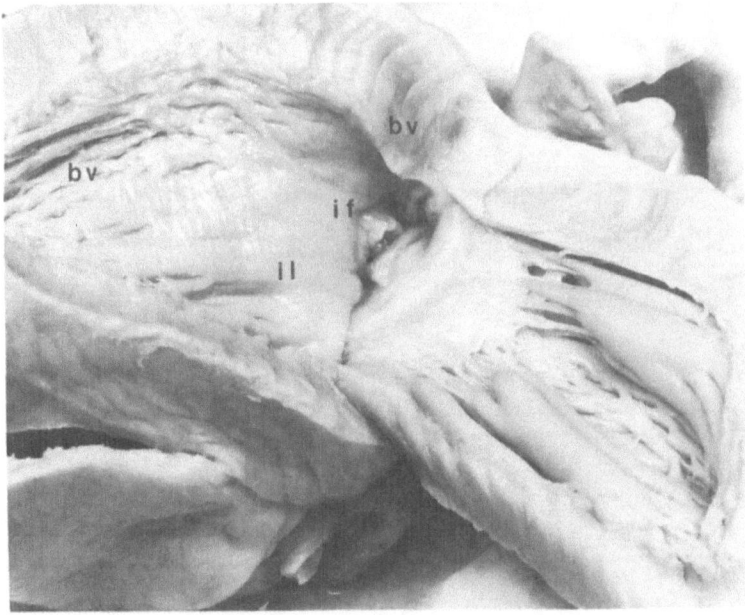

Fig. 2. Normal left ventricle. The incision has been made in a plane parallel to the main part of the ventricular septum and therefore the sinistroventricular curve in the basilar part of the bulboventricular septum has been cut. The anterior portion of the anterior mitral leaflet extends to the anterior border of the left ventricle, and is in this specimen continuous with part of the left coronary cusp and with the noncoronary cusp. Abbreviations as in Figure 1.

4

septum. In normal hearts, these three components are merged imperceptibly with one another and in particular the left ventricular side does not offer much additional guidance for distinguishing among them (Fig. 2). The inlet septum can partially be identified, namely, its basilar rim, because the posterior portion of the anterior mitral leaflet is attached to this rim by means of its annulus. It is worth noting that the anterior portion of the anterior mitral leaflet together with the membranous septum belongs to the nonmuscular wall of the left ventricular outflow tract: it is continuous with the left coronary aortic semilunar cusp – or part of it, especially in cases with an anterolateral muscle – with the noncoronary cusp, and with the membranous septum. The anterolateral muscle, present in about 40% of normal hearts as a derivative of the left extremity of the bulboventricular fold, extends from the left coronary cusp into the anterolateral wall of the left ventricular outflow tract (Fig. 3).

The whole left ventricular septal surface can hemodynamically be considered to belong to the left ventricular outflow tract, the inflow tract being guarded by the mitral valve and its anterolateral and posteromedial papillary muscles, which are not attached to the septal surface. The subaortic part of the outflow tract is a slender fibromuscular tunnel, the basilar portion of the bulboventricular septum and the infundibular septum form the muscular

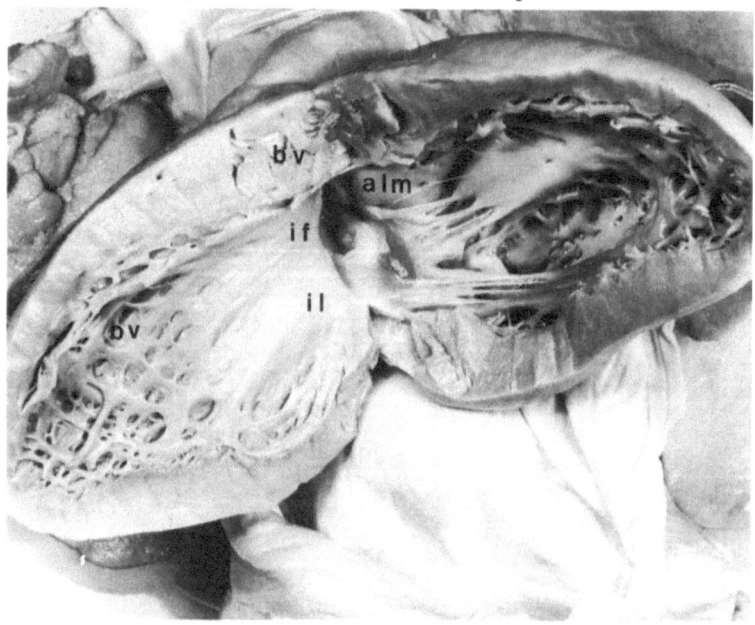

Fig. 3. Normal left ventricle with anterolateral muscle (alm) bordering on the left coronary cusp; the anterior mitral leaflet consequently does not reach the anterior border of the left ventricle. Further abbreviations as in Figure 1.

wall, while membranous septum and anterior mitral leaflet constitute the fibrous wall.

The architecture of the right ventricular septal surface is greatly influenced by the facts that in the right ventricle the inflow and the outflow regions are two distinct entities, and that the tricuspid valvular apparatus has a close anatomical relationship with the inlet septum (Figs. 1b and 4).

The inflow tract is anatomically separated from, and hemodynamically communicates with, the outflow tract by a more or less horseshoe-shaped muscular zone, embryologically related to part of the bulboventricular fold (Wenink, Chapter 3 of this book). It is formed by the rim of the crista supraventricularis, the trabecula septomarginalis and the anterior papillary muscle, which supports the anterior tricuspid valve leaflet. The rim of the crista supraventricularis and the trabecula septomarginalis is an important landmark with respect to the extension of the sites of insertion of papillary muscles. The tricuspid valve apparatus is part of the inflow region and the

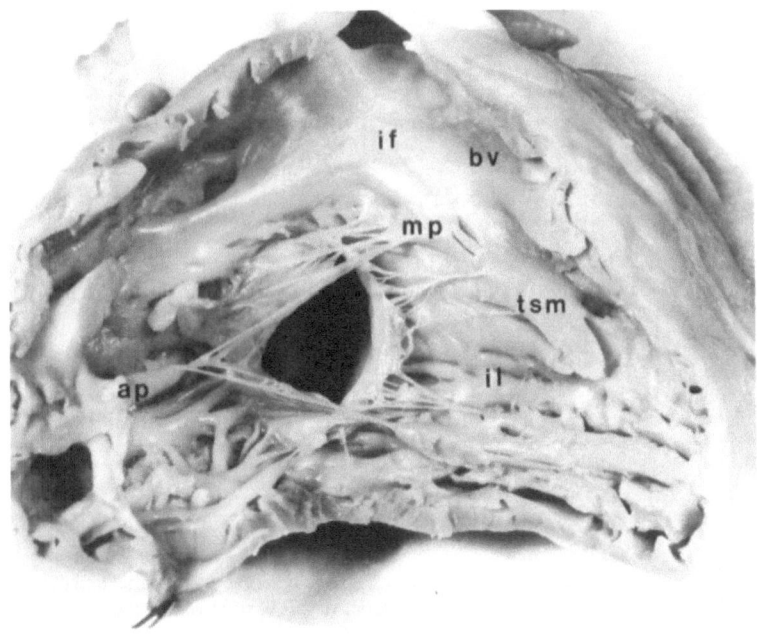

Fig. 4. Normal right ventricle: mp, medial papillary muscle; ap, anterior papillary muscle, artificially separated from the trabecula septomarginalis (tsm) by the incision in the right ventricle, which has been made parallel to the ventricular septum. Further abbreviations as in Figure 1. In this heart the trabecula septomarginalis has no proximal limb toward the left anterior cusp of the pulmonary orifice.

6

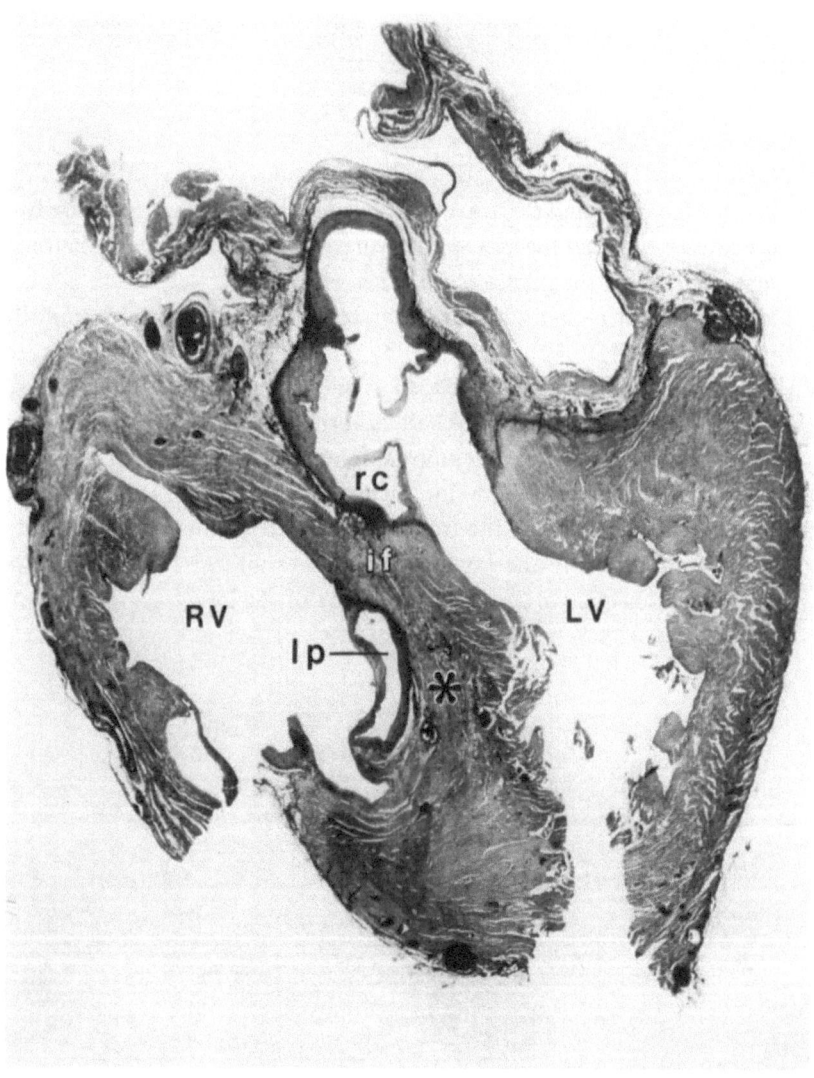

Fig. 5. Transverse section of neonatal human heart at the level of the aortic orifice and the lowest part of the pulmonary orifice: LV, left ventricular cavity; RV, right ventricular cavity; lp, left anterior pulmonary semilunar cusp; rc, right coronary aortic semilunar cusp; if, infundibular septum; asterisk, bulboventricular septum.

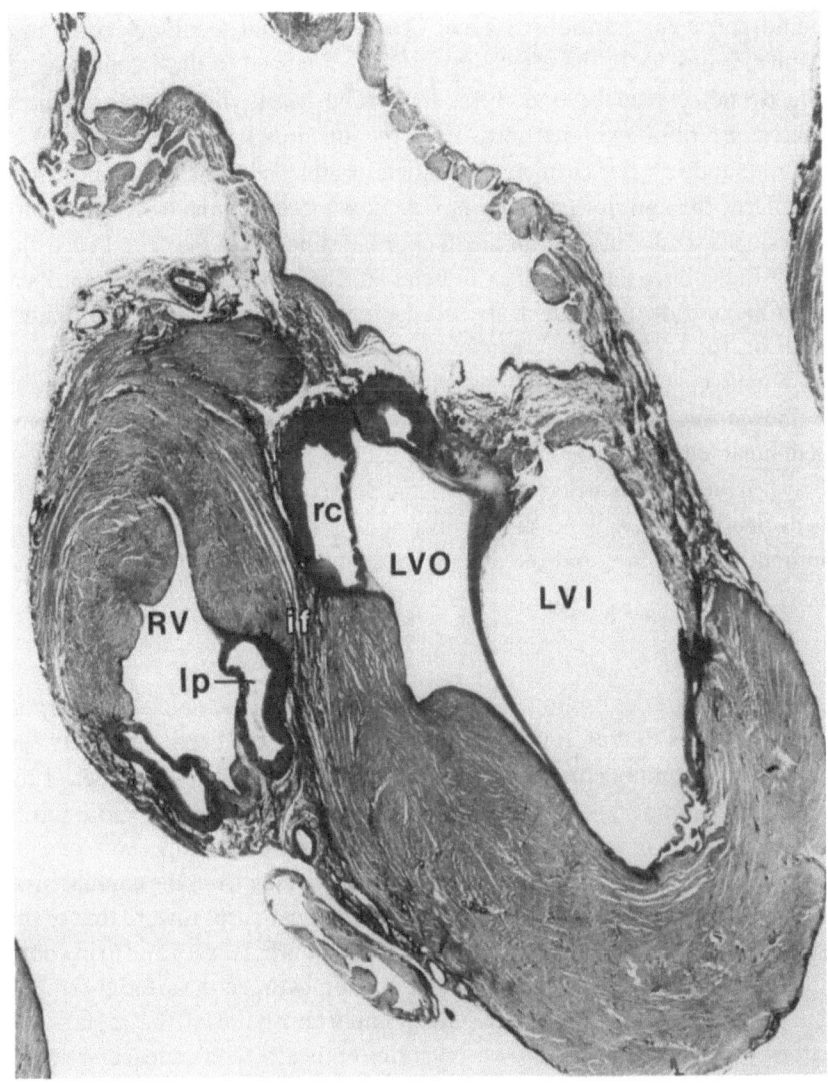

Fig. 6. Transverse section of neonatal human heart at the level of the lower parts of the arterial orifices: RV, right ventricular cavity; LVI, left ventricular inflow portion; LVO, left ventricular outflow portion; lp, left anterior pulmonary semilunar cusp; rc, right coronary aortic semilunar cusp; if, infundibular septum. The bulboventricular septum is not present in this picture because the plane of sectioning of this heart slopes down from anterosuperior to posteroinferior as compared with Figure 5.

bulboventricular transitional zone. This implies that tendinous cords and papillary muscles of the tricuspid valves are attached to these components, i.e., do not extend beyond them. In normal hearts, the medial papillary muscle, bearing tendinous cords from the junctional zone (commissure) of anterior and septal tricuspid valve leaflets, is attached to the crista supraventricularis, the anterior papillary muscle is connected to the trabecula septomarginalis, and a number of small chordae supporting the septal tricuspid valve leaflet have their papillary muscles attached to the inlet septum proper.

In the outflow tract, the trabecula septomarginalis may have a proximal limb on the septal surface extending toward the base of the left anterior semilunar cusps are continuous with each other. Usually the borderline bulboventricular septum, bordering on the posterior and the left anterior semilunar cusps are continuous with each other. Usually the borderline between the bulboventricular septum and the ventral wall of the outflow tract is distinct, but there is no sharply distinguishable demarcation between the infundibular septum and the external, parietal (lateral) wall of the outflow tract.

From the above description, it can be concluded that inspection of the septal surfaces leaves us with several questions regarding the borderlines between the various components of the ventricular septum. Microscopic serial investigation of normal fetal and neonatal hearts provides some more information, so far mainly concerning the infundibular septum. This can be recognized as a bundle of myocardial fibers extending from the commissural region of the right and left coronary aortic semilunar cusps toward that of the posterior and left anterior pulmonary semilunar cusps (Figs. 5 and 6) in about the same location as the so-called conal tendon between the arterial orifices, but at a somewhat lower level. Other important data on the septal constituents can be derived from observations on hearts with ventricular septal defects (cf. Chapter 5 of this book).

2. VENTRICULAR SEPTAL GEOMETRY: A SPECTRUM WITH CLINICAL RELEVANCE

CHARLES J.F.M. MIDDELHOFF AND ANTON E. BECKER

INTRODUCTION

The ventricular septum is a complex structure both from embryological [1–3] and anatomical [4] viewpoints. The complexity is particularly apparent in hearts with congenital malformations such as univentricular hearts with rudimentary chambers and hearts with malalignment ventricular septal defects, such as Fallot's tetralogy and double-outlet right ventricle. Observations in such hearts strongly suggest that the ventricular septum is composed of "building blocks", a concept familiar to embryologists.

The normal ventricular septum, furthermore, is not a straight shelf but an angular structure possessing curvatures in different planes [4]. In general, one may say that the greater part of the inlet septum is almost in the frontal plane, while the trabecular part bends toward the horizontal plane and the outflow part curves toward the sagittal plane. Knowledge of this geometry has clinical relevance. The angiocardiographer and the echocardiographer, for instance, have to know that projections or ultrasound "cuts" from different angles can visualize different parts of the septum. In other words, statements such as "the ventricular septum is present" need further specification, particularly in case of complex congenital malformations.

The hearts of elderly people, moreover, almost invariably show a distinct subaortic bulge, while this convexity in the young usually is either absent or less distinct. Thus, the shape of the septum appears also to be related to age.

On the basis of these empirical observations, the question was raised as to whether the geometry of the ventricular septum in normal hearts might constitute a spectrum with functional implications.

MATERIALS AND METHODS

The hearts were obtained from autopsies on patients who had died of diseases not related to the cardiovascular system. Inspection of these hearts revealed no gross abnormalities. Hearts were selected that shared a similar state of mild contraction. The atria were opened, and blood clots removed from the ventricular chambers. The cavities were then passively filled with formalin and further processing (see below) was performed only after complete fixation of at least one week.

Two groups of hearts were distinguished. The first group comprised hearts of patients less than 20 years of age (eight specimens: $2\frac{1}{2}$, 3, 4, 4, 9, 9, 17, and 19 years, respectively). The second group comprised hearts of patients over 60 years of age (seven specimens: 61, 62, 71, 74, 77, 79, and 91 years of age, respectively).

A step-by-step dissection of the hearts was performed so that various geometric measurements could be obtained. The first step was to remove the two atria, thus exposing both atrioventricular valve rings. The aorta was

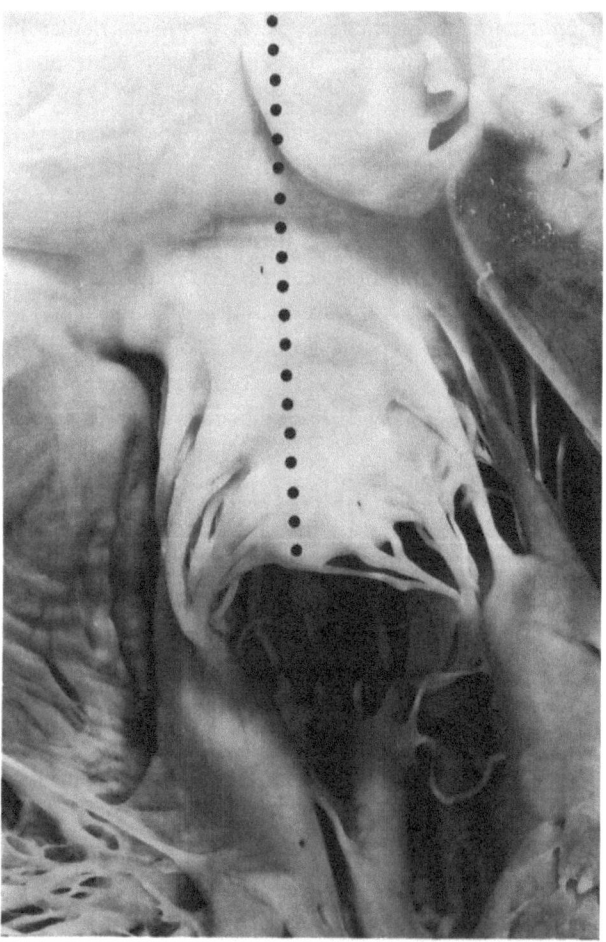

Fig. 1. Aortic-mitral valve relationship viewed from the left ventricular outflow tract. The mitral valve midline is indicated by the dotted line. In this particular specimen the midline cuts through the left coronary cusp, just aside of the commissure with the noncoronary cusp.

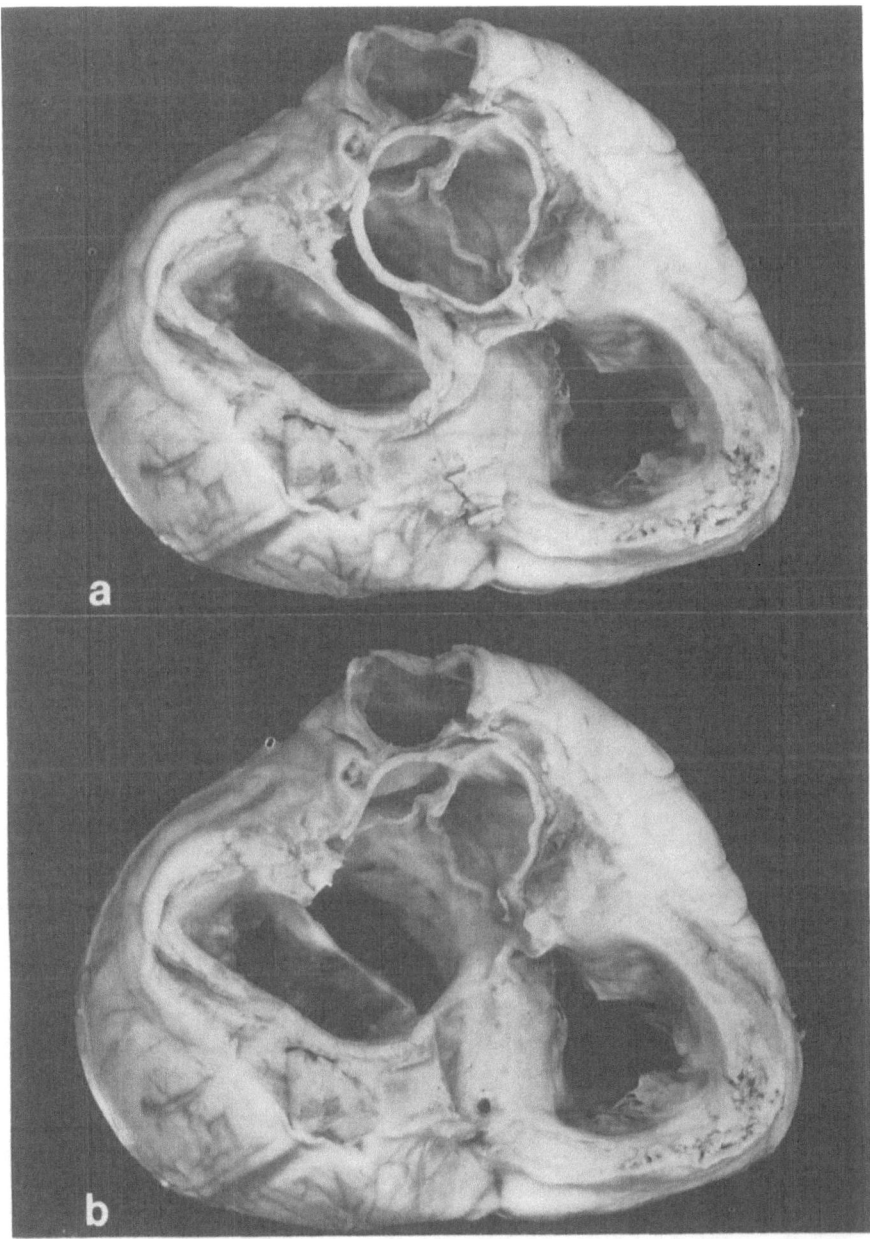

Fig. 2. Heart specimen, after removal of atria, looked at from above. (*a*) The specimen with the aortic valve ring still in place, although the area of aortic-mitral valve continuity has already been severed. The lower part of the atrial septum is left intact. (*b*) Further dissection of the same specimen after removal of the atrial septum and part of the aortic valve ring. These dissections were used to measure the angulation between inlet and outlet parts of the ventricular septum, along a "short-axis" line, and to determine the position of the aortic ostium in relation to these septal structures.

trimmed down to the level of the semilunar valves. At this stage, the relationship between the mitral valve and the aortic valve was determined. A line was drawn through the middle of the anterior leaflet of the mitral valve and its precise point of intersection with the semilunar valves of the aorta was then established (Fig. 1). The next step was to remove the area of aortic-mitral valve continuity (Fig 2a). Thereafter, the septal atrioventricular junctional region was dissected down until the top of the inlet part of the ventricular septum was exposed (Fig. 2b). At this stage, the position of the aortic ostium was determined both with regard to the inlet part of the ventricular septum and with respect to the outlet part of the ventricular septum. For both measurements, a line was drawn along the left ventricular aspect of these septa. The aortic ostium was then projected on the same plane and the percentages of the ostial circumferences to the left or right of the septal lines were approximated. The same stage of dissection also allowed measurement of the angle between the inlet and outlet parts of the ventricular septum. The orientation of the septal lines was again determined by using the endocardial geometry. The heart was then sectioned in the left ventricular long axis, comparable to an echocardiographic parasternal left ventricular long-axis view (Fig. 3). The section was used to measure the angle between the outlet and trabecular

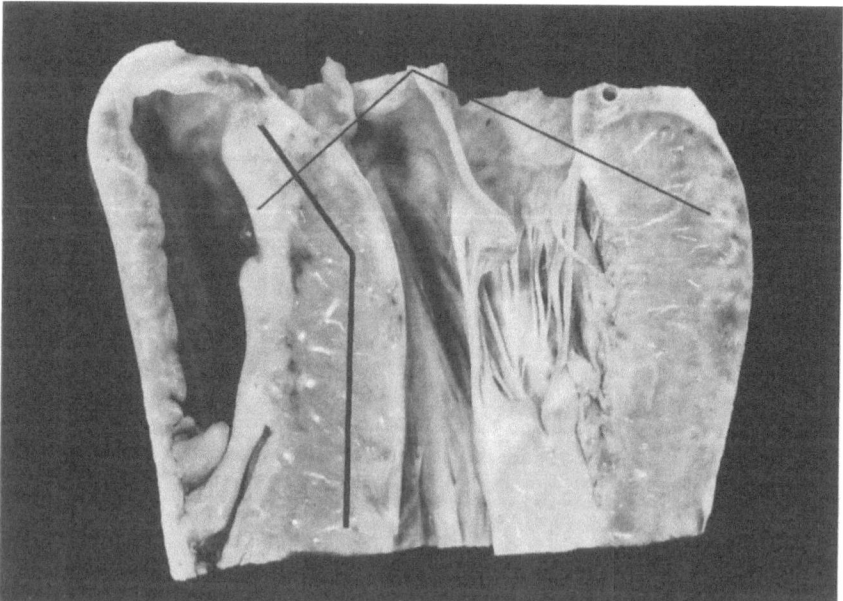

Fig. 3. Long-axis cut, comparable to a parasternal left ventricular long-axis echographic section, through a heart specimen after removal of the atria and the apical part of the ventricles. The angulation between outlet and trabecular parts of the ventricular septum is indicated by the thick solid lines. The angulation between the mitral and aortic valve planes is indicated by the thin solid lines.

parts of the ventricular septum, using an approach similar to that described for previous measurements of septal angulations. Finally, the angle between the planes of the mitral and aortic ostia was measured, taking the fibrous annuli as points of reference (Fig. 3).

RESULTS

Throughout the results, a distinction will be made between the two groups, that is, hearts of patients less than 20 years of age and those of over 60 years of age. For reasons of brevity, these groups will also be referred to as "young" and "elderly", respectively.

Aortic-mitral valve relationship. The intersection of the midline drawn through the anterior leaflet of the mitral valve with the semilunar valve cusps, for the 15 specimens, is shown in Figure 4. In elderly hearts, the line passed through the commissure between the noncoronary and left coronary cusps in six cases and through the left coronary cusp in only one instance. In young hearts, six of the eight specimens showed the line through the noncoronary cusp, while two hearts had this intersection at the site of the commissure with the left coronary cusp.

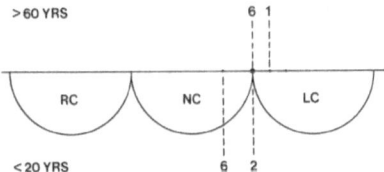

Fig. 4. Drawing illustrating the relationship between the anterior mitral valve leaflet and the semilunar aortic valve cusps. The intersection at the level of the semilunar cusps is indicated. In hearts over 60 years of age the line cuts through the commissure between the noncoronary (NC) and left coronary (LC) cusp in six hearts. In one instance the line went through the left coronary cusp. In specimens under 20 years of age the majority had the line passing through the non-coronary cusp; RC, right coronary cusp.

Aortic ostium-inlet septum relationship. All eight young specimens had the aortic circumference projected to the left side of the line drawn through the inlet parts of the ventricular septum (Fig. 5). In elderly specimens, on the other hand, only three hearts presented an aortic ostium completely to the left of that line. In one heart an almost 25% rightward shift had occurred and in the three remaining hearts almost 50% of the aortic ostium projected to the right of the septal line (Fig. 5).

14

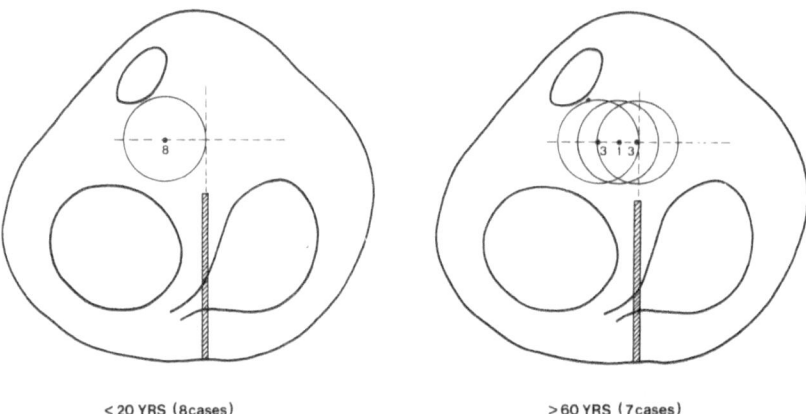

< 20 YRS (8cases)   > 60 YRS (7cases)

Fig. 5. Drawing of the aortic ostium in relation to the underlying inlet part of the ventricular septum. In young hearts the circumference of the aortic ostium projected completely to the left of the line through the inlet septum. In the seven elderly hearts, only three showed the ostium solely committed to the left ventricular cavity. In one instance approximately 25% of the ostial circumference was astride the septum and in three other hearts almost 50% of the circumference projected to the right.

Aortic ostium-outlet septum relationship. The projected position of the aortic ostium in relation to the line drawn through the outlet part of the ventricular septum showed a range of positions in both groups (Fig. 6). In the eight young hearts, two showed an override with the main circumference still projecting over the left ventricular outflow tract. In three instances approximately 50% was still confined to the left ventricle, whereas in the remaining three cases the major part of the ostial circumference projected to the right. In the seven elderly hearts, all specimens presented the major part of the ostial circumference to the right of the septal line, except for two hearts where approximately 50% was still confined to the left ventricular outflow tract (Fig. 6).

Inlet-outlet septum angulation. The results are shown in Figure 7. In young specimens the angle varied between 20° and 32°, while in elderly specimens the angle varied between 28° and 48°. However, 11 of the 15 specimens were confined to a narrow zone between 28° and 32°. In two young hearts a decreased angulation was present and in two elderly specimens an increased angulation was found.

Outlet-trabecular septum angulation. The measurements of the angle between the outlet part of the ventricular septum and the trabecular part of the ventricular septum revealed striking differences between the two groups (Fig. 8). In hearts under 20 years of age the angle varied between 135° and 180°,

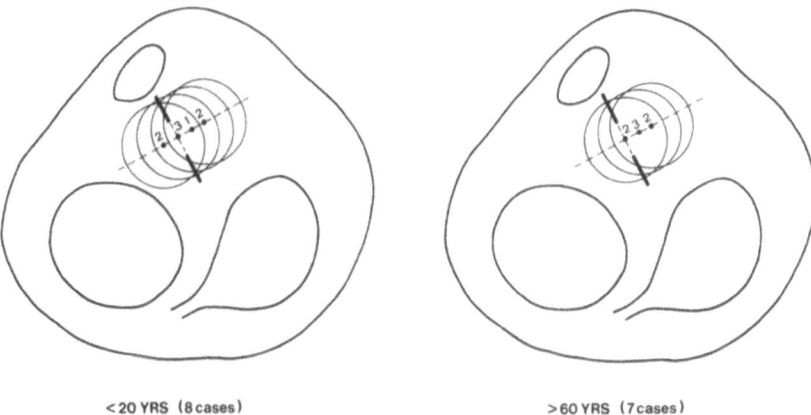

<20 YRS (8 cases)　　　　　　　　　　>60 YRS (7 cases)

Fig. 6. Drawing of the aortic ostium in relation to the underlying outlet part of the ventricular septum. In hearts under 20 years of age, two showed the major part of the circumference on the left side of the septal line. Of the remaining six cases, three showed an almost 50% override, one an almost 75% override, and two specimens projected for almost all of the circumference to the right of the septal line. Among elderly specimens there was not a single case in which the major part of the aortic ostium projected to the left of the septal line.

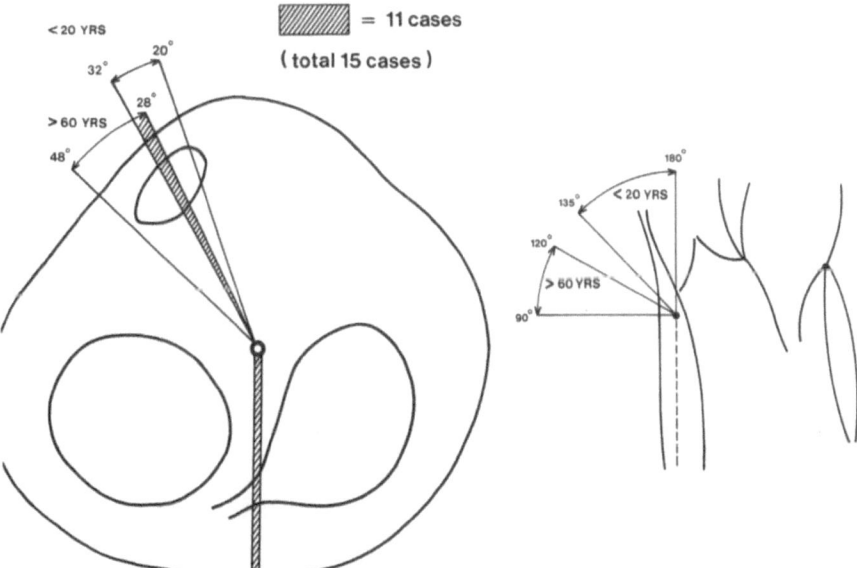

Fig. 7. Drawing of the angle between inlet and outlet parts of the ventricular septum in the "short axis" view. The angle varied in elderly hearts between 28° and 48° and in young hearts between 20° and 32°. The shaded area of overlap contained 6 young and 5 elderly cases.

Fig. 8. Drawing of the angle between the trabecular and outlet parts of the ventricular septum in a "long-axis" view. Specimens over 60 years of age showed a range between 90° and 120°. Those under 20 years of age ranged from 135° to 180°. There was no overlap between the two groups.

while in hearts over 60 years of age the angle varied between 90° and 120°. There was no overlap between the two age groups in this respect.

Aortic-mitral ostium angulation. In young hearts the angle varied between 110° and 150° while elderly hearts showed an angle varying between 100° and 135°. The overlap zone between 110° and 135° contained ten hearts, five out of each group (Fig. 9). Two elderly specimens showed an *in*creased angulation and three young presented a *de*creased angulation. The relationship between the aortic-mitral ostium angulation and the long-axis septal angulation is relevant in that lesser degrees of septal angulation, which are reflected in a more pronounced left-sided bulge, are related to lesser degrees of aortic-mitral valve angulation (Fig. 10).

DISCUSSION

The empirical observations that the shape of the ventricular septum may vary from the one individual to the other and that age-related changes occur have now a firm basis on the geometric data obtained in this study. Firstly, it appears that, within a given age group, fluctuations do occur, albeit often within a narrow range. Nevertheless, some features stand out, such as the position of the aortic ostium in relation to the outflow part of the ventricular

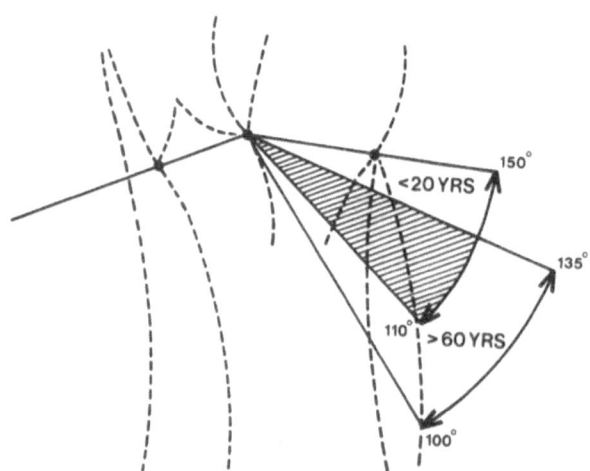

Fig. 9. Drawing of thh angle between the aortic and mitral valve planes (the aortic-mitral valve tilt). In hearts over 60 years of age the angle varied between 100° and 135°. In hearts under 20 years of age the angle varied between 110° and 150°. The shaded area of overlap contained ten hearts, five from each group.

SEPTAL ANGULATION

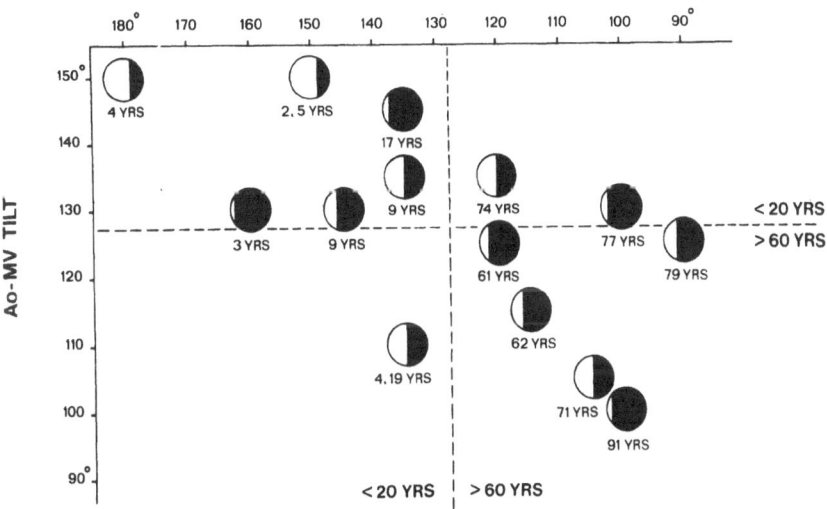

Fig. 10. Graft showing the raltionship between the aortic-mitral valve tilt and the septal angulation between the outlet and trabecular parts of the ventricular septum. The graft also shows the projected position of the aortic ostium onto the outlet septum. The dark area is the zone to the right side of the line representing the position of the outlet septum.

septum, the subaortic angulation, and the angulation between the aortic and mitral valve planes. Even in the young, that is, under 20 years of age, it appears that hearts occur in which the left ventricular outflow tract shows features similar in nature to those seen in elderly patients, the main difference being that in the latter group these features are more universally present and almost always more pronounced. The question cannot be solved as to whether the basic anatomical features of the left ventricular outflow tract architecture actually play a role as points of departure for further molding with age. However, from a hemodynamic point of view, it is obvious that in a proportion of young hearts the outflow tract is not a natural elongation of the left ventricular cavity, but instead curves to the right, thus producing an angled outlet. It is tentative to speculate that the rheological circumstances evoked by this architecture could eventually lead to characteristic sigmoid-shaped outflow as commonly seen in the elderly [5] (Fig. 11). Indeed, the differences between young and elderly hearts are striking. This applies in particular to the subaortic septal bulge, where the measurements showed no overlap between young and elderly specimens. This is an important observation with clinical relevance, as judged from a recent report by Fowles and co-workers [6], who pointed out that the occurrence of an "angled inter-

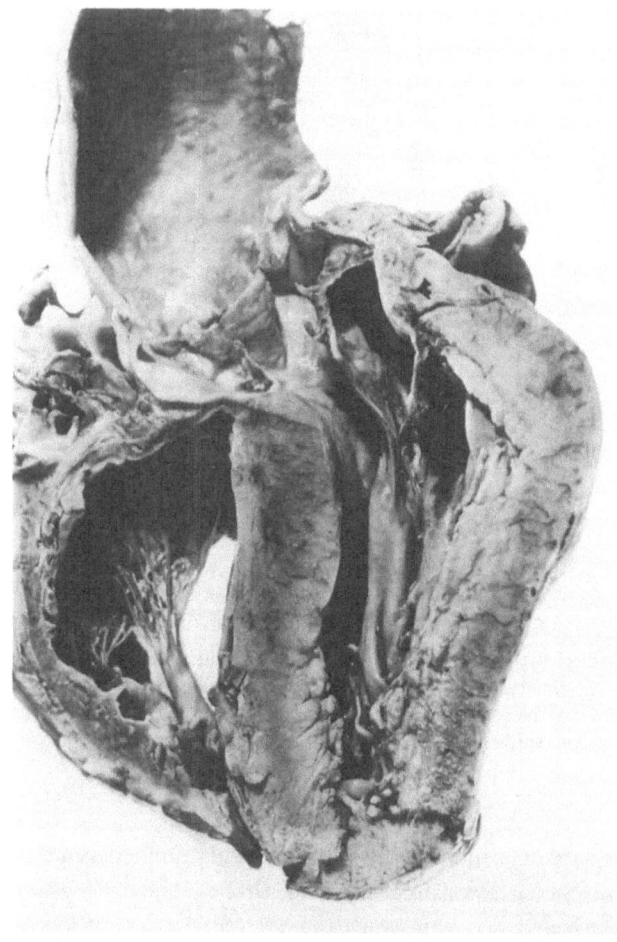

Fig. 11. Example of a sigmoid-shaped ventricular septum in the heart of a 67-year-old patient.

ventricular septum" in otherwise normal hearts could mislead the echocardiographer in diagnosing asymmetric septal hypertrophy.

There is another functional consequence that relates to this process of outflow tract molding. The study of the angle between the aortic and mitral valve planes reveals that the angle tends to become less obtuse with aging. This feature, together with the increased septal bulge, creates a setting in which the mitral ostium tends to face the septum rather than the left ventricular apical part. One may speculate about the possible functional significance of this phenomenon with regard to the mitral and aortic valve function, but there is no doubt that it can jeopardize the outcome of valve replacement

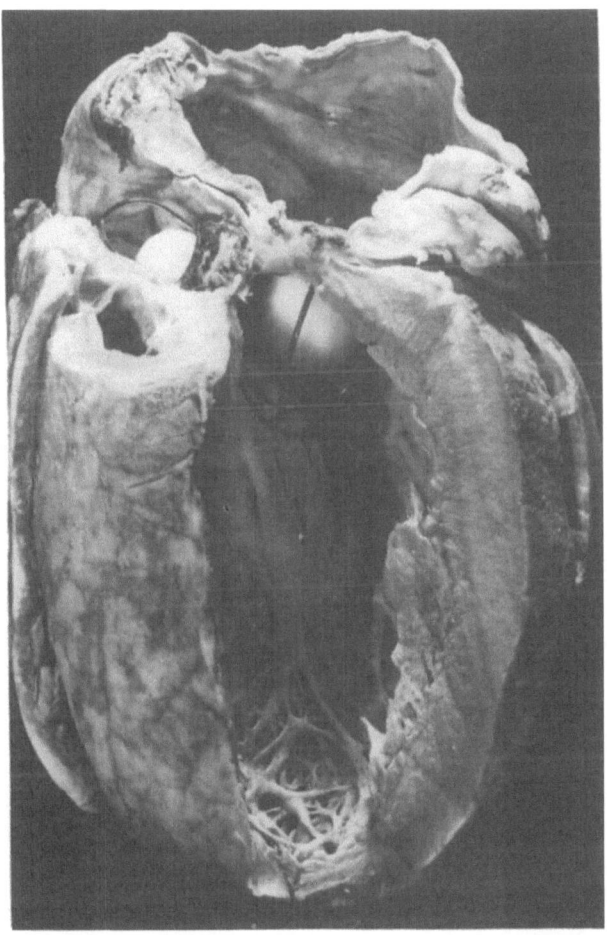

Fig. 12a. Heart exhibiting the consequences of a change in the geometry of the aortic-mitral valve planes for the left ventricular outflow tract. The opened left ventricle in a patient with caged ball prostheses in aortic and mitral positions. The prosthesis in the mitral ring points to the outflow part of the ventricular septum and the cage with ball definitely obstructs the left ventricular outflow tract.

procedures. Indeed, it has long been known that a caged ball prosthesis in the mitral position may occasionally obstruct the left ventricular outflow tract (Fig. 12a) and may induce septal endocardial fibrosis due to continuous rubbing. However, particularly in hypertrophied hearts, the aforementioned geometry may also affect other artificial valves placed in the mitral position. We recently came across a case of a patient of 71 years of age in whom a Carpentier bioprosthesis in the mitral position had led to outflow tract obstruction and death (Fig. 12b). Moreover, we have seen similar problems

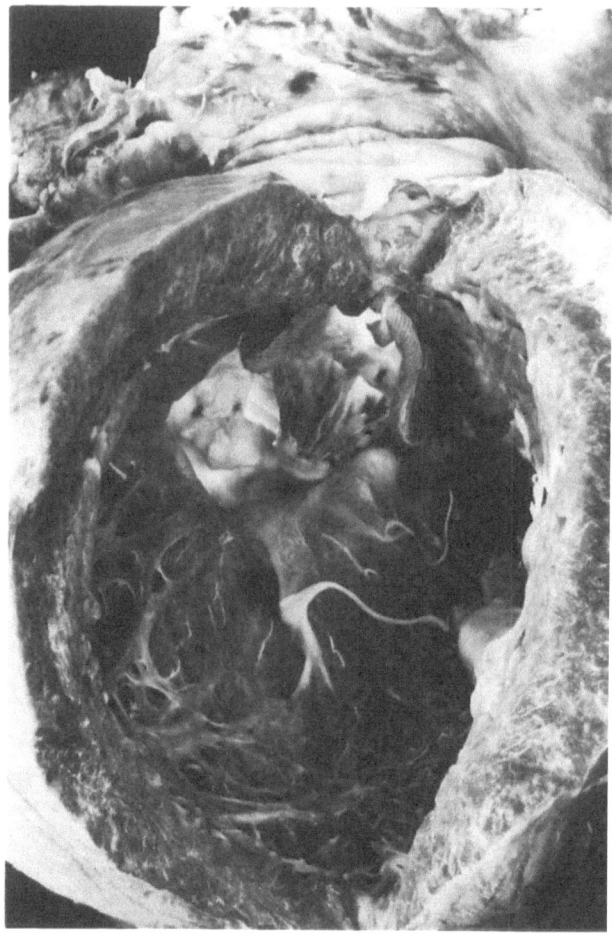

Fig. 12b. Heart exhibiting the consequences of a change in the geometry of the aortic mitral valve planes for the left ventricular outflow tract. The heart of a patient 71 years of age with a Carpentier bioprosthesis in the mitral valve position. Note how the struts of the prosthetic valve obstruct the left ventricular outflow.

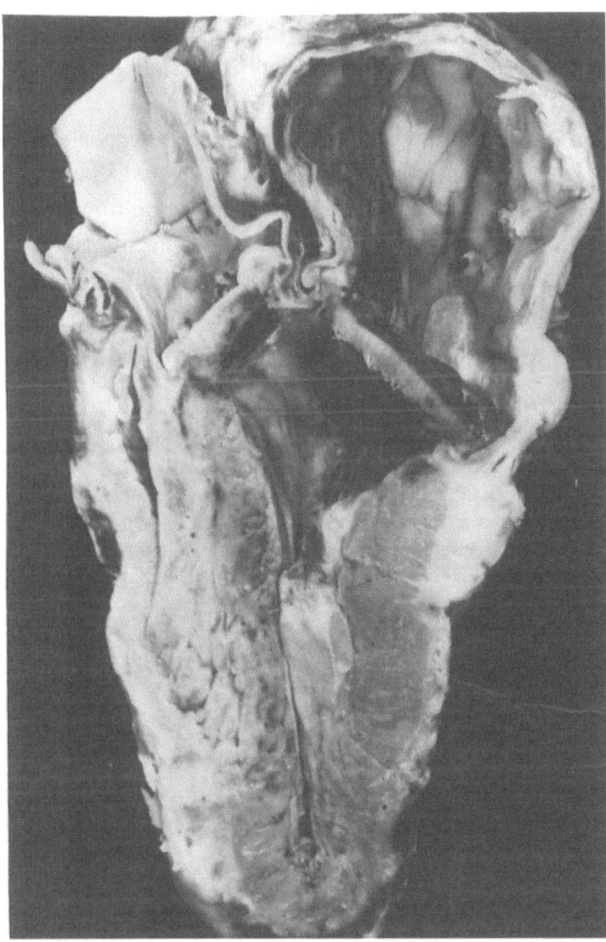

Fig. 12c. Heart exhibiting the consequences of a change in the geometry of the aortic-mitral valve planes for the left ventricular outflow tract. The heart of a patient 61 years of age with disc valve in aortic and mitral positions. The mobility of the disc in the mitral valve ring is hampered because of the altered geometry of the mitral valve plane.

with disc valves in the mitral position (Fig. 12c) mainly due to an intimate relationship between the disc and the septal wall as a consequence of the altered geometry.

Whether or not the geometry of the septum in the young, and its extremes in particular, play a role in enhancing the typical septal shape of the elderly remains to be established. However, there is as yet no doubt that the septal geometry normally constitutes a spectrum and that age-dependent changes of similar nature as occasionally seen in the young occur in the elderly and that these may have important clinical implications.

REFERENCES

1. Goor DA, Edwards, JE, Lillehei CW: The development of the interventricular septum of the human heart: correlative morphogenetic study. Chest 58:453–467, 1970.
2. Wenink ACG: Development of the ventricular septum (this volume, Chapter 3).
3. Wenink ACG: Embryology of the ventricular septum. Virchows Arch [Pathol Anat] 390:71–79, 1981.
4. Anderson RH, Becker AE: Cardiac anatomy. An integrated text and colour atlas. London, Gower Medical, 1980.
5. Goor D, Lillehei CW, Edwards JE: The "sigmoid septum". Variation in the contour of the left ventricular outlet. Am J Roentgenol Radium Ther Nucl Med 107:366–376, 1969.
6. Fowles RE, Martin RP, Popp RL: Apparent asymmetric septum hypertrophy due to angled interventricular septum. Am J Cardiol 46:386–392, 1980.

3. DEVELOPMENT OF THE VENTRICULAR SEPTUM

ARNOLD C.G. WENINK

INTRODUCTION

A description of the development of the ventricular septum should be linked directly to an account of that of the left and right ventricular cavities. In the early stages, where there is still no ventricular septum, there are also no left and right ventricles. Nevertheless, in these stages, the part of the heart tube that contributes to the ventricular portion of the adult heart is subdivided into two distinct cavities: a left-sided cavity receives all the blood from the as yet undivided atrium, while the right-sided cavity drains into the arterial trunk. These two cavities communicate via an ostium that is indicated externally by a constriction.

The use of different terms for the same part of the embryonic heart and of similar terms for different cardiac constituents has produced much confusion [1]. It has therefore become necessary to define each term before use. Since the anatomy of the heart in the preseptation stage, as described above, conforms with the account given by Davis [2], I feel quite comfortable with his terms "ventricle" and "bulbus". The embryonic ventricle is the left-sided cavity receiving all the atrial blood, and it drains into the right-sided bulbus which itself is below the arterial trunk. The latter segment will eventually give rise to the two great arteries. The ostium between the ventricle and the bulbus is called the bulboventricular ostium. The groove that indicates the site of this ostium externally is called the bulboventricular groove and it corresponds to an internal elevation in the cardiac wall called the bulboventricular fold.

Formation of the ventricular septum will be described on the basis of this anatomy and terminology (Fig. 1).

EMBRYOLOGICAL OBSERVATIONS

Before the ventricular septum is present, distinction can be made between the left-sided embryonic ventricle and the right-sided bulbus. The bulboventricular orifice is defined by a shallow internal ridge, the bulboventricular fold. It is important to note that this fold completely encircles the looped heart tube (Figs. 1 and 2). Posteriorly, it is directly to the right of the atrioventricular

24

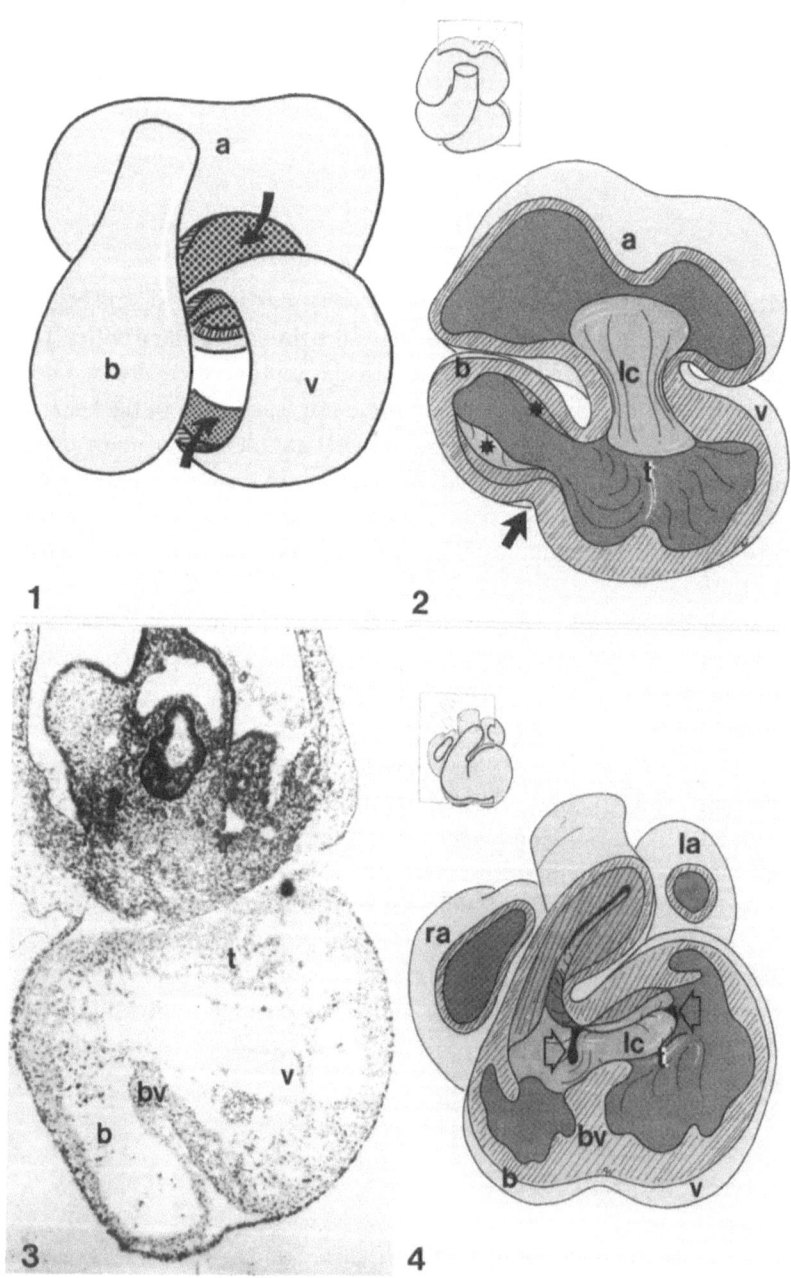

Figs. 1–4. (1) Exploded view of the embryonic heart to show the three constituents dealt with in this chapter: a, atrium; v, ventricle; b, bulbus. The atrioventricular and bulboventricular orifices are arrowed.

orifice. Here, it forms the sole boundary between the atrioventricular orifice and the bulbus. Thus, the blood coming from the atrium enters the ventricle and then has to pass the bulboventricular fold to reach the bulbus.

In histological sections (Fig. 3), the embryonic ventricle appears more trabeculated than the bulbus, particularly on its posterior wall. Reconstruction of these posterior ventricular trabeculations shows that they together form an elevation that commences at the lower atrioventricular endocardial cushion and gradually disappears in an apical direction (Fig. 2). Obviously, the reconstruction shown in Figure 2 is an oversimplification. It does not show the important difference between the posterior ventricular "ridge" and the bulboventricular fold. The latter is a double structure and it is relatively smooth. The ridge in the ventricle is built up of extremely loose trabeculations. This would also appear to be a criterion for distinguishing between the ridge and the fold in later stages.

In more advanced developmental stages, the bulboventricular fold has become larger and particularly its anterior portion forms a septum between the ventricle and the bulbus. Concurrently, the posterior ventricular trabeculations have accumulated to form a more or less concrete ridge. This ridge corresponds to the lower atrioventricular cushion and, therefore, its posterior portion is to the left of the bulboventricular fold. More anteriorly, the accumulated trabeculae coalesce with the anterior portion of the bulboventricular fold (Fig. 4).

No change has taken place in the relationships of the atrioventricular orifice and the bulbus. The blood coming from the right side of the atrioventricular orifice still drains into the embryonic ventricle, but now this portion of the ventricle has become a distinct entity. To the right, it is still separated from the bulbus by the bulboventricular fold. To the left, it is separated from the rest of the ventricle by the posterior ridge. This posterior ridge separates the left and right atrioventricular bloodstreams and may be called the "inlet septum". The anterior portion of the bulboventricular fold, with which the inlet septum fuses, is called the "bulboventricular septum".

---

(2) Graphic reconstruction of the heart of a human embryo of 3.6-mm CR length. The anterior part has been removed (see inset): a, atrium; v, ventricle; b, bulbus; lc, lower atrioventricular endocardial cushion; asterisks, endocardial bulbar ridges. The posterior ventricular ridge (t) is to the left of the bulboventricular transition (arrow). From reference 26.

(3) Transverse section of the heart of a human embryo of 3.6-mm CR length: v, ventricle; b, bulbus; bv, bulboventricular fold. The posterior ventricular ridge (t) consists of loose trabeculations. From reference 26.

(4) Reconstruction of the heart of a human embryo of 7.5-mm CR length. The anterior part has been removed (see inset): la, left atrium; ra, right atrium; v, ventricle; b, bulbus; bv, bulboventricular fold; t, posterior ventricular ridge; lc, lower atrioventricular endocardial cushion. The left and right atrioventricular orifices are arrowed. From reference 26.

26

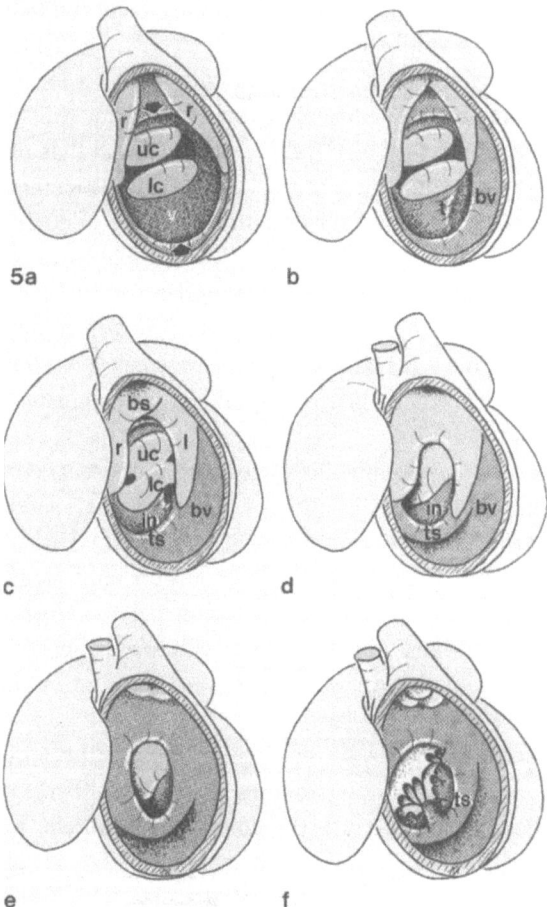

5a   b

c   d

e   f

Fig. 5. Diagrams to show ventricular septation. Right-lateral view. The right parietal wall of the bulbus has been removed.

(*a*) Preseptation stage. The bulboventricular fold (arrows) encircles the bulboventricular orifice, through which the ventricular cavity (v) is seen. Part of the fold is hidden by the endocardial bulbar ridges (r). The atrioventricular orifice is guarded by the upper (uc) and lower (lc) atrioventricular endocardial cushions.

(*b*) Outgrowth of the bulbar and ventricular cavities leads to accentuation of the bulboventricular fold (bv). From individual trabeculations a ridge (t) is formed on the posterior ventricular wall.

(*c*) The posterior ventricular ridge has grown out to form the inlet septum (in), and the anterior portion of the bulboventricular fold has formed the bulboventricular septum (bv). The cranial portion of the bulboventricular fold is nearly completely hidden by the bulbar septum (bs), resulting from fusion of the bulbar ridges. The upper (uc) and lower (lc) atrioventricular cushions have fused to separate the left and right atrioventricular orifices. The right and apical portion of the bulboventricular fold persists to form the trabecula septomarginalis (ts). Note that the so-called interventricular foramen is bounded by the following structures: inlet septum, lower atrioventricular cushion, upper atrioventricular cushion, right bulbar ridge (r), bulbar septum, left bulbar ridge (l).

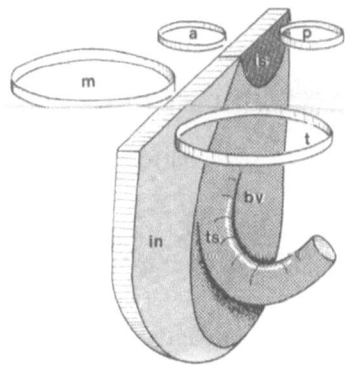

Fig. 6. Diagram to show the three components of the ventricular septum. Right-posterior view: in, inlet septum; bv, bulboventricular (trabecular) septum; is, infundibular (outlet) septum; ts, trabecula septomarginalis; a, aortic annulus; p, pulmonary annulus; m, mitral annulus; t, tricuspid annulus. From reference 26.

Up to the stage of 11-mm CR length, the bulboventricular septum is the most conspicuous of the two septal components. Being a double structure, it develops from both bulbar and ventricular walls and its appearance is probably caused by outgrowth of the bulbar and ventricular cavities to its sides.

The more lateral and posterior portions of the bulboventricular fold remain relatively inconspicuous and thus there remains ample communication between the part of the ventricular cavity that receives the right atrioventricular bloodstream and the bulbus. The general architecture of the adult right ventricle is already present. There is an inlet portion that belongs to the embryonic ventricle. Its downstream boundary is the bulboventricular fold. The rim of this fold remains recognizable at the site of fusion with the inlet septum as well as more laterally. This rim is the anlage of the trabecula septomarginalis.

The remainder of the bulboventricular fold, i.e., its more basal portion, is bound to become a left ventricular structure. This is effected by the septation process within the bulbus. The endocardial bulbar ridges fuse to form the bulbar septum, which is the third component of the ventricular septum and in adult hearts is known as infundibular ("outlet") septum (Figs. 5 and 6). This

(*d*) The interventricular communication is closed. The trabecula septomarginalis (ts) indicates the boundary between inlet septum (in) and bulboventricular septum (bv).

(*e*) Muscularization of the endocardial bulbar ridges makes further distinction between bulboventricular fold and bulbar (i.e., adult infundibular) septum impossible. Together they surround the ostium between inlet and outlet portions of the right ventricle.

(*f*) Mature right ventricle. The inlet part, containing the tricuspid valve, is separated from the outlet part, containing the pulmonary valve, by the trabecula septomarginalis (ts).

28

septum forms to the right of the basal portion of the bulboventricular fold. To close off the final interventricular communication, it fuses mainly with that part of the bulboventricular fold that had developed into the bulboventricular septum.

As is mentioned above, the right ventricle of the 11-mm embryo is quite comparable with that of the adult heart. The most striking difference is the dimension of the inlet septum. It is still a very short structure, so that the right atrioventricular bloodstream may seem to reach the bulbar cavity directly. However, from this stage onward, the inlet septum grows out, and in the heart of a 25-mm embryo there is an inlet septum of considerable dimensions. This is, of course, connected with the fact that the inlet component of the ventricular cavity has grown considerably.

This growing process takes place in the same period in which other anatomical changes are seen. The 11-mm embryo does not possess any atrioventricular valves. There are, of course, the endocardial cushions which undoubtedly function as valves, but there are no fibrous leaflets and there is no tension apparatus. The invagination of the sulcus and the undermining of inner myocardium, to form the valve leaflets, the chordae tendineae, and the papillary muscles [3], take place later. In the 25-mm embryo this process has advanced to the stage of a mainly muscular valvular apparatus.

The myocardium involved in the elaboration of the valvular apparatus belongs to the embryonic ventricle. The anatomical boundary of this undermining process is formed by the bulboventricular fold. Thus, contributions to the valves and papillary muscles come from this fold and from ventricular myocardium. In other chapters of this book, it will be shown that these embryological observations are of great importance to our concept of straddling atrioventricular valves.

The formation of the ventricular septum out of different embryonic sources is summarized in Figure 5. In Figure 6, the three main constituents are shown schematically. It has to be pointed out that the present term of "bulboventricular septum" largely covers the alternative term of "trabecular septum" [4]. However, I believe there is a major advantage in the use of the embryological term. It underlines its embryonic origin and that of the cavities to its left and right. This septum is part of the bulboventricular fold, which is a unique landmark in cardiac development [5, 6]. In many congenital malformations, observation of this fold or its remnants may lead to an understanding of the nature of the anomaly.

THE BULBOVENTRICULAR FOLD IN NORMAL AND MALFORMED HEARTS

The main point of the above description is to show that partitioning of the bulboventricular part of the embryonic heart tube occurs in more than one plane. It is therefore necessary to realize fully the actual topography of the bulboventricular fold. In Figure 7, the separate structures that collaborate in the partitioning processes are shown schematically. It follows that only the anterior (bulboventricular, "trabecular") septum coincides with the plane of the embryonic bulboventricular transition. Development of the infundibular (embryonic bulbar) septum takes place in another plane. Thus, part of the bulboventricular fold ends up lying to the left of the infundibular septum, that is, in the left ventricle. Alternatively, the inlet septum originates to the left of the bulboventricular fold. Therefore, part of this fold comes to lie in the right ventricle.

It is now possible to make conclusions about the embryonic background of the ventricular cavities. Unequal partitioning of the embryonic ventricle causes part of this cavity to contribute to the adult right ventricle, while septation of the bulbus contributes another part to the adult left ventricle.

It has been stated [7] that part of the primary interventricular foramen is never closed, because it is used to carry the left ventricular bloodstream into the aorta. "Transfer of the aorta to the left ventricle" is the term used for this phenomenon [8]. If the term primary interventricular foramen is changed into

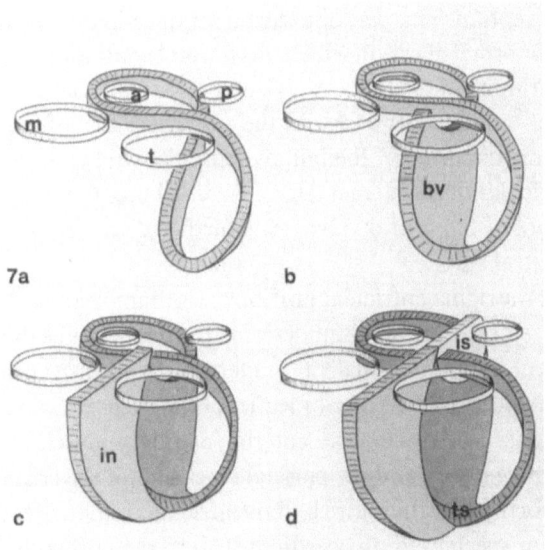

Fig. 7. (*a*) Diagram to show the full extent of the bulboventricular fold in the mature heart. Right-posterior view: a, aortic annulus; p, pulmonary annulus; m, mitral annulus; t, tricuspid annulus. (*b*) The same, with addition of that portion of the fold that has grown out to form the bulboventricular septum (bv). (*c*) The same, with addition of the inlet septum (in). (*d*) Completed diagram of septal components, including the infundibular septum (is); ts, trabecula septomarginalis.

"bulboventricular ostium", then this concept of transfer has still to be amplified, as another portion of this communication is needed to lead the blood from the right atrioventricular orifice into the outflow tract of the right ventricle. A process of "rightward migration of the atrioventricular canal" [9–11] has been described to explain the asymmetric partitioning of the inlet portion of the heart. Recently, this latter concept has been modified in that it was stated [12] that the ventricular septum itself, after having been split off from the bulboventricular fold, migrates and not the atrioventricular canal. This so-called migration may be explained by the fact that the inlet portion of the right ventricle enlarges relatively late and the inlet septum may only seem to be "split off" from the bulboventricular fold.

What portion, then, of the bulboventricular communication does close in normal hearts? If any at all, it can only be a very small portion, and must be expected to lie at the site of the membranous septum of the adult heart.

A greater part of the bulboventricular fold has been described as corresponding to the "left interventricular sulcus" [13]. Part of the fold was considered to contribute to the crista supraventricularis and this view was supported by Bersch and Doerr [14]. It is essential to recognize that the bulboventricular fold does not primarily continue from the trabecula septomarginalis (i.e., the posterior rim of the bulboventricular septum) into the parietal extension of the crista supraventricularis. The muscular arch in the roof of the normal right ventricle is only completed by the interposition of the infundibular septum. This was one reason for questioning the use of the term "crista" in abnormal hearts in which this normal continuity may be disrupted [15]. The continuity of the bulboventricular fold is not traceable in its entirety in the roof of the right ventricle. At the site where the infundibular septum effects a "short-circuiting", the bulboventricular fold is diverted to encircle the left ventricular outflow tract. Here, it contributes to the formation of the anterior leaflet of the mitral valve, as is further discussed in the chapter on straddling mitral valve.

The fate of the right ventricular portion of the bulboventricular fold is more readily understood. Part of it is undermined and remains as the loose portion of the trabecula septomarginalis ("moderator band"). Another portion of this fold contributes to the anterior leaflet of the tricuspid valve, and thus the ring can be closed by tracing the anterior papillary muscle and its chordae toward the valve leaflet and the parietal extension of the crista.

It is noteworthy that the entire bulboventricular fold carries the bulboventricular ring of specialized myocardium [16]. In the normal heart, the atrioventricular bundle is found on the rim of the bulboventricular septum. But other portions of the bulboventricular fold may also carry the bundle, which may then be related to the right atrioventricular orifice [17–20] and may or may not encircle the posterior great artery [21].

In general, all three components may be deficient or relatively displaced. If the individual components are not obvious in all instances, it should be borne in mind that the primarily malformed heart may still have a long path of development ahead and the general architecture may be influenced by adaptive changes [22].

Displacement of the infundibular septum relative to the bulboventricular septum may cause a characteristic "malalignment defect" [23], as is schematically shown in Figure 8. By this malalignment, it is often easy to follow that part of the bulboventricular fold that encircles the posterior great artery. Persistence of this portion of the fold may be obvious in many hearts with

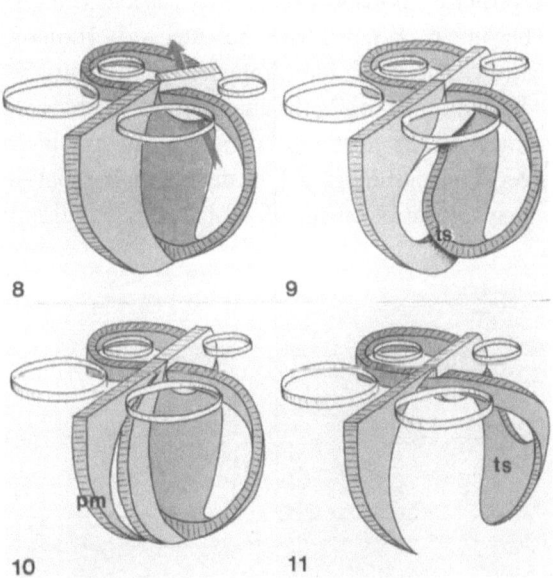

Figs. 8–11. (*8*) Septal components in an infundibular malalignment defect. The arrow passes the defect between infundibular and bulboventricular septa.

(*9*) Septal components in a central muscular defect. From the right, this defect is just posterior to the trabecula septomarginalis (ts).

(*10*) Septal components in a posterior muscular defect. Note that the defect is situated within the inlet septum. The posterior portion of the inlet septum is seen as the posteromedial muscle (pm) in the left ventricle.

(*11*) Septal components in a univentricular heart of left ventricular type with complete double inlet. The normal bulboventricular septum has not fully grown out to fuse with the inlet septum. Instead there has been overgrowth of the more lateral portion of the bulboventricular fold (ts), which forms a septum between the main chamber (embryonic ventricle) and the outlet chamber (bulbus).

double-outlet right ventricle. There is probably only one underlying malformation, as is suggested by the typical anatomy of the Taussig–Bing heart.

Other infundibular defects may be caused by simple deficiency of the infundibular septum and/or lack of coaptation of this septum with the bulboventricular septum.

Similar malformations may be seen at the site of fusion of the bulboventricular septum with the inlet septum. In Figure 9, it is shown how malalignment in this region may lead to a central muscular defect [24], although this malalignment is never as obvious as it may be in the case of the infundibular septum.

Above, it was shown how the inlet septum originates from initially loose trabeculations. It was further shown that this part of the myocardium continues to exhibit these early features of loose myocardium in that it is secondarily undermined to contribute to the atrioventricular valves and their tension apparatus. This probably also explains the occurrence of defects within the inlet septum, which were described as posterior muscular defects [24] (Fig. 10). Here, the posterior portion of the inlet septum (the "posteromedial muscle") may become malaligned with the anterior portion of the inlet septum and is always visible in the morphologically left ventricle. This kind of pathology will be elaborated on in the chapter on straddling tricuspid valve.

Gross deficiency of the inlet septum is seen in hearts with an atrioventricular defect. This pathology will be dealt with in separate chapters.

A final example of derangement of ventricular septation combines de-

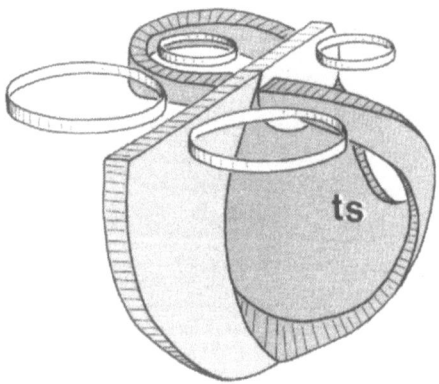

Fig. 12. Septal components in two-chambered right ventricle. In addition to normal septation, the lateral portion of the bulboventricular fold (ts) has grown out to separate inlet and outlet portions of the right ventricle.

ficiencies, displacements, and undue overgrowth. This is found in uni-ventricular hearts of left ventricular type with an outlet chamber (Fig. 11). The normal fusion of the inlet and bulboventricular septa is absent. The remnant of the inlet septum is present as a ridge between the two atrio-ventricular valves in the main chamber. In addition, that portion of the bulboventricular fold that normally forms the trabecula septomarginalis is present as a thick septum and separates the main chamber from the outlet chamber. Such an uninhibited growth of what was only meant to be trabecula septomarginalis can also occur independently. A two-chambered right ven-tricle [25] then results (Fig. 12).

REFERENCES

1. Laane HM: The arterial pole of the embryonic heart. I. Nomenclature of the arterial pole of the embryonic heart. II. Septation of the arterial pole of the embryonic chick heart. Thesis, University of Amsterdam, Swets and Zeitlinger, 1978.
2. Davis CL: Development of the human heart from its first appearance to the stage found in embryos of twenty paired somites. Contrib Embryol 19–107:247–293, 1927.
3. Van Gils FAW: The development of the human atrioventricular heart valves. J Anat 128:427, 1979.
4. Anderson RH: Embryology of the ventricular septum. In: Anderson RH, Shinebourne EA (eds) Paediatric cardiology 1977. Edinburgh–London–New York, Churchill Livingstone, 1978, pp 103–112.
5. Doerr W: Über ein formales Prinzip der Koppelung von Entwicklungsstörungen der ve-nösen und arteriellen Kammerostien. Z Kreislaufforsch 41: 269–284, 1952.
6. Bersch W: On the importance of the bulboauricular flange for the formal genesis of con-genital heart defects, with special regard to the ventricular septum defects. Virchows Arch Pathol Anat 354:252–267, 1971.
7. Van Mierop LHS, Alley RD, Kausel HW, Stranahan A: Pathogenesis of transposition complexes. I. Embryology of the ventricles and great arteries. Am J Cardiol 12:216–225, 1963.
8. Mall FP: On the development of the human heart. Am J Anat 13: 249–298, 1912.
9. Tandler J: Die Entwicklungsgeschichte des Herzens. In: Keibel F, Mall FP (eds) Handbuch der Entwicklungsgeschichte des Menschen, IIa + IIb. Leipzig, Hirzel, 1911, pp 517–551.
10. De la Cruz MV, Miller BL: Double-inlet left ventricle. Two pathological specimens with comments on the embryology and on its relation to single ventricle. Circulation 37:249–260, 1968.
11. Los JA: Embryology. In: Watson H (ed) Paediatric cardiology. London, Lloyd-Luke, 1968, pp 1–28.
12. Dor X, Corone P, Cabral C: Création expérimentale de ventricules uniques chez l'embryon de poulet. Étude au microscope électronique à balayage. Coeur 9:1131–1156, 1978.
13. Meredith MA, Hutchins GM, Moore GW: Role of the left interventricular sulcus in for-mation of the interventricular septum and crista supraventricularis in normal human cardio-genesis. Anat Rec 194:417–428, 1979.
14. Bersch W, Doerr W: Reitende Gefässe des Herzens. Homologiebegriff und Reihenbildung. Sitzungsberichte der Heidelberger Akademie der Wissenschaften. Mathematisch-natur-wissenschaftliche Klasse. 1. Abhandlung, 1976.
15. Anderson RH, Becker AE, Van Mierop LHS: What should we call the crista? Br Heart J 39:856–859, 1977.

16. Wenink ACG: Development of the human cardiac conducting system. J Anat 121:617–631, 1976.
17. Anderson RH, Arnold R, Thapar MK, Jones RS, Hamilton DJ: Cardiac specialized tissue in hearts with an apparently single ventricular chamber (double inlet left ventricle). Am J Cardiol 33:95–106, 1974.
18. Anderson RH, Becker AE, Arnold R, Wilkinson JL: The conducting tissues in congenitally corrected transposition. Circulation 50:911–923, 1974.
19. Baissus C, Latour H, Puech P, Grolleaux-Raoux R: Dualité embryologique des voies nodo-hisiennes: son rôle en pathologie. Arch Mal Coeur 68:953–959, 1975.
20. Bharati S, Lev M: The course of the conduction system in single ventricle with inverted (L-)loop and inverted (L-)transposition. Circulation 51:723–730, 1975.
21. Wenink ACG: The conducting tissues in primitive ventricle with outlet chamber. Two different possibilities. J Thorac Cardiovasc Surg 75:747–753, 1978.
22. Somerville J: Congenital heart disease – changes in form and function. Br Heart J 41:1–22, 1979.
23. Moulaert AJ: Anatomy of ventricular septal defect. In: Anderson RH, Shinebourne EA (eds) Paediatric cardiology 1977. Edinburgh–London–New York, Churchill Livingstone, 1978, pp 113–124.
24. Wenink ACG, Oppenheimer-Dekker A, Moulaert AJ: Muscular ventricular septal defects: a reappraisal of the anatomy. Am J Cardiol 43:259–264, 1979.
25. Anderson RH, Becker AE, Wilkinson JL, Gerlis LM: Morphogenesis of univentricular hearts. Br Heart J 38:558–572, 1976.
26. Wenink ACG: Embryology of the ventricular septum. Separate origin of its components. Virchows Arch [Pathol Anat] 390:71–79, 1981.

4. COMPARATIVE ANATOMY OF THE VENTRICULAR SEPTUM

LODEWIJK H.S. VAN MIEROP AND LYNN M. KUTSCHE

INTRODUCTION

All vertebrates possess a well-developed heart which represents a specialized section of the vascular system located mediocentrally near the cranial end of the body. Primitively the heart consists of a caudocranial series of four expansions of blood vessel, the cardiac chambers, the walls of which contain contractile elements consisting of typical cross-striated, branched myocardial cells. Caudally the sinus venosus receives the great veins and discharges its blood into the atrium through the sinoatrial ostium. The atrioventricular canal gives access to the ventricle which is the main pumping chamber of the heart and which discharges its blood into the arterial system by way of the more or less cone-shaped fourth chamber, the conus arteriosus. (There continues to be disagreement and confusion concerning the nomenclature of the arterial pole of the heart. The term "conus arteriosus" is used by most recent authors.)

The sinoatrial ostium is usually flanked by a bicuspid valve; the atrioventricular canal contains a valvar apparatus of variable morphology consisting of one or more pad- and/or cusp-like structures. The conus arteriosus also contains valves, which vary tremendously in number of cusps and morphology among different vertebrate species.

The primitive condition in which the four cardiac chambers are arranged in a caudocranial series exists only in very young embryos, and is not found in adults of any living vertebrate species. During ontogeny, the tubular heart forms a loop directed to the right and anteriorly which results in a shift of the sinoatrial part of the heart from its initial far-caudal position to one dorsal or even dorsocranial to the ventricle. The sinus venosus and the conus arteriosus lose their identity in higher vertebrates (birds, mammals) because the former is incorporated into the atrium, the latter into the ventricle. Since, however, in birds and mammals the atrium and the ventricle are each divided by a septum into two compartments, the heart in higher vertebrates again consists of four chambers.

In gill-breathing aquatic vertebrates, the newly oxygenated blood from the gills is led directly to the dorsal aorta by the epibranchial arteries. None is returned to the heart prior to entering the systemic arterial system and no

A.C.G. Wenink et al. (eds.) The Ventricular Septum of the Heart, *35–46. All rights reserved.*
Copyright ©1981 by Martinus Nijhoff Publishers, The Hague/Boston/London.

cardiac septa are needed under these conditions.

Whenever respiration by means of lungs (or lung homologues) occurs, oxygenated blood is returned to the heart by one or more pulmonary veins. Pulmonary respiration may supplement gill breathing, as in some fishes and amphibians, or is used (almost) exclusively as in most amphibians and all amniotes (in all amphibians and some reptiles, gas exchange also takes place through the skin and pharynx). Throughout phylogeny, we see the development of a number of provisions aimed at keeping oxygenated and deoxygenated blood separate as much as possible. This involves not only the creation of partial or complete septa in the atrium, the ventricle, and the conus arteriosus, but also changes in the shape of the heart and other modifications. These structural changes, in conjunction with certain patterns of sequential cardiac contraction, tend to keep the two kinds of blood separate by producing streaming effects. Such mechanisms can be quite effective, even if cardiac septation is only partial and may be far more appropriate and advantageous than the apparently more advanced condition of complete septation as seen in birds and mammals. Incomplete cardiac septation therefore should not necessarily be considered primitive in the sense of it being less sophisticated. In fact, it permits much greater flexibility to changing environmental conditions and must be looked upon as a perfect adaptation to the life style of the particular animal species.

There are many excellent accounts in the literature on the comparative anatomy and physiology of the cardiovascular system, such as those by Benninghoff[1], Foxon[2], Goodrich[3], Greil[4], Holmes[5], Johansen and Martin[6], Romer[7], Vorstman[8], Webb et al.[9], and White[10].

The present study on the comparative anatomy of the ventricular part of the heart and of the ventricular septum was undertaken as part of a larger investigation of the phylogeny and embryology of the heart. The specimens available for study included the hearts of elasmobranchs (sharks, rays), holosteid (Lepisosteus, Amia) and teleost fishes, amphibians (frogs, toads), reptiles (turtles, snakes, alligators), and birds. All hearts were fixed in the distended state under slight pressure in alcoholic formalin, Carnoy's or Bouin's fixative, and either cut transversely in two or more parts or windows were made in the chamber walls.

THE VENTRICULAR SEPTUM IN NONMAMMALIAN VERTEBRATES

The ventricular septum in fishes

In all species of fish examined, the ventricle has the shape of a three-sided pyramid the base of which faces anteriorly (cranially) and the apex points posteriorly (caudally) (Fig. 1). The base contains the atrioventricular and the ventriculoconal ostia. The right and left ventral sides of the pyramid are almost equal in size and each is smaller than the dorsal side. The ventricle therefore is somewhat flattened dorsoventrally.

In elasmobranchs the ventricle is asymmetric in that the atrioventricular ostium is located dorsally and on the left side, adjacent to the ventriculoconal ostium which is ventral and on the right. The two ostia are separated from each other by a well-developed bulboventricular fold which is oriented obliquely from right dorsal to left ventral. Dorsally it is continuous with a large muscle bundle which does not quite reach the cardiac apex. From this muscle bundle originate trabeculae which fan out radially toward the periphery. The trabeculae are higher than wide and are imperforate, i.e., the shark heart does not contain the randomly oriented mass of trabeculae with intratrabecular spaces as seen in the mammalian heart. The radial septa are connected with each other by somewhat lower and smaller ones giving the ventricular wall a honeycombed appearance as seen from the interior (Fig. 2B).

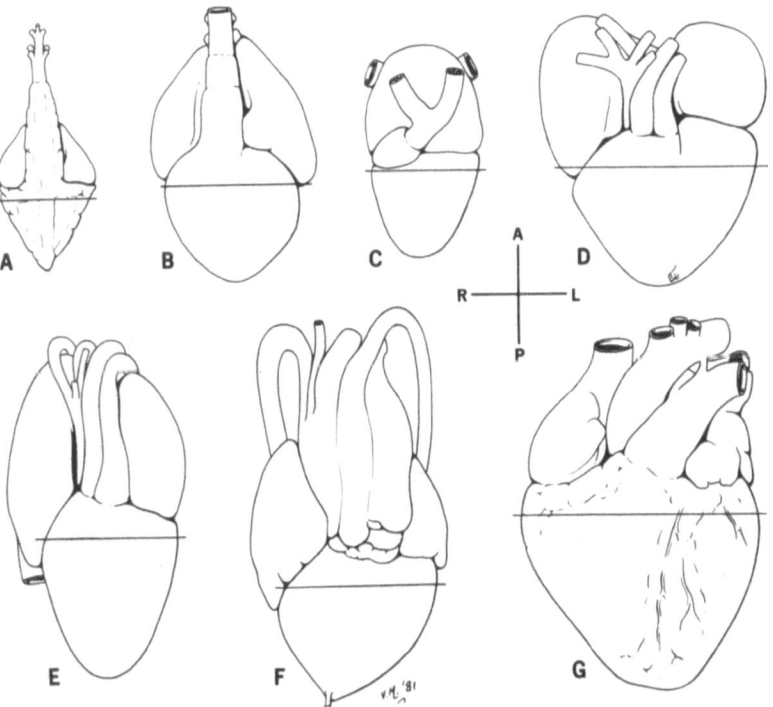

Fig. 1. Ventral view of the heart of (*A*) a gar (*Lepisosteus spatula*), (*B*) a shark (*Negaprion brevirostris*), (*C*) a frog (*Rana grylio*), (*D*) a turtle (*Chelonia mydas*), (*E*) a snake (*Python molurus*), (*F*) an alligator (*Alligator mississippiensis*), and (*G*) man; A, anterior; P, posterior; R, right; L, left.

38

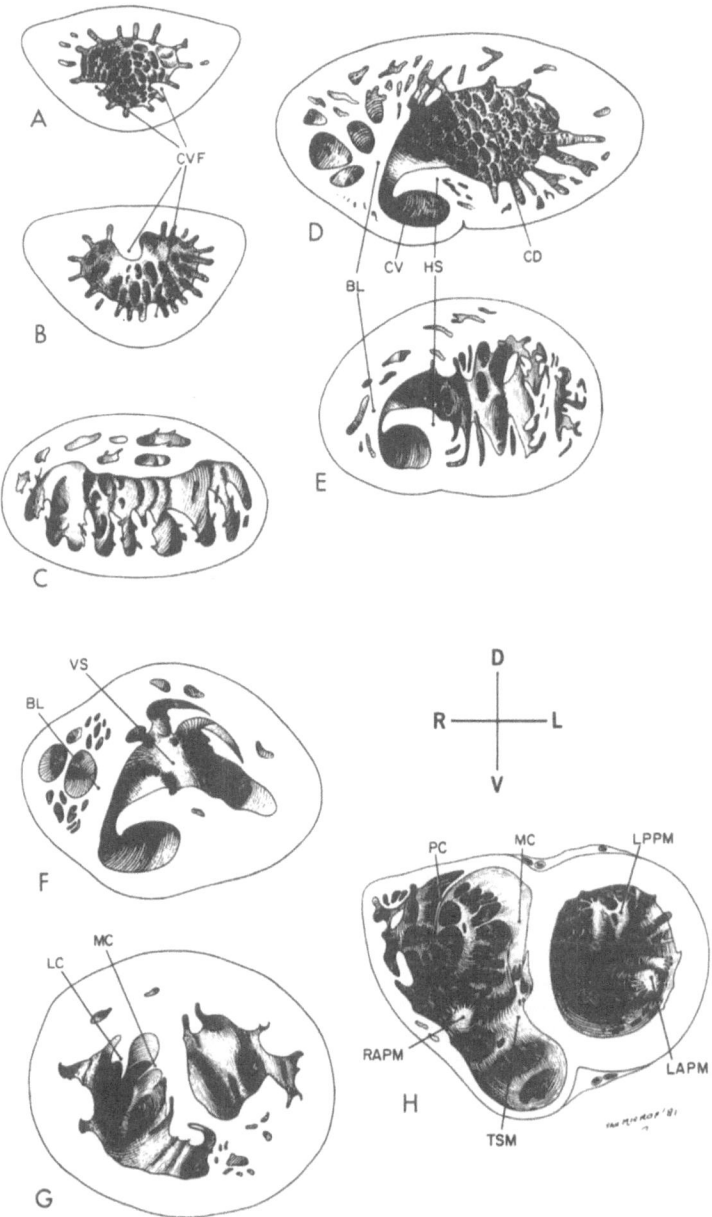

Fig. 2. Interior of the ventricle(s) of (*A*) a gar, (*B*) a shark, (*C*) a frog, (*D*) a turtle, (*E*) a boa constrictor, (*F*) a python, (*G*) an alligator, and (*H*) man. Plane of section as indicated in Figure 1. Anterior view of posterior (apical) part of the heart; BL, bulbus lamelle; CD, cavum dorsale; CV, cavum ventrale; CVF, conoventricular fold; HS, horizontal septum; L(R)APM, left (right) anterior papillary muscle; L(M,P)C, lateral (medial, posterior) cusp of right atrioventricular valve; LPPM, left posterior papillary muscle; MPM, medial papillary muscle; TSM, trabecula septomarginalis; VS, vertical septum.

The atrioventricular ostium is elliptical with the long axis oriented some-what obliquely from dorsomedial to ventrolateral. It is guarded by four well-developed, thin fibrous cusps: a large ventromedial cusp related to the bul-boventricular fold, an equally large dorsolateral one, and two smaller cusps alternating with the others. The edge of each cusp is attached to the ventric-ular myocardium by chorda-like slips. The elasmobranch heart rather strik-ingly resembles that of a mammalian embryo of Streeter's developmental Horizon XIV [11].

In actinopterygian fish the heart is bilaterally symmetric: the ventriculo-conal ostium is ventral to the atrioventricular ostium and the conus arteriosus lies in a midsagittal plane rather than slightly to the right as in sharks and in early vertebrate embryos (Figs. 1 and 2A). The bulboventricular fold there-fore lies in a horizontal rather than in an oblique plane and is less prominent. Even more than in elasmobranchs, the very thick ventricular wall has a honeycombed appearance (Fig. 2A) and the cells of the honeycomb are quite deep. The free lumen of the ventricle is correspondingly very small. The ventral and largest atrioventricular valve cusp associated with the bulbo-ventricular fold is well developed, thin, and fibrous. The other three are equally well developed in teleosts, but in holosteid fish they are little more than fibrous pads.

In lungfish, not available to us for study, the ventricular septum is reported to be well developed but incomplete [12]. It is muscular and almost as thick as the ventricular wall. The atrioventricular ostium in these fish does not contain valve cusps; instead there is a large fibrous or fibrocartilaginous plug. This structure, highly characteristic for lungfish, appears to be homologous to the embryonic posterior (inferior in man) atrioventricular endocardial cushion. No ventricular septum is apparently present in *Latimeria chalumnae*, the only other extant sarcopterygian fish [13].

The ventricular septum in amphibians

An atrial septum is present in all anurans (frogs, toads) and many urodeles (tailed amphibians, e.g., salamanders) and a rather complicated mechanism aimed at separating pulmonary from systemic blood flows is present in the arterial pole of the heart. However, a ventricular septum is not present in any living amphibian species. The very thick spongy layer consists of numerous muscular partitions and, as in fish, has essentially a honeycomb-like ap-pearance. The sagittally (dorsoventrally) oriented septa, however, tend to be higher and thicker, thus dividing the interior of the ventricle in a number of more or less parallelly oriented compartments (Fig. 2C).

The atrioventricular ostium contains two pad-like cusps, one dorsal and one ventral, attached to the interior of the ventricle by numerous short chordae tendineae. Both are bisected by the atrial septum, the free border of which extends slightly beyond the level of the valve and into the ventricle. Thus the atrioventricular ostium is divided into right and left components. The two lateral cusps are so tiny as to be nearly nonexistent. In aquatic, gill-bearing urodeles and lungless salamanders, the atrial septum is poorly developed or absent, and the arterial pole of the heart occupies a more medial position as in fishes.

The ventricular septum in reptiles

All reptiles are air-breathing animals in which the oxygenated blood from the lungs is carried to the left atrium by means of a common pulmonary vein. The atrium is always divided into right and left atria by a complete septum and there are two atrioventricular ostia, each of which in noncrocodilian reptiles is guarded by a large fibrous cusp arising from the base of the atrial septum. The left atrioventricular ostium has a small lateral cusp; no corresponding right lateral cusp is present.

In all reptiles, three great arteries arise from the ventricular part of the heart: a pulmonary trunk, and a left and a right aorta each with a bicuspid valve. (The terms "left" and "right" refer to the location of the aortic arches, not the valves.) At least one partial ventricular septum is present in all noncrocodilian reptiles. Septation of the ventricle is least advanced in turtles. In these animals an incomplete septum divides the ventricle into a smaller dextroventral cavum ventrale (also referred to as cavum pulmonale) and a much larger dorsal chamber, the cavum dorsale (Figs. 2 and 3D). The septum originates from the ventral ventricular wall where it extends from apex to base and runs dorsolaterally to join the right posterior ventricular wall. The anterolateral border of the septum is free. Ventral and dorsal chambers communicate with each other over this free border. Because of its almost horizontal position the septum has been referred to as the horizontal septum [14], a term which for a number of reasons deserves preference over the German word *Muskelleiste* introduced by Brücke [15] and subsequently adopted by Greil [4] and others. Opposite the free septal border the ventricular wall is thickened. This ridge is referred to as *Bulbuslamelle* by German authors. The pulmonary trunk originates from the small ventral chamber, while the large cavum dorsale receives both atrioventricular ostia and gives rise to the two aortae. The valve of the left aorta is located to the right of the pulmonary valve, but is separated from it by the horizontal septum. The right aortic valve is directly adjacent and dorsal to that of the left aorta. In the green turtle (*Chelonia mydas*) the very thick ventricular wall has a striking honeycomb-like appearance and the cells of the honeycomb are very deep (Fig. 2D). Toward the center of the heart the walls of the cells are thin,

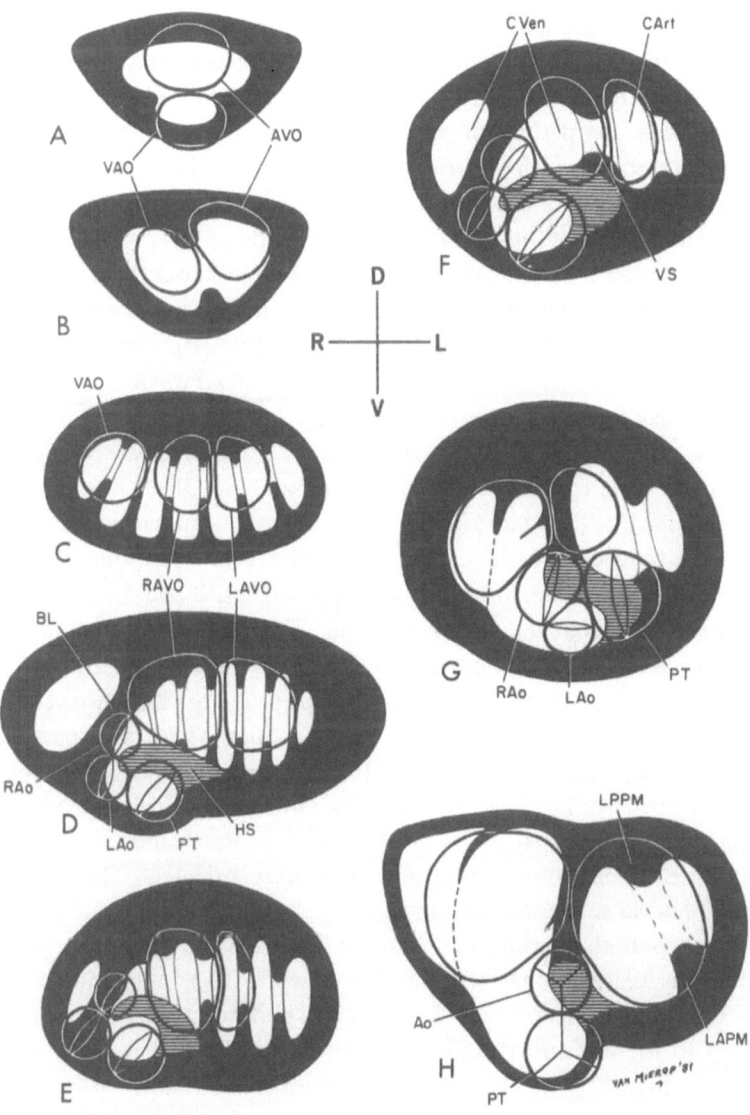

Fig. 3. Same sections as in Figure 2, diagrammatic, to show phylogeny of the ventricular septum and relationships between the atrioventricular and arterial ostia. Horizontal septum in non-crocodilian reptiles and its presumed homologue in the alligator and human heart is cross-hatched; AVO, atrioventricular ostium; CArt, cavum arteriosum; CVen, cavum venosum; L(R)Ao, left (right) aorta; L(R)AVO, left (right) atrioventricular ostium; VAO, ventriculoar-terial ostium; other abbreviations as before.

delicate, and perforated: peripherally, however, they gradually become thicker. In other turtles, e.g., the cooter (*Chrysemys floridana*), the differences between central and peripheral parts of the ventricular walls are greater and more abrupt: the central parts of the cell walls are reduced to a few lace-like strands while the peripheral parts rather suddenly become much thicker, particularly those which are oriented dorsoventrally. Thus six to eight sagittally oriented septa divide the dorsal chamber in a number of parallel compartments, similar to those seen in the frog heart.

In lizards and snakes the dorsal chamber contains fewer septa and in some the medial-most septa become clearly dominant while the others tend to regress, particularly those on the right side [1] (Fig. 3E). This is particularly evident in some lizards (*Varanus*) and snakes (*Python*) where a condensation of trabeculae forms a partial septum, the vertical septum, which originates from the dorsal aspect of the horizontal septum and runs between the atrioventricular ostia to the dorsal ventricular wall (Fig. 3F). Thus, the cavum dorsale is partly divided into a right-sided cavum venosum which receives the right atrioventricular ostium and a left-sided cavum arteriosum with which the left atrioventricular ostium is associated (Figs. 2 and 3). Both aortae, however, arise from the cavum venosum. The remaining communication between cavum venosum may be quite small, e.g., in *Python*.

In crocodilians the cardiac septum is complete and there are two ventricles, each of which receives an atrioventricular ostium. The basilar part of the ventricular septum, below the arterial ostia, is mostly thin and fibrous and contains cartilage. The honeycomb-like or compartmentalized appearance of the posterior (apical) part of the heart has become nearly unrecognizable; the trabeculae carneae are much more randomly oriented. The left atrioventricular valve is essentially bicuspid with a large medial and a smaller lateral cusp, both of which are thin and fibrous. The right atrioventricular ostium has a large, thin, fibrous medial or septal cusp, and a muscular flap serves as a lateral cusp (Figs. 2 and 3G). The three arterial ostia have all shifted to the left and therefore occupy a more medial position than in noncrocodilian reptiles. The pulmonary trunk and left aorta arise from the right ventricle, but the right aorta originates from the left ventricle. There is a distinct subpulmonary conus with a muscular wall which is separate from the right ventricle. A ring of nodules is present within the conus proximal to the pulmonary valve. An interesting feature of the crocodilian heart is the presence of an opening, the foramen of Panizza, between the two aortae at the level of their valves.

The ventricular septum in birds

In birds the ventricular septum is also complete and bulges rather strongly to the right. The right ventricular aspect is smooth and the right ventricle is almost devoid of trabeculae. The left ventricular aspect is trabeculated, particularly its apical two-thirds, and the trabecular pattern resembles that seen in mammals. The left atrioventricular ostium consists of a large medial or aortic cusp and a smaller lateral cusp. Both are fibrous but are somewhat thicker and stiffer than those of mammals. Chordae tendineae attach the valve cusps to barely elaborated anterior and posterior papillary muscles. The right atrioventricular ostium, as in Crocodilia, has a very large muscular flap laterally which corresponds in position to the anterior and posterior cusps of the mammalian tricuspid valve, but has no chordae tendineae. The medial or septal cusp is extremely thin and translucent and consists of a tiny ventral and a somewhat larger dorsal component separated by a gap of bare ventricular septal surface. Both components of the septal cusp are attached to the ventricular septum by means of short and delicate chordae tendineae. As in mammals, only two great arteries are present, each of which has three semilunar valve cusps.

DISCUSSION

It comes as no surprise that a ventricular septum is not present in fish in which gas exchange takes place exclusively or primarily by means of gills. Even in phylogenetically archaic actinopterygian fish (*Polypterus, Lepisosteus, Amia*) in which a primitive lung or lung-like swim bladder is present in addition to gills, the blood returning from these accessory respiratory organs is returned to the systemic venous system, not directly to the atrium [1, 2]. Only Dipnoi (lungfishes) possess a well-developed but incomplete ventricular septum. These sarcopterygian fish live in an environment which is subjected to long periods of drought which makes gill breathing impossible for part of the year and air breathing by means of lung(s) is substituted. Their hearts show other unusual anatomical features which very probably represent specializations rather than ancestral conditions. The absence of a ventricular septum in *Latimeria chalumnae*, also a sarcopterygian and belonging to the Crossopterygii, an order until recently considered to have become extinct during the Paleozoicum and containing forms broadly ancestral to land vertebrates, may be related to the fact that the animal is a deep-sea dweller. Its swim bladder is filled with fatty tissue and has no respiratory function.

The organization of the very thick ventricular wall of lower vertebrates in a number of radially disposed compartments might be expected to limit the free movement of blood within the ventricle. While in gill-breathing fish this compartmentalization of the ventricle does not seem to offer any particular benefit for the animal, it theoretically should make at least partial separation of oxygenated and unoxygenated blood possible in air-breathing amphibians. According to the "classic hypothesis" [15, 16], disputed by some [2, 8], blood from the left atrium will tend to be sequestered in the left side of the single ventricle and that from the right atrium in the right side. The far-rightward position of the conus cordis in amphibians, and the complex arrangement in the conus consisting of proximal and distal sets of pocket valves with a spiral fold or septum [6] in between, favors venous blood to enter the pulmocutaneous channel early in ventricular systole and arterial blood to be discharged subsequently into the carotid arteries and dorsal aortae.

A similar mechanism appears to be operative in noncrocodilian reptiles [6, 10]. Here the horizontal septum of the ventricle functions in a manner analogous to that of the amphibian spiral fold. During the early phases of ventricular contraction, venous blood which has entered the cavum ventrale and right side of the cavum dorsale (the cavum venosum in reptiles which have a vertical septum) is ejected into the pulmonary trunk. At some time during ventricular contraction the free edge of the horizontal septum will contact the opposite, thickened ventricular wall (the *Bulbuslamelle* of German authors), thus preventing further entry of blood into the cavum ventrale and arterial blood from the left side of the cavum dorsale (cavum arteriosum) is ejected into the aortae. It has been demonstrated by physiological studies [6, 10] that the separation of arterial and venous blood is quite complete even in turtles and other reptiles which do not have a vertical septum. It is quite possible that in reptiles, as in birds and mammals, resistance to flow in the pulmonary circuit is less than in the systemic circulation, thus aiding the separation of unoxygenated and oxygenated blood by sequential ejection.

Complete septation of the ventricles prevents mixing of blood in crocodilians, birds, and mammals, and the blood from both sides of the heart is ejected into the pulmonary and the systemic circulations simultaneously. Even in crocodilians, where both the left aorta and the pulmonary trunk arise from the right ventricle, this ventricle ordinarily ejects its blood only into the pulmonary trunk. This is because the right ventricular pressure in normally active animals does not, at any time during the cardiac cycle, exceed the diastolic pressure in the two aortae and the left aortic valve therefore does not open. Oxygenated blood from the right aorta flows into the left aorta through the foramen of Panizza and separation of oxygenated and unoxygenated blood is complete, as in birds and mammals. Under certain circumstances, however (diving?), the resistance to flow into the pulmonary trunk is increased, apparently due to contraction of the subpulmonary circular muscle of the right ventricular outflow tract. This narrows down the circularly arranged subpulmonary nodules, causing stenosis of the right ventricular outflow tract. The right ventricular pressure rises and, once it has reached systemic levels, the left ventricular aortic valve can open. Part of the right ventricular blood is ejected into the systemic circulation, rather than into the lungs which in the submerged animal are nonfunctioning.

There continue to be disagreements about comparative anatomical nomenclature and concerning the homologies between the reptilian horizontal and vertical septa, on the one hand, the components of the complete ventricular septum of crocodilians, birds, and mammals, on the other. These problems have recently been reviewed in detail by Webb et al. [9] and by Holmes [5]. The term *Muskelleiste* has been translated by some authors into the English "muscular ridge". Others, however, use this same term for the vertical septum. The ventricular septum in crocodilians, birds, and mammals, according to some authors, has evolved from the vertical septum, according to others from the horizontal septum, while again others believe that it is derived from both. To complicate matters further, it has been suggested that the ventricular septum in birds and crocodilians is not homologous with that of mammals. Holmes [5] believes that the avian and crocodilian and probably also the mammalian septum is derived from the horizontal septum of reptiles, completed by a new addition derived from the atrioventricular endocardial cushions.

On the basis of our studies carried out thus far, we believe, as do others [1, 3, 14], that the anterior part of the mammalian ventricular septum is probably homologous to the anterior portion of the reptilian horizontal septum and that the posterior part of the septum in mammals, except for a small basilar part where in man the membranous septum is located, is homologous to the vertical septum of reptiles (Fig. 3). We consider the trabecula septomarginalis and associated trabeculae in the apical part of the right ventricle to be remnants of the posterolateral portion of the horizontal septum which, with the development of a complete ventricular septum, has lost its function as a septum, has regressed, and has become perforated. These tentative conclusions will have to be substantiated by embryological studies currently going on in our laboratory.

REFERENCES

1. Benninghof A: Herz. In: Bolk L, Göppert E, Kallius E, Lubosch W (eds) Handbuch der vergleichenden Anatomeder Wirbeltiere, vol 6. Berlin–Vienna, Urban and Schwarzenberg, 1933, pp. 467–556.
2. Foxon, GEH: Problems of the double circulation in vertebrates. Biol Rev 30:196–228, 1955.
3. Goodrich ES: Studies on the structure and development of vertebrates. London, Macmillan, 1930, pp. 553–561.
4. Greil A: Beiträge zur vergleichenden Anatomie und Entwicklungsgeschichte des Herzens und des Truncus arteriosus der Wirbeltiere. Morphol Jahrb 31:123–310, 1903.
5. Holmes EB: A reconsideration of the phylogeny of the tetrapod heart. J Morphol 147:209–228, 1975.

6. Johansen K, Martin AW: Comparative aspects of cardiovascular function in vertebrates. In: Hamilton WF, Dow P (eds) Handbook of physiology, section 2: Circulation, vol 3, Washington DC, Am Physiol Soc, 1965, pp 2583–2614.

7. Romer AS: The vertebrate body. Shorter version. Philadelphia–London, WB Saunders, 1971, pp 295–325.

8. Vorstman AG: Het bloed- en lymphvaatstelsel. In: Ihle JEW (ed) Leerboek der vergelijkende ontleedkunde van de vertebraten. Utrecht, A Oosthoek, 1947, pp 229–300.

9. Webb GJW, Heatwole H, de Bavay J: Comparative cardiac anatomy of the reptilia. II. A critique of the literature on Squamata and Rhynchocephalia. J Morphol 142:1–20, 1974.

10. White FN: Functional anatomy of the heart of reptiles. Am Zool 8:211–219, 1968.

11. Streeter GL: Developmental horizons in human embryos. Description of age group XIII, embryos about 4–5 mm long, and age group XIV, period of indentation of the lens vesicle. Contrib Embryol 31:27–63, 1945.

12. Robertson JI: The development of the heart and vascular system of *Lepidosiren paradoxa*. Q J Microsc Sci 59:53–132, 1913.

13. Antony J, Millot J, Robineau D: Le coeur et l'aorte ventrale de *Latimeria chalumnae* (*Poisson coelacanthidè*). CR Acad Sci (Paris) 273:689–692, 1971.

14. Leene JE Vorstman AG: Note on the structure of the heart of *Varanus* as compared with other reptilian hearts. Tijdschr Ned Dierkd Ver 2:62–66, 1930.

15. Brücke E: Beiträge zur vergleichenden Anatomie und Physiologie des Gefässsystems. Denkschr Akad Wiss Wien 3:335–367, 1852.

16. Sabatier A: Études sur le coeur et la circulation centrale dans la série des vertébrés. Ann Sci Nat Zool [Ser 3] 18:1–89, 1873.

5. SEPTAL ARCHITECTURE IN HEARTS WITH VENTRICULAR SEPTAL DEFECTS

ARENTJE OPPENHEIMER-DEKKER

INTRODUCTION

In discussing the septal architecture in hearts with ventricular septal defects, it is neither the aim to adhere to one or other of the existing classifications of septal defects [1, 2] nor to introduce a new one. Rather is it the purpose to focus attention on certain characteristics of the anatomical and the spatial relationships – or maybe lack of relationships – of septal components, which arise during and after the developmental derangement underlying the evolution of ventricular septal defects. Such an approach can take advantage of the available embryological data and at the same time, if handling matters very cautiously, can be an aid in filling some gaps, for instance in the identification and demarcation of septal components as defined in Chapter 1 of this book.

Starting with the right and left ventricular outflow tracts, various anomalies can be selected which provide useful information on the mature and macroscopically visible derivations and aberrations of the infundibular and bulboventricular components of the ventricular septum. But it becomes equally apparent that, in particular in hearts with lack of coaptation between septal components, considerable overlap of outflow and inflow pathology may be found, with participation of the inlet septum. Therefore in this context a subdivision in outflow and inflow defects appears to be impractical, if not confusing. The following notes and observations will exemplify the occurrence of such overlapping in several of the malformations.

TRUNCUS ARTERIOSUS PERSISTENS (Fig. 1a and b)

In this malformation it is the infundibular septum which has failed to develop properly. This fact defines the defect as indicating the presumed site of this septal component. In the normal heart the infundibular septum, as seen from the right ventricular side, borders posteriorly on the external, parietal (lateral) wall of the outflow tract (i.e., at the right ventricular aspect it represents the posterior edge of the septum); anteriorly it is continuous with the bulboventricular septum. This implies that in the right ventricle of hearts with truncus arteriosus persistens, septal myocardium borders the defect anteriorly only and this myocardium has its source in the bulboventricular septal

A.C.G. Wenink et al. (eds.) The Ventricular Septum of the Heart, *47–56. All rights reserved.*
Copyright ©1981 by Martinus Nijhoff Publishers, The Hague/Boston/London.

48

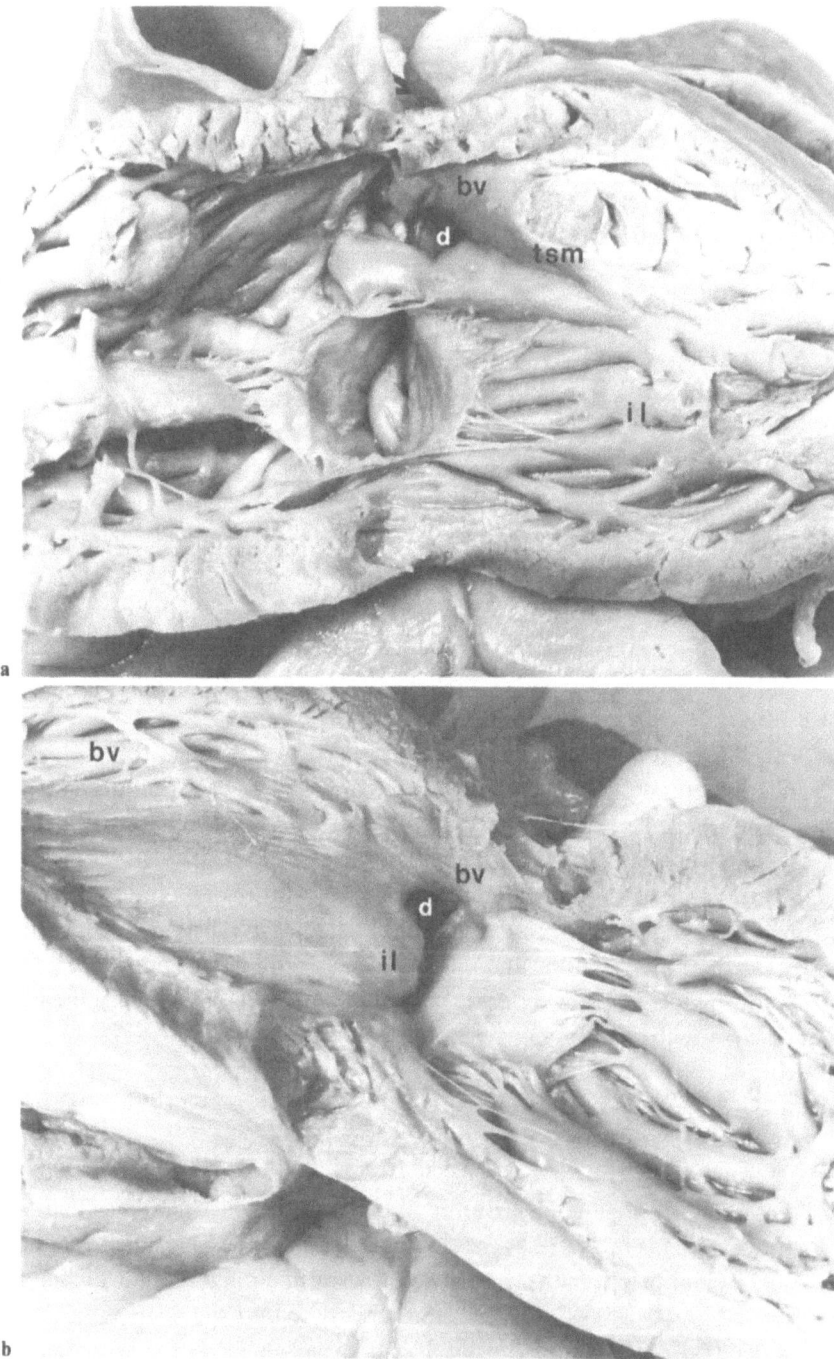

Fig. 1. (*a*) Right ventricle in a case of truncus arteriosus persistens. The small ventricular septal defect (d) immediately underneath the truncal orifice indicates the presumed site of the infundibular septum, which in this malformation has failed to develop properly; bv, bulboventricular septum; il, inlet septum; tsm, trabecula septomarginalis. (*b*) Left ventricle in a case of truncus arteriosus persistens. Abbrevations as in Figure 1a.

component. At the left ventricular side the infundibular septum is wedged between the bulboventricular component anteriorly, and the membranous septum and the inlet septum posteriorly. This adequately describes the sources of the left ventricular septal components surrounding the defect in truncus arteriosus persistens.

MALALIGNMENT INFUNDIBULAR SEPTAL DEFECTS (Figs. 2–4)

In this group the infundibular septum is deprived of its normal junctions because of a faulty development in the final stages of the right and left ventricular outflow tract formation. In this situation the infundibular septal component seeks and finds various other meeting points by developing extensions either toward the right parietal or the anterior wall of the right ventricle (Figs. 2 and 3a), or toward the left ventricle, usually in the direction of the left anterior parietal wall (and the anterolateral muscle [3], if present

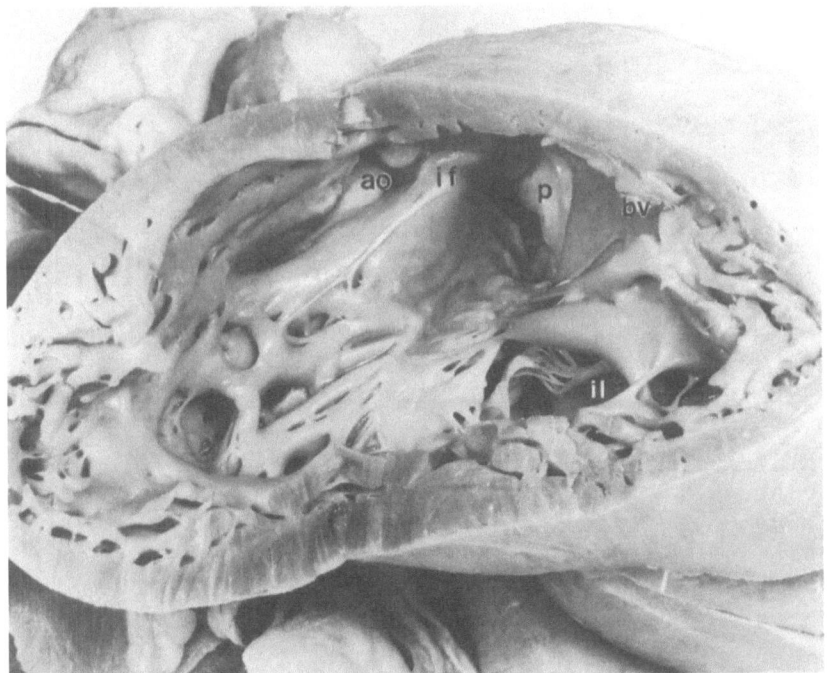

Fig. 2. Right ventricle in a case of transposition with malalignment septal defect. Between the aortic orifice (ao) and the pulmonary orifice (p) is the infundibular septal component (if), which in this case extends toward the parietal right ventricular wall; bv, bulboventricular septum; il, inlet septum.

50

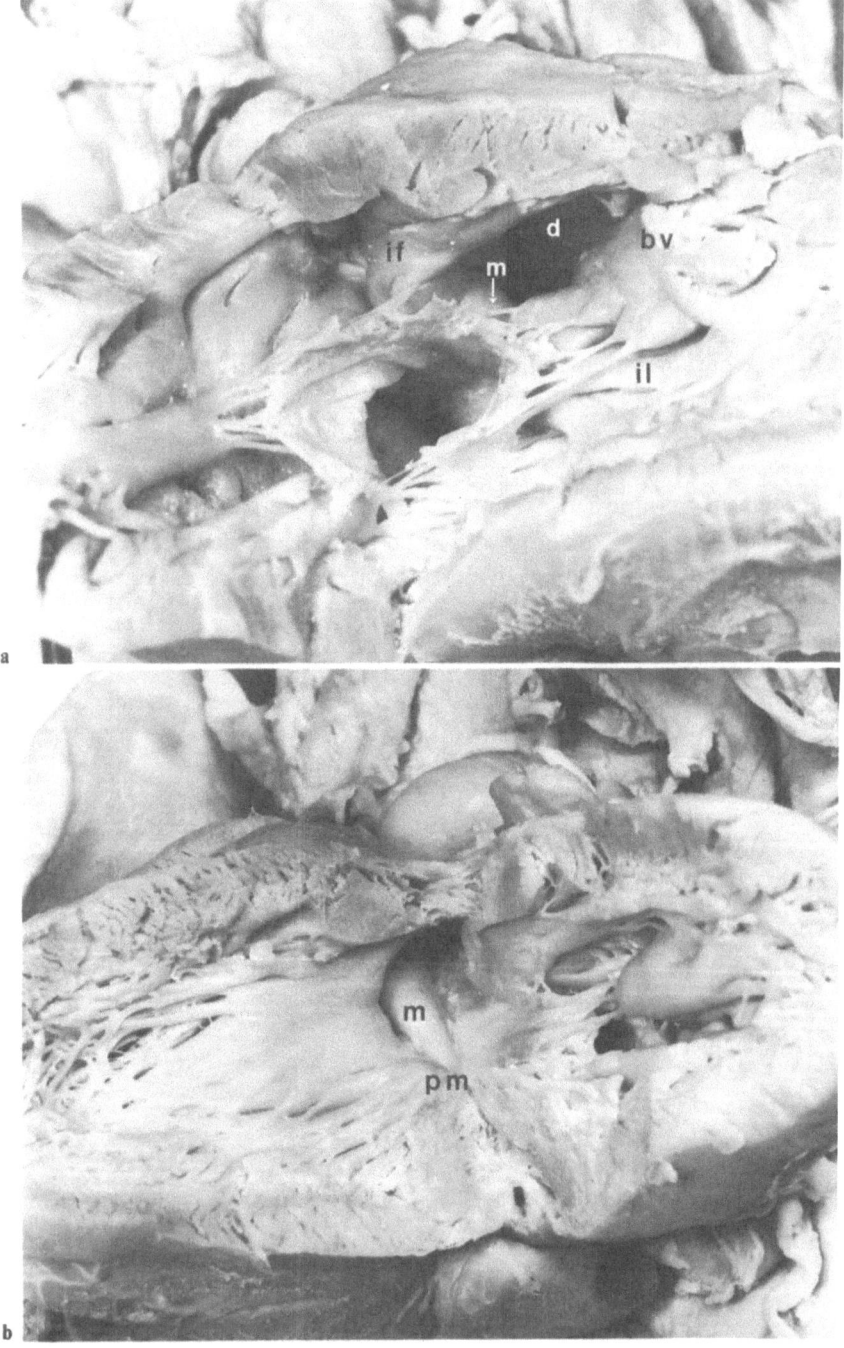

Fig. 3. (*a*) Right ventricle in a case of transposition with malalignment septal defect; if, infundibular septal component, attached to the anterior right ventricular wall; m, extension of the malaligned infundibular septum toward the posteromedial muscle (cf. Fig. 3b); bv, bulboventricular septum; d, ventricular septal defect; il, inlet septum. (*b*) Same specimen as in Figure 3a, left ventricle, showing the malaligned infundibular septum (m) extending toward the posteromedial muscle (pm).

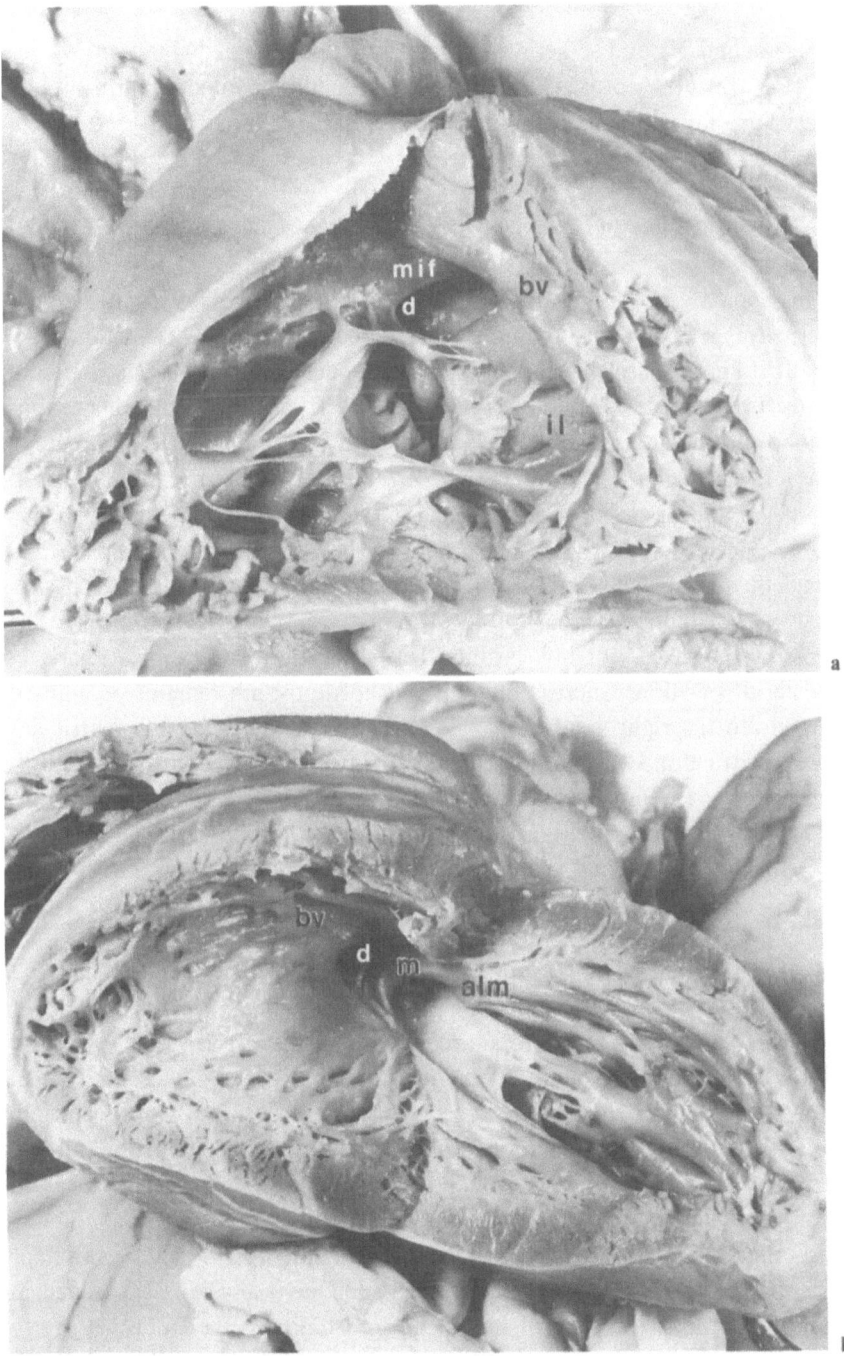

Fig. 4. (*a*) Right ventricle in a case with malalignment infundibular septal defect (d); mif, malaligned infundibular septum, extending toward left ventricle; further abbreviations as in previous figures. (*b*) Same specimen as in Figure 4a, left ventricle. Extension of the malaligned infundibular septum (m) toward the anterolateral muscle (alm); d, ventricular septal defect; further abbreviations as in previous figures.

[Fig. 4a and b]), and sometimes also toward a posteromedial muscle [4], i.e., part of the inlet septum (Fig. 3b). These secondary contacts can result in a very large infundibular septal derivative.

EISENMENGER VENTRICULAR SEPTAL DEFECT (Fig. 5a and b)

This anomaly is well known as far as the right ventricular aspects are concerned (Fig. 5a) and it is commonly considered, anatomically and embryologically, to be a relatively simple type of septal defect. However, inspection of the left ventricular morphology reveals that we are dealing with a conspicuous bulboventricular septal maldevelopment with great impact on the buildup of the left ventricular outflow tract (Fig. 5b). The anteroseptal portion of the left ventricle appears to be very abnormal in that it consists of a disproportionately thick mass of myocardium. This is the result of an insufficient and inadequate elaboration of the left ventricular outflow tract in the left basilar part of the bulboventricular fold (Wenink, Chapter 3 of this book). The anteroseptal excess of myocardium leaves the mitral valve in a relatively posterior position, whereas the adjacent aortic ostium remains committed largely to the right ventricle. Most probably the deficient left ventricular outflow tract must be considered to be the primary developmental disturbance in the Eisenmenger anomaly. In this context and with reference to Chapter 10 of this book, it should be mentioned that the combination of the Eisenmenger defect and atrioventricular defect is not rare.

CENTRAL MUSCULAR VENTRICULAR SEPTAL DEFECT (Fig. 6a and b)

A grossly disturbed myocardial architecture in the left ventricular outflow tract is also found in many of the hearts with a central muscular type of ventricular septal defect (defined according to the criteria of Wenink et al. [5]). Before analyzing the striking features in the subaortic part of the outflow tract, it should be emphasized that, for various reasons, this malformation confronts the cautious and open-minded examiner with several conflicting observations. These are related to the fact that indeed in the right ventricular view the central muscular septal defect can unequivocally be called a defect in the inflow tract (because of its position posterior to the trabecula septomarginalis and its close relationship with septal tricuspid papillary muscles), whereas in the left ventricular view this is not at all self-evident. Using the morphological and hemodynamic approach, one can define the left ventricular inflow tract as guarded by the mitral valve and its anterolateral and posteromedial papillary muscles, which are not inserted on the septal surface

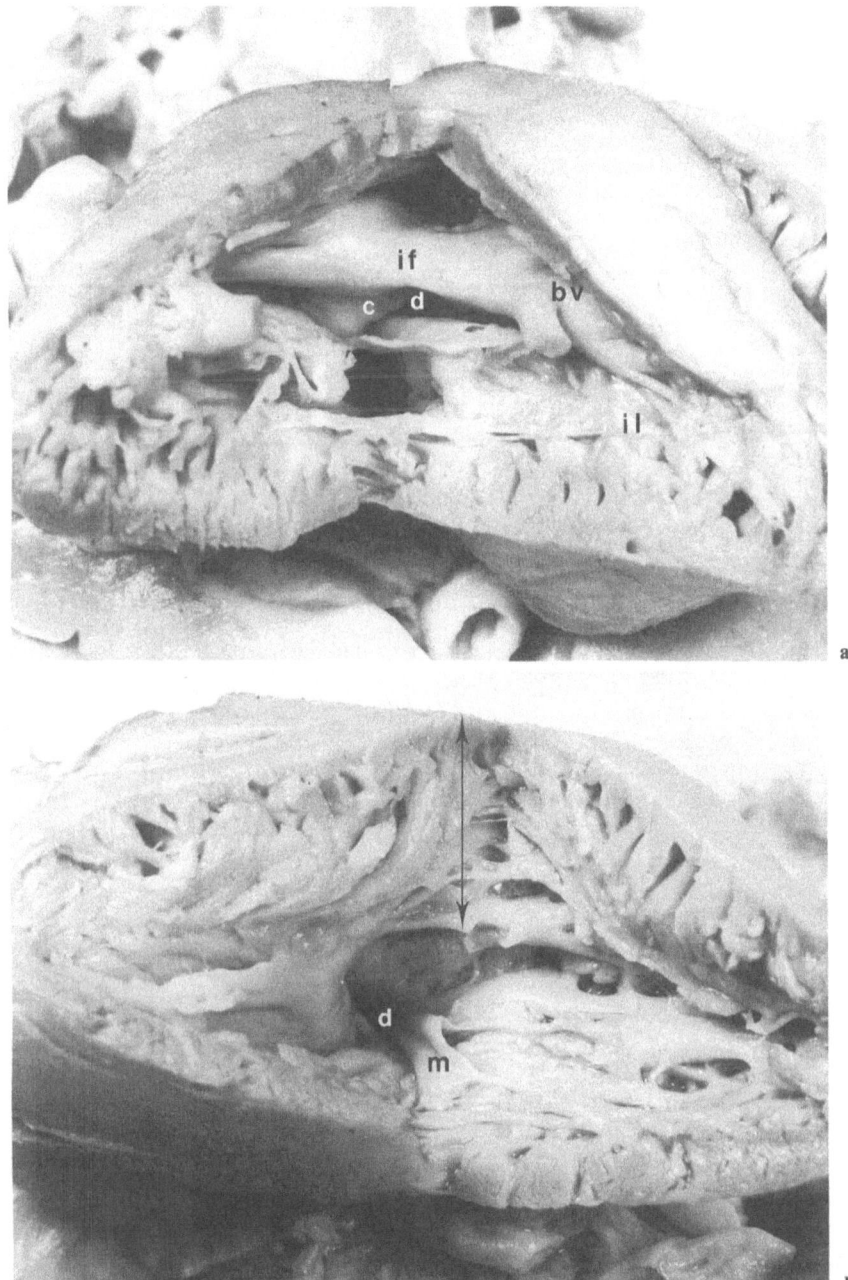

Fig. 5. (*a*) Right ventricle of a case with Eisenmenger ventricular septal defect (d), showing one of the semilunar cusps (c) of the overriding aortic orifice; further abbreviations as in previous figures. (*b*) Same specimen as in Figure 5a, left ventricle. The anteroseptal portion consists of a disproportionately thick mass of myocardium (indicated by double-headed arrow), which leaves the mitral valve (m) in a relatively posterior position, whereas the aortic ostium remains committed largely to the right ventricle; d, ventricular septal defect.

54

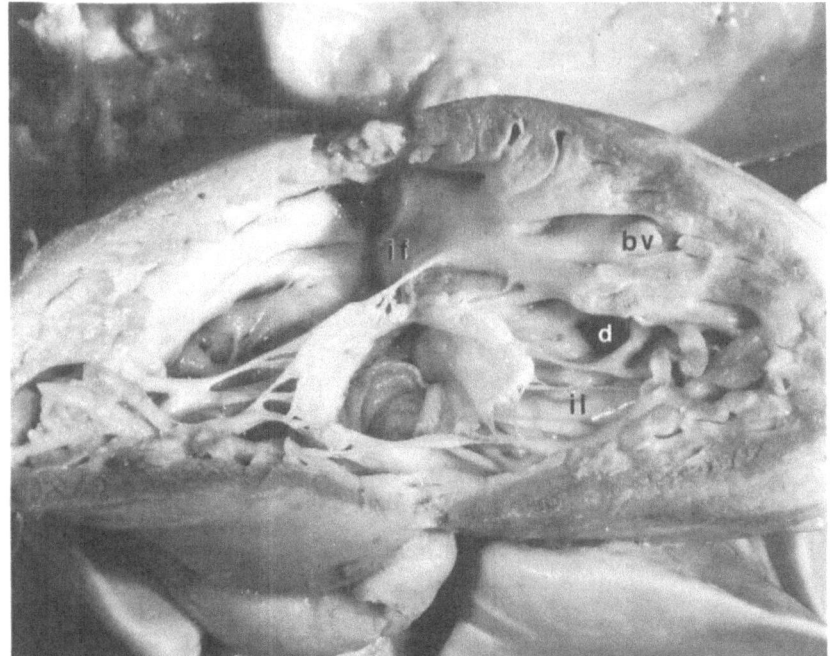

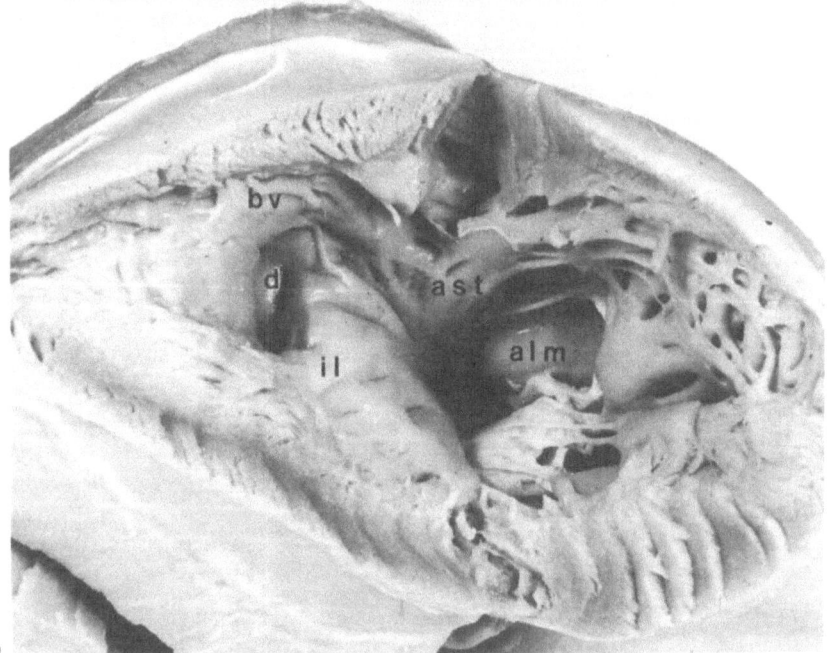

Fig. 6. (*a*) Right ventricle of a case with central muscular ventricular septal defect (d); abbreviations as in previous figures. (*b*) Same specimen as in Figure 6a, left ventricle; alm, anterolateral muscle; ast, anteroseptal twist; further abbreviations as in Figure 6a.

(Chapter 1, Fig. 1a). This definition implies that the whole left ventricular septal surface, and consequently a defect in it, belongs to the outflow tract, except for the malformations with atrioventricular defect or with tricuspid straddling (Chapters 10 and 13 of this book). But also if one tries to bring forward the embryogenetic approach, this would, at the most, allow the term inlet (not inflow) septal defect in specimens with malaligned inlet septal components (posterior muscular septal defect) [5] or with an incomplete inlet septum as in atrioventricular defects. This all adds up to the conclusion that many defects in the left ventricular outflow tract communicate with the right ventricular inflow tract.

This kind of inconsistency and discrepancy can be avoided by abstaining from the notions inflow and outflow tract, and by using the data gained from Wenink's embryological observations (Chapter 3 of this book) for the description of the characteristics and the site of the central muscular defects. They are usually oval and, seen from the left, bordered by two crescent-shaped septal structures: an anterior and apical one with trabeculations, and a posterior and basal one with a relatively smoother surface. They are obliquely fitted to each other and many of them show a remarkable malformation which can be described as "anteroseptal twist" [6] (Fig. 6b). The twist consists of leftward bending and thickening of the anterior part of the interventricular septum (bulboventricular septum) and of the anterior left ventricular wall, thus displacing the aortic ostium posteriorly. There is a high incidence of a prominent anterolateral muscle, and moreover a frequent association with aortic bicuspidy and mitral valve anomalies. Combining these data on left ventricular abnormalities with the data on embryonic development, it is evident that we are dealing with a complex developmental disturbance in the bulboventricular fold: the bulboventricular septum has inadequately fused with the inlet septum (central muscular defect; this lack of correspondence factually places the hole in the right ventricular inflow tract, posterior to the trabecula septomarginalis); an excessive myocardial growth has taken place in the left basal curve of the bulboventricular fold (anteroseptal twist) and in the left extremity of the fold (prominent anterolateral muscle). This portion of the bulboventricular fold partly represents the boundary between aortic and mitral orifices, eventually forming the anterior mitral leaflet with its tension apparatus, which can explain the frequent association with mitral valve anomalies and the involvement of the adjacent aortic valve.

Summing up. The ventricular septal defect of the central muscular type is by no means an isolated anomaly consisting of merely a hole in the ventricular septum. Commonly it is part of a complex developmental aberration involving primarily the bulboventricular fold, resulting in abnormal septal architecture and associated inflow and outflow pathology, in which the central muscular septal defect might even be nor more than a secondary outcome of a grossly disturbed development. This complex is discussed here rather extensively as it illustrates so clearly the importance of a sound knowledge of embryonic development for application in a careful and effective analysis of abnormal septal and related myocardial and even valvular architecture.

REFERENCES

1. Moulaert AJ: Anatomy of ventricular septal defect. In: Anderson RH, Shinebourne EA (eds) Paediatric cardiology 1977. Edinburgh, Churchill Livingstone, 1978, pp 113–124.
2. Soto B, Becker AE, Moulaert AJ, Lie JT, Anderson RH: Classification of ventricular septal defects. Br Heart J 43:332–343, 1980.
3. Moulaert AJ, Oppenheimer-Dekker A: Anterolateral muscle bundle of the left ventricle, bulboventricular flange and subaortic stenosis. Am J Cardiol 37: 78–81, 1976.
4. Wenink ACG: Considerations pertinent to the embryogenesis of transposition. In: Van Mierop LHS, Oppenheimer-Dekker A, Bruins CLDC (eds) Embryology and teratology of the heart and the great arteries. Leiden, Leiden University Press, 1978, pp 129–135.
5. Wenink ACG, Oppenheimer-Dekker A, Moulaert AJ: Muscular ventricular septal defects: a reappraisal of the anatomy. Am J Cardiol 43:259–264, 1979.
6. Moene RJ, Oppenheimer-Dekker A, Wenink ACG: The relationship between aortic arch hypoplasia of variable severity and central muscular ventricular septal defects: emphasis on associated left ventricular abnormalities. Am J Cardiol (in press).

6. TWO-DIMENSIONAL ECHOCARDIOGRAPHIC LOCALIZATION OF ISOLATED VENTRICULAR SEPTAL DEFECTS

GERTJAN VAN MILL, ANDRÉ J. MOULAERT, AND ERIC HARINCK

INTRODUCTION

Isolated ventricular septal defects (VSDs) can vary in size, shape, and localization. To obtain adequate information about these different aspects, cardiac catheterization including shunt measurements and angiocardiography is usually indicated. Recent data show that with the noninvasive two-dimensional sector echocardiography (2D Echo), VSDs can be visualized, localized, and measured directly [1–3]. To understand 2D Echo of VSDs, extensive knowledge of the cardiac anatomy is necessary together with a clear understanding of the various echocardiographic cross-sectional planes obtained from different views [4].

THE INTERVENTRICULAR SEPTUM – ANATOMICAL DESCRIPTION

A practical classification of the VSDs can be obtained if the interventricular septum (IVS) is divided into four parts: an inlet (posterior), a trabecular (bulboventricular), an outlet (infundibular), and a membranous part [5] (Fig. 1). The first three parts together constitute the muscular ventricular septum. The membranous septum is situated in the medial wall of the left ventricular outflow tract (LVOT) just beneath the aortic valve. In the right ventricle this part of the IVS is situated at the site where the anterior and the septal tricuspid leaflet meet on the IVS. The three parts of the muscular septum converge toward and, therefore, border on the membranous septum. The inlet septum divides the ventricular inflow tracts and the outlet septum separates the ventricular outflow tracts. The trabecular septum is located between in- and outlet septum, and is demarcated posteriorly by the trabecula septomarginalis (Fig. 1). The right ventricular inflow tract is situated on the right and adjacent to the left ventricle. Therefore, the inlet septum extends in an anterior-posterior direction one way and in a left-inferior to right-superior direction the other way. On account of this, the inlet septum can be passed perpendiculary by the echo beam only from the upper abdomen. The outlet septum and the trabecular septum separate the left ventricle from the anteriorly situated part of the right ventricle. Hence, these parts of the muscular

58

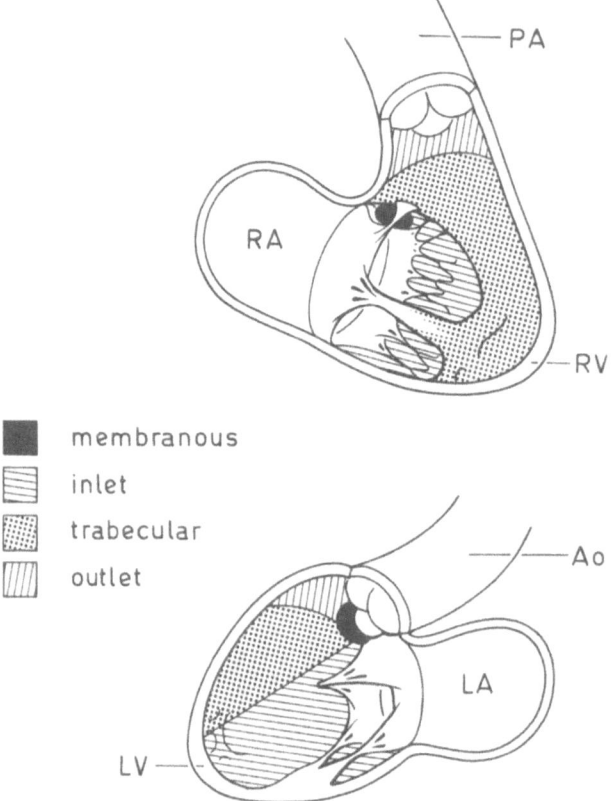

Fig. 1. Diagrammatic representation of the right side and the left side of the IVS, which is divided into its four parts; RA, right atrium; RV, right ventricle; PA, pulmonary artery; LA, left atrium; LV, left ventricle; Ao, aorta.

septum extend into a plane more or less parallel to the frontal plane and can be passed perpendicularly by the precordial approach.

ANATOMICAL CLASSIFICATION OF THE VSDS

The membranous VSD is the most frequently occurring VSD. Hemodynamically important VSDs are never limited to the small membranous septum. They extend into the different parts of the muscular septum. Soto et al. [6] classified the VSDs as follows:

1) Perimembranous with extension to inlet, outlet, and/or trabecular septum.
2) Muscular, inlet, outlet, or trabecular.

3) Subarterial-infundibular. This VSD borders the semilunar valve rings and, therefore, is deprived of a complete muscular rim.
4) Mixed defects.

Two-dimensional echocardiographic approach to the VSD requires the following ultrasonic "windows": subcostal, apical, and parasternal. During the subcostal investigation the transducer is positioned in the subxiphoid area (Fig. 2). The subcostal four-chamber view is an important cross section which provides a simultaneous visualization of right atrium, right ventricular inflow tract, left atrium, and left ventricular inflow tract.

Angulation of the transducer anteriorly provides a longitudinal view of the left ventricle with the aorta originating as the posterior great artery. Anterior to the aorta the inflow part of the right ventricle with tricuspid valve remains visible. This cross section is important for visualizing the medial wall of the LVOT and specifically for locating the site where the membranous septum is limited to a small area just below the tricuspid valve ring. The rest of the IVS that remains visible lies at the transition between inlet and trabecular septum. A similar four-chamber view, as previously mentioned, with the subcostal approach can also be obtained from the apex of the heart. The transducer is placed on the chest at the site of the apex beat. Four-chamber views visualize simultanously the inflow tracts of the right and left heart. In these cross sections the inlet septum is particularly visualized together with the atrioventricular septum. The latter part of the IVS is situated between the insertion of the mitral valve and the tricuspid valve and separates the left ventricle from the right atrium.

As far as the parasternal window is concerned, the transducer is placed immediately left of the sternum. Long- and short-axis views of the left ventricle are routinely made (Fig. 3). In the cross section along the long axis of the ventricle, the following parts of the heart are visualized simultaneously: the ascending aorta, the left atrium, the left ventricle, and the right ventricular outflow tract. The anterior parts of the IVS only are visualized in this cross section, i.e., the outlet septum situated directly under the aortic valve and more distally the trabecular septum. Shifting the transducer to the left, a sagittal cross section of the pulmonary artery is visualized. This also shows the subpulmonic part of the outlet septum. When the transducer is rotated through 90°, short-axis views of the left ventricle can be obtained allowing a review of the various parts of the ventricular septum. A transverse cross section through the LVOT shows the anticipated site of the membranous septum and the outlet septum. At the level of the mitral valve, the posterior inlet septum and the anterior trabecular septum can be seen.

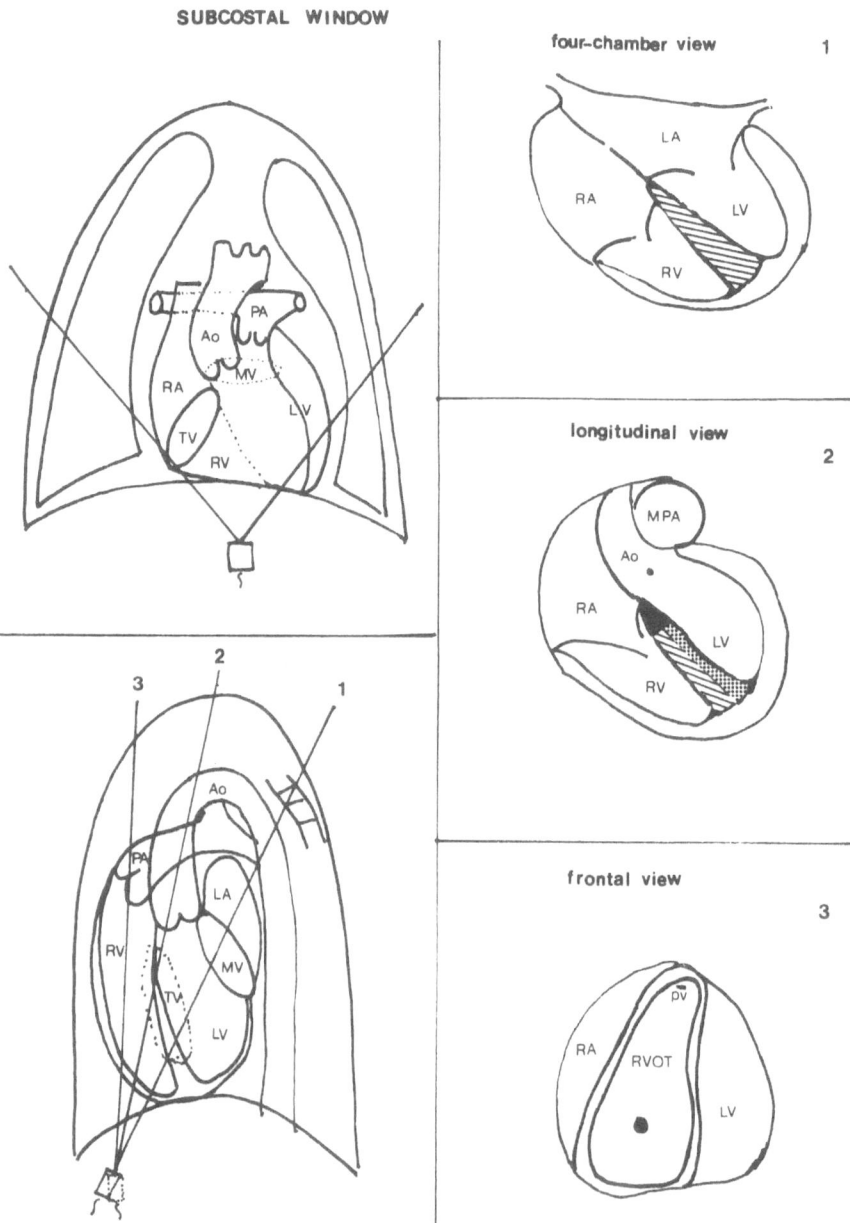

SUBCOSTAL WINDOW

four-chamber view 1

longitudinal view 2

frontal view 3

Fig. 2. Diagrammatic representation of the use of the subcostal window. The posterior four-chamber view is indicated by number *1* and in this cross section the posterior inlet septum is visualized with its atrioventricular part between the insertion of septal tricuspid and mitral leaflets. Angulation of the transducer to plane *2* gives a longitudinal view of the left ventricle with the originating posterior great artery. In this plane the upper part of the interventricular septum represents the membranous septum and the larger lower part the transition zone between inlet and trabecular septum. In the frontal view *3* no part of the IVS is visible; MV, mitral valve; TV, tricuspid valve; PV, pulmonary valve; MPA, main pulmonary artery; RVOT, right ventricular outflow tract; other abbreviations as in Figure 2.

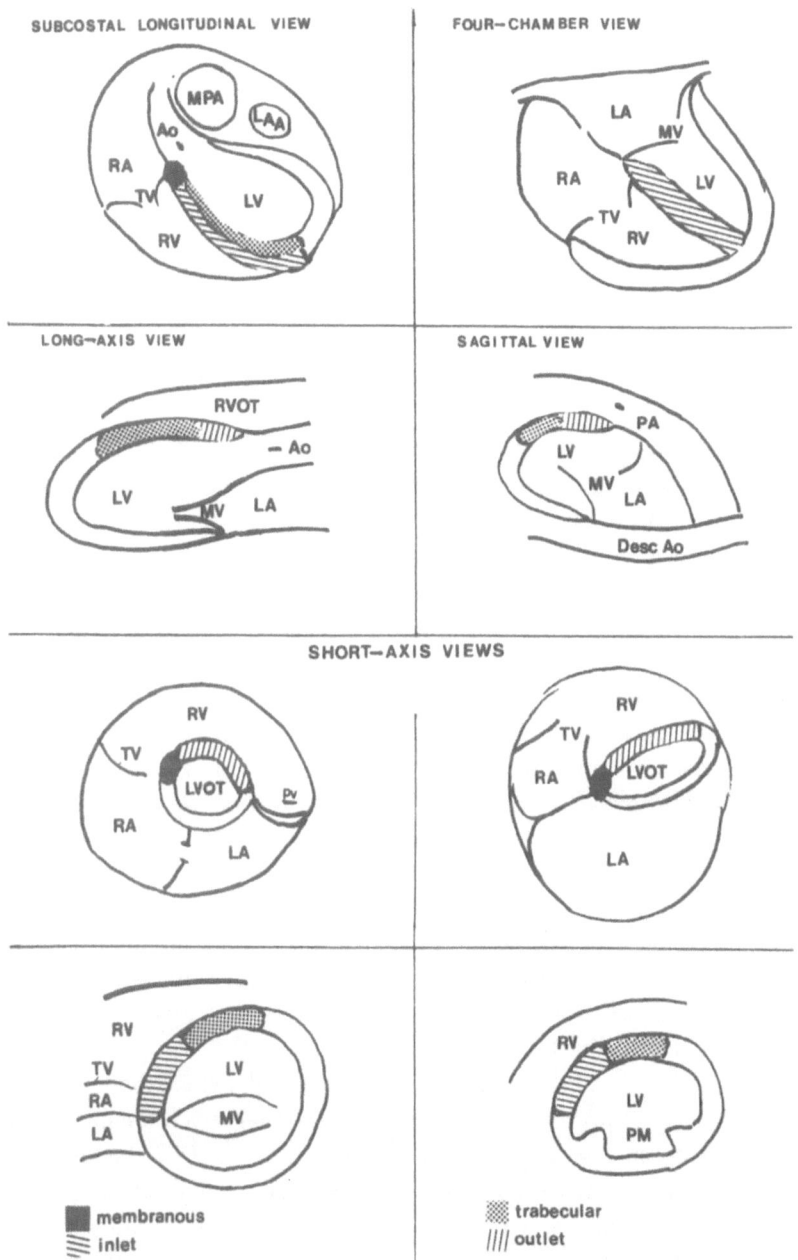

Fig. 3. Diagrammatic representation of all the matching cross-sectional planes showing the different parts of the IVS. Short-axis views are shown at the level of the left ventricular outflow tract, the mitral valve, and the papillary muscles in the left ventricle; LAA, left atrial appendage; Desc Ao, descending aorta; LVOT, left ventricular outflow tract; PM, papillary muscles; other abbreviations as in previous figures.

ECHOCARDIOGRAPHIC RECOGNITION OF THE VSDS

The previously described approach is routinely carried out in all our 2D Echo investigations. VSDs of several millimeters to sometimes more than 1 cm become visible as a constant interruption of the continuity of the IVS. The size of the VSD can vary during the cardiac cycle [3]. The existence of an interruption must be visualized in the corresponding part of the septum in different cross sections. Hemodynamically important membranous VSDs can be shown or excluded by the subcostal longitudinal view. Using the same subcostal transducer position, an extension of the defect into the inlet septum can be determined by angulating posteriorly to the subcostal four-chamber view.

The short-axis view across the LVOT confirms the existence of a large membranous VSD and allows the assessment of anterior extension. Posterior or inlet VSDs only can be seen in the four-chamber views and in the short-axis view at the level of the mitral valve. Anteriorly located VSDs only can be detected with the parasternal transducer positions, unless the examination can be completed with the subcostal sagittal views. When the results obtained from different views are combined, the presence, localization, and size of a hemodynamically important VSD can be established.

In 20 consecutive patients, mainly infants under one year of age, with hemodynamically important VSDs, it was possible to visualize the VSD directly by the above-described method. The observations were confirmed by cardiac catheterization, left ventricular angiocardiography, echocontrast studies with "contrast" injections into the left ventricle, and in most cases also at operation (Figs. 4 and 5). False positive findings did not occur.

The following types of VSDs were recognized: "localized" perimembranous 11; perimembranous with extension to anterior (outlet and/or trabecular) 3; perimembranous inlet 1; muscular inlet 2; muscular trabecular 1; muscular outlet 1; subarterial-infundibular 1.

Figure 6 shows the parasternal two-dimensional echocardiogram of a patient with a large perimembranous ventricular septal defect extending in an anterior direction. The catheter is passed through the VSD in the long-axis and the sagittal view. In the sagittal view there is an obvious distance between the VSD and the pulmonary valve. In the short-axis view the VSD is located on the right side of the left ventricular outflow tract. It starts at the insertion of the tricuspid valve and extends from that point into an anterior direction.

In Figure 7, the two-dimensional echocardiograms are shown of a perimembranous inlet septal defect. The subcostal longitudinal view exhibits a large membranous defect and the many septal attachments of the tricuspid valve which covers the defect. The four-chamber view shows a distinct deficiency of the upper part of the inlet septum including the atrioventricular

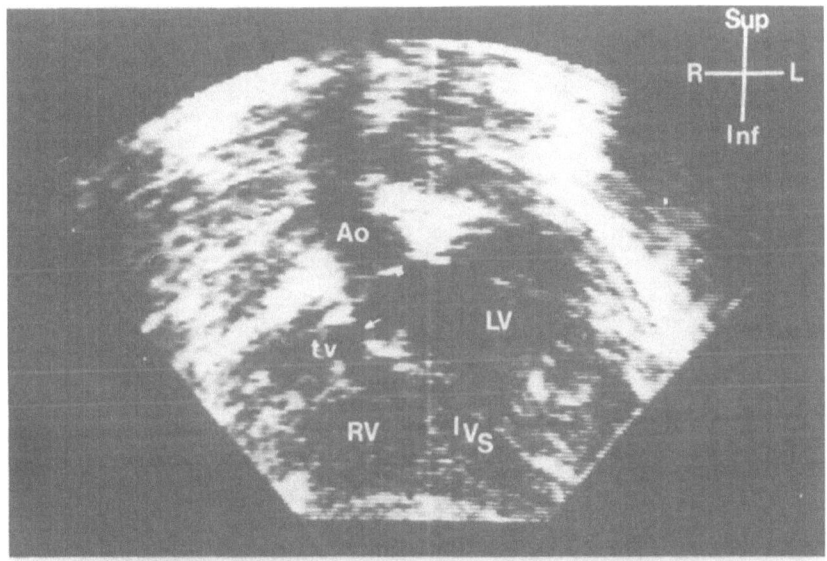

Subcostal Longitudinal View

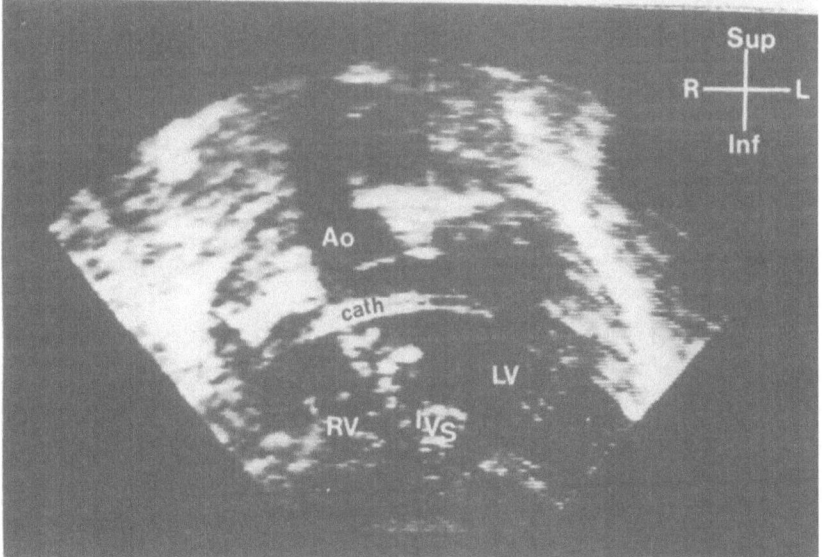

Fig. 4. (*Top*) Two-dimensional echocardiogram showing a membranous VSD as indicated by the arrow. From the right side the tricuspid valve covers the defect. (*Bottom*) During cardiac catheterization, it was possible to put a catheter through the VSD from the right ventricle to the left ventricle; IVS, interventricular septum; cath, catheter; other abbreviations as in previous figures.

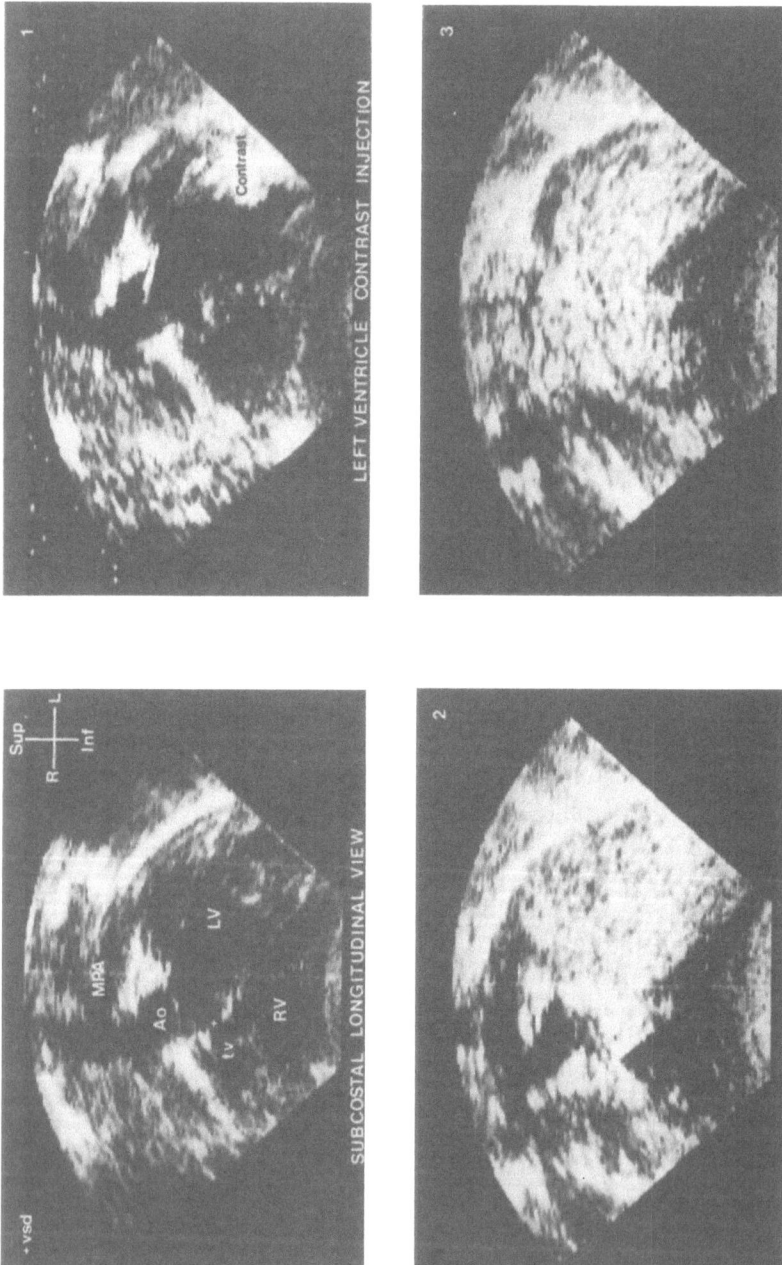

Fig. 5. Two-dimensional echocardiogram from the same patient as Figure 4. During cardiac catheterization the left ventricle was also reached *via* the foramen ovale. An echo contrast injection was done with some saline. The contrast appeared first in the apex of the left ventricle (*1*). A moment later (*2*) the whole left ventricle was filled with contrast and through the VSD there was already some contrast against the septal tricuspid leaflet. Finally the right ventricle was filled with contrast (*3*) as the result of a large left to right shunt.

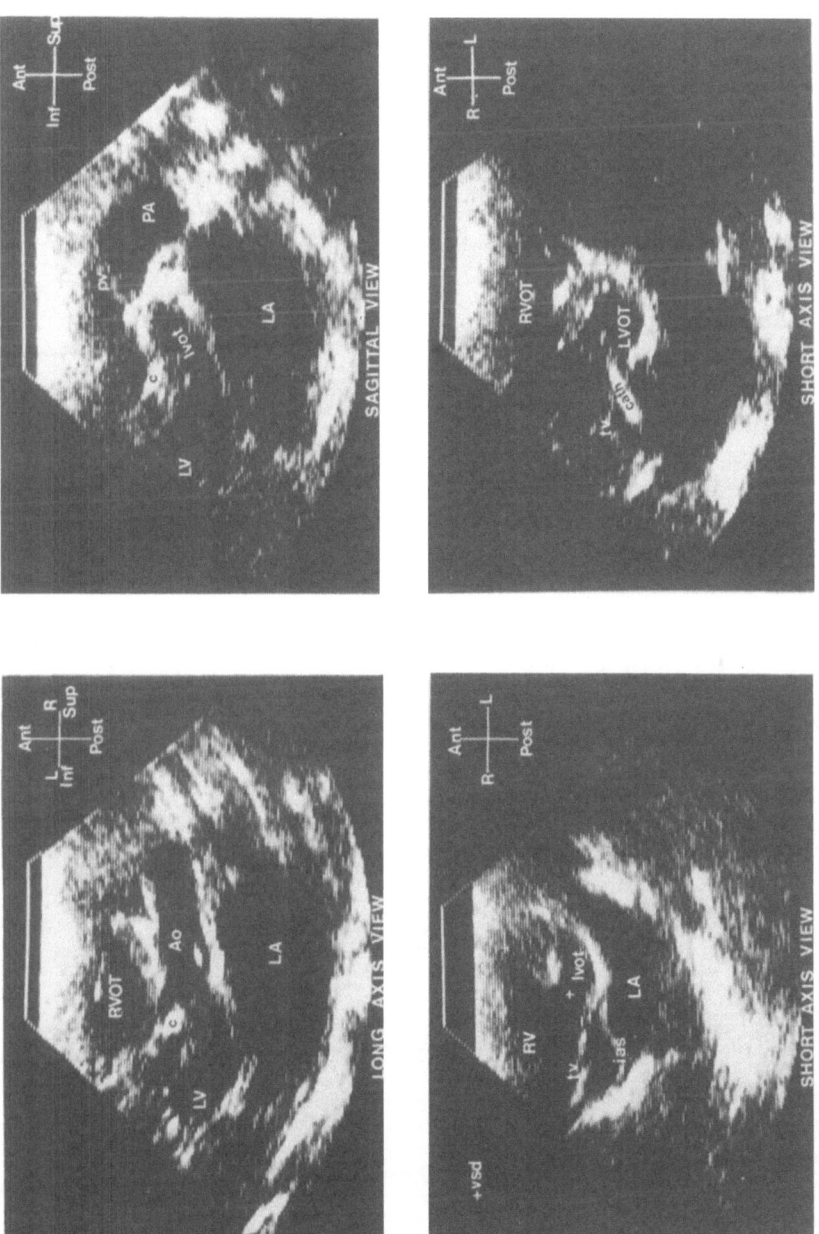

Fig. 6. Parasternal two-dimensional echocardiogram showing a large perimembranous VSD; ias, interatrial septum; cath, catheter; other abbreviations as in previous figures.

66

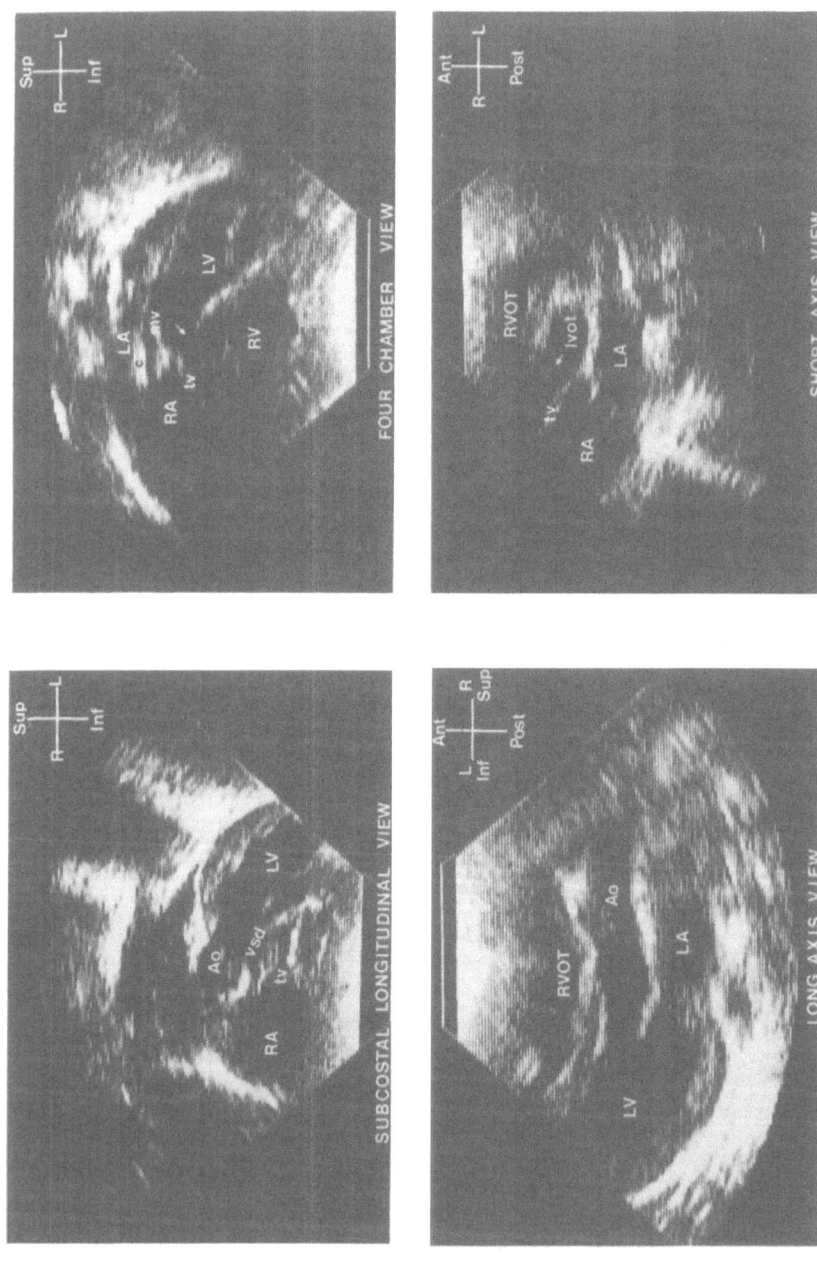

Fig. 7. Two-dimensional echocardiograms of a perimembranous inlet septal defect; vsd, ventricular septal defect; other abbreviations as in previous figures.

septum as indicated by the arrow. Therefore, the membranous defect extends into the inlet septum. In the short-axis view the defect is on the right side of the left ventricular outflow tract. There is not enough anterior extension to visualize the VSD in the long-axis view. This VSD is also called isolated atrioventricular canal type VSD (7). The 2D echocardiograms of a muscular inlet septal defect are shown in Figure 8. In the subcostal longitudinal view the membranous septum is intact. In the four-chamber view, however, a large defect is present in the upper part of the inlet septum between the septal leaflets of tricuspid and mitral valve. In the short-axis view, at the level of the mitral valve, the defect can also be clearly seen in the posterior part of the IVS. The anterior septum is also intact in the long-axis view.

Figure 9 portrays the two-dimensional echocardiograms of two defects in the muscular inlet septum. In the subcostal longitudinal view the membranous septum is intact. More distally a defect is visible in the transition zone of inlet and trabecular septum as indicated by the arrow. The subcostal four-chamber view revealed a large inlet defect. In the short-axis view, at the level of the mitral valve, two VSDs became visible, an anterior defect and a larger posterior defect (see arrows). In the second short-axis view on the right, the transducer was slightly shifted to the apex of the heart.

The two-dimensional echocardiograms of a patient with a large trabecular VSD are shown in Figure 10. The subcostal longitudinal view indicates the intact membranous septum. More distally a defect is visible in the transition zone of inlet and trabecular septum. Angulation to the four-chamber view excluded extension into the inlet septum. In the short-axis view the posterior septum is intact and the defect is situated in the anterior part. The distal and anterior localization of the large trabecular defect is also clearly shown in the long-axis view. This muscular VSD which lies at the transition between inlet and trabecular septum has also been called a central muscular defect [8]. Figure 11 shows the two-dimensional echocardiograms of a patient with a ventricular septal defect and pulmonary hypertension. The long-axis view exhibits a large defect of the outlet septum just beneath the aortic valve. The size of the defect hardly changed throughout the cardiac cycle. The anterior wall of the aorta is located more anteriorly than the IVS, which indicates some degree of overriding. This outlet VSD is also called a Fallot-like VSD.

A subarterial-infundibular VSD can be seen in Figure 12. In the long-axis view the defect is located at the level of the aortic valve (arrow). In the short-axis view the defect (arrow) is on the left side of the aortic ring and shows a close relation to the pulmonary valve. The sagittal view also exhibits the close relation of the defect with the subpulmonic area (arrow). The long-axis view to the right shows a right-to-left shunt through the VSD, visualized by an intravenous "contrast" injection. This VSD has been called a supracristal or subpulmonic VSD [9].

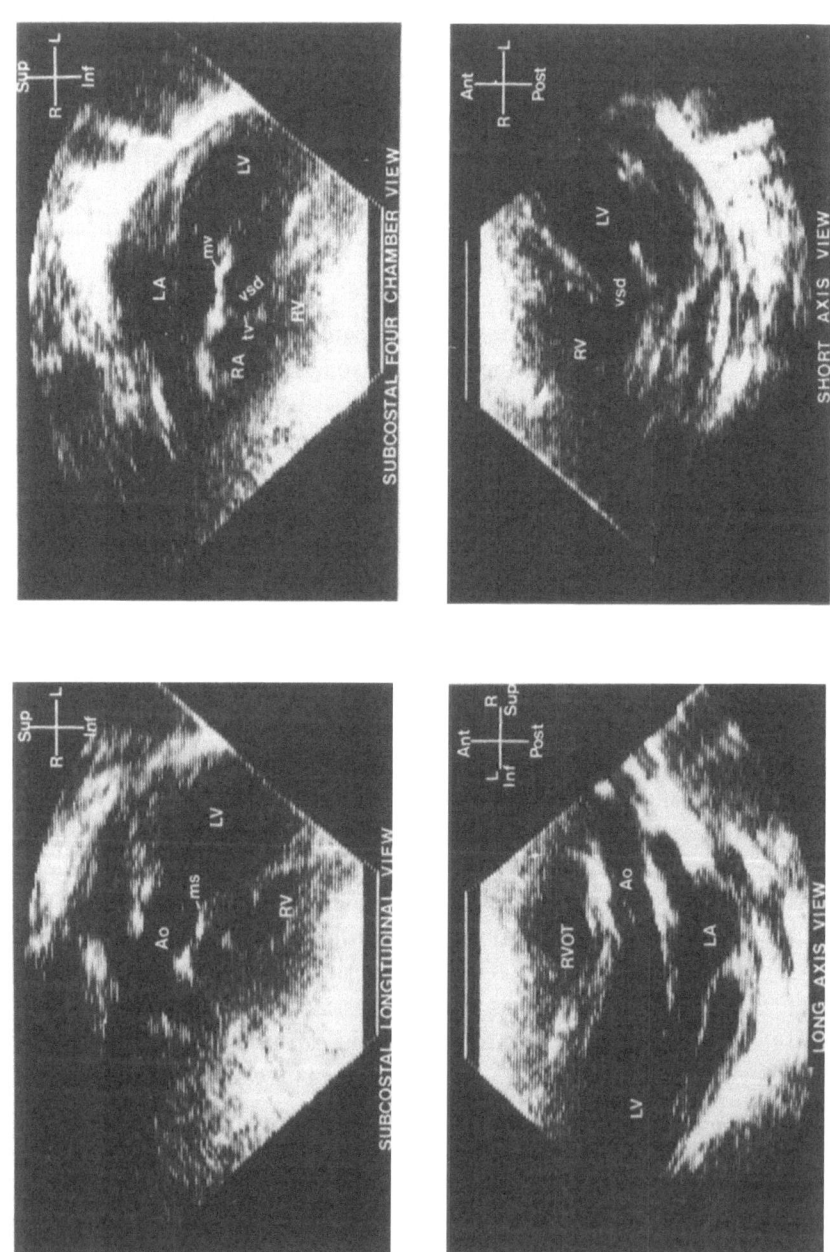

Fig. 8. Two-dimensional echocardiograms of a large muscular inlet septal defect; ms, membranous septum; other abbreviations as in previous figures.

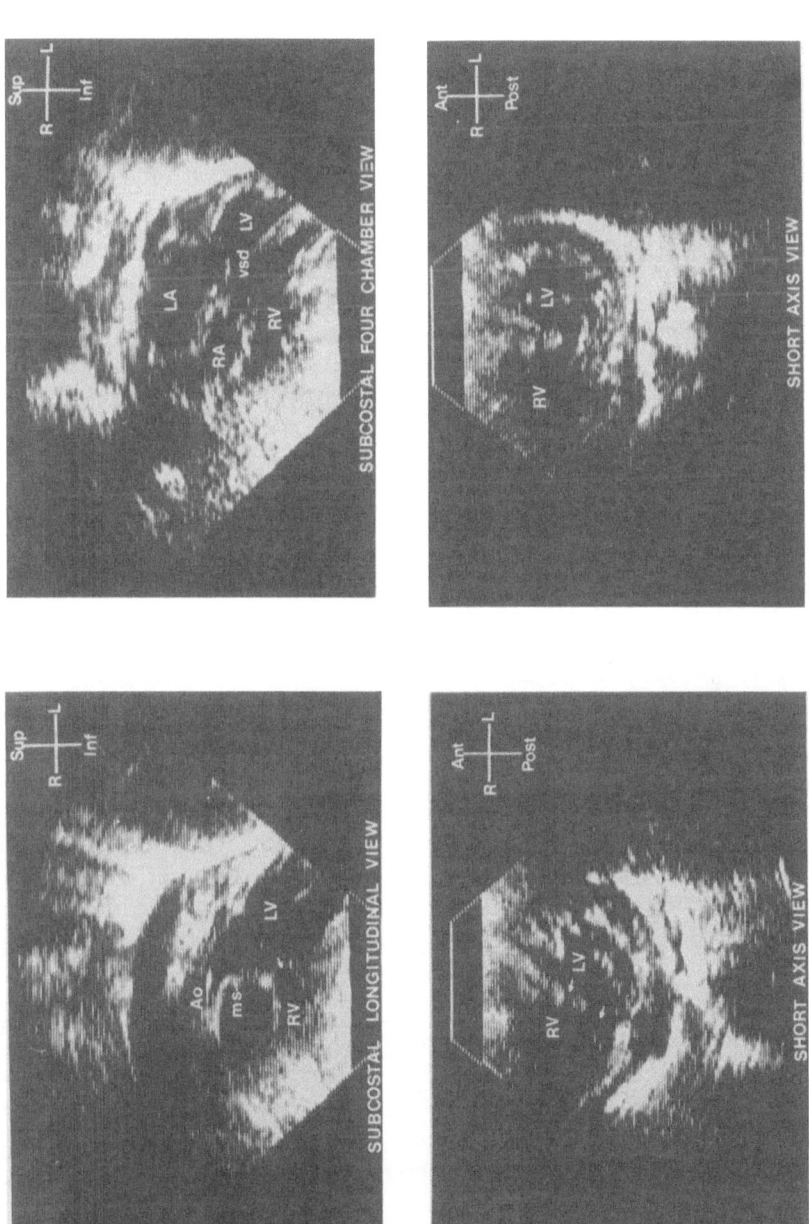

Fig. 9. Two-dimensional echocardiograms of a patient with two VSDs in the muscular inlet septum; abbreviations as in previous figures.

70

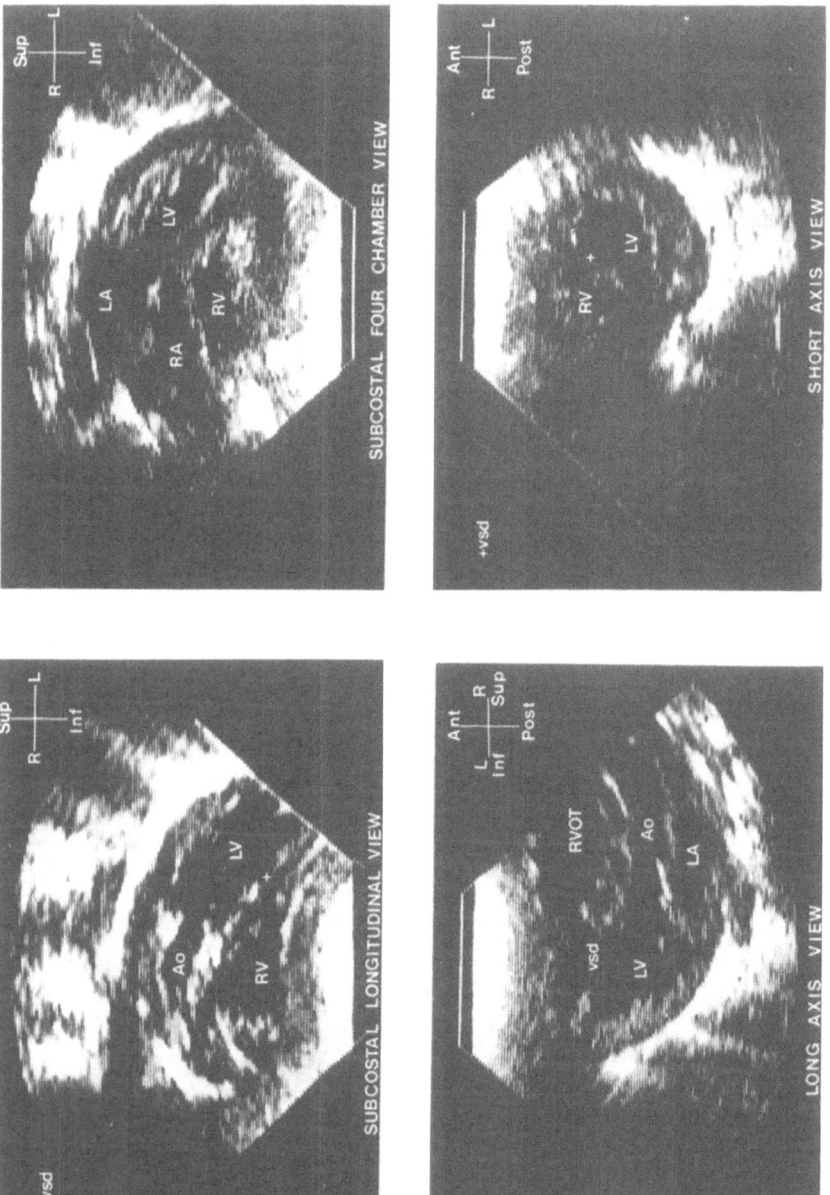

Fig. 10. Two-dimensional echocardiograms showing a large trabecular VSD; abbreviations as in previous figures.

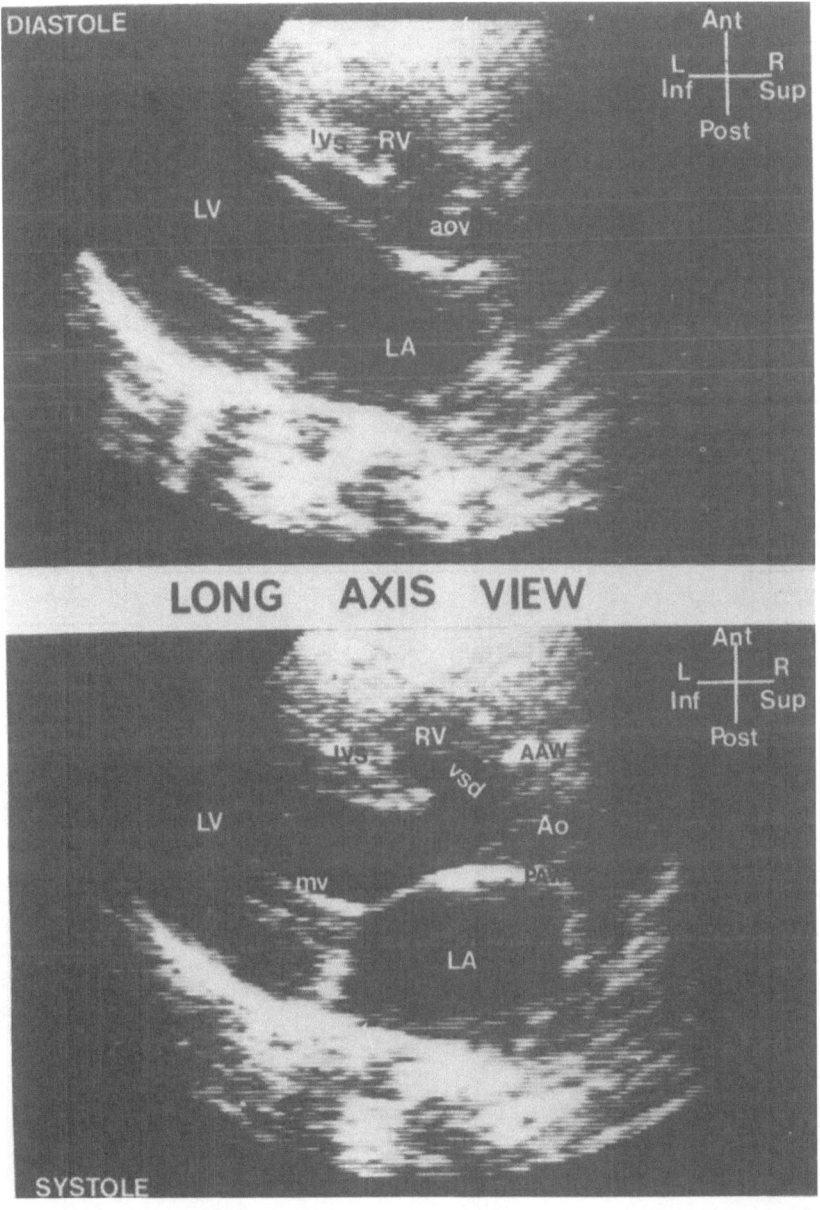

Fig. 11. Two-dimensional echocardiograms of a patient with a Fallot-like VSD; aov, aortic valve; AAW, anterior aortic wall; other abbreviations as in previous figures.

72

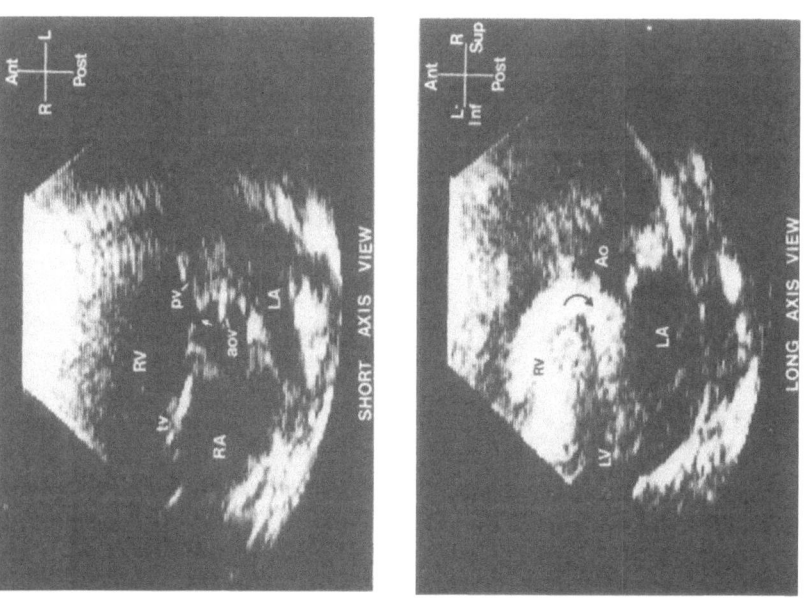

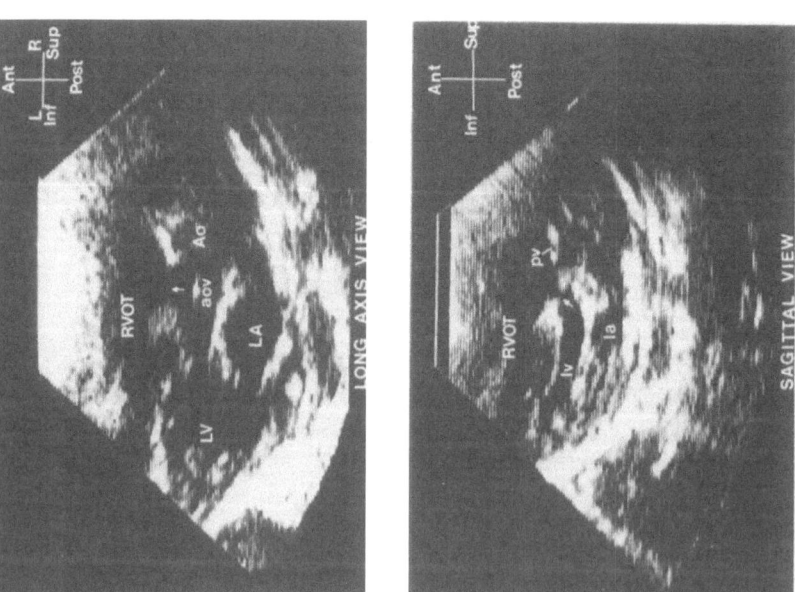

Fig. 12. Two-dimensional echocardiograms showing a subarterial-infundibular VSD; abbreviations as in previous figures.

CONCLUSIONS

The number of patients described does not allow irrefutable conclusions, but nevertheless the information obtained indicates that the two-dimensional echocardiogram is an important acquisition for the diagnosis of hemodynamically important VSDs. Size and localization of those defects can be reliably, accurately, and noninvasively determined. The concept of a division of the IVS into four distinct parts in combination with the anatomical classification of the VSDs as described by Soto et al. [6] simplifies the understanding of the several types of VSD.

REFERENCES

1. Cheatham JP, Latson LA, Gutgesell HP: Ventricular septal defect in infancy: detection by two-dimensional echocardiography [abstr]. Circulation 60:112, 1979.
2. Bierman FZ, Williams RG: Prospective diagnosis of ventricular septal defects in infants by subxiphoid two-dimensional echocardiography [abstr]. Circulation 60:112, 1979.
3. Canale JM, Sahn DJ, Allen HD, Goldberg SJ: Factors affecting real-time cross-sectional echocardiographic imaging of ventricular septal defects [abstr]. Am J Cardiol 45:467, 1980.
4. Tajik AJ, Seward JB, Hagler DJ, Mair DD, Lie JT: Two-dimensional real-time ultrasonic imaging of the heart and great vessels. Mayo Clin Proc 53:271–203, 1978.
5. Anderson RH: Embryology of the ventricular septum. In: Anderson RH, Shinebourne EA (eds) Paediatric cardiology 1977, Edinburgh, Churchill Livingstone, 1978, pp 103–112.
6. Soto B, Becker AE, Moulaert AJ, Lie JT, Anderson RH: Classification of isolated ventricular septal defects. Br Heart J 43:332–343, 1980.
7. Neufeld NH, Titus JL, Dushane JW, Burchell HB, Edwards, JE: Isolated ventricular septal defect of the persistent common atrioventricular type. Circulation 23:685–696, 1961.
8. Wenink ACG, Oppenheimer-Dekker A, Moulaert AJ: Muscular ventricular septal defects: a reappraisal of the anatomy. Am J Cardiol 43:259–264, 1979.
9. Steinfeld L, Dimich I, Park SC, Baron MG: Clinical diagnosis of isolated subpulmonic (supracristal) ventricular septal defect. Am J Cardiol 30: 19–23, 1972.

7. HEMODYNAMIC CONSIDERATIONS IN VENTRICULAR SEPTAL DEFECT

CAROLINE L.D.C. BRUINS

INTRODUCTION

The conventional methods of hemodynamic assessment of ventricular septal defect (VSD) are well known. They pertain to the measuring of pressure and oxygen, the latter as saturation, content, or partial pressure. They include the calculation of systemic, pulmonary, and effective flow, and of pulmonary and systemic vascular resistance, either in mutual relation or in absolute figures. A few grains of salt on the applicability of data may be reviewed.

METHODS AND CALCULATIONS

Considerations of pressure

To use pressure data in the calculations in cases of VSD, various influences have to be taken into account, for instance the influence of flow on pressure.

Pulmonary artery pressure gradients. A secondary hypertrophy around the right ventricular (RV) outflow tract may be present or may develop, causing a subvalvular or infundibular pressure gradient (Fig. 1). After closure of the VSD, it is slowly, and at least partially, reversible.

A very large flow through the pulmonary orifice, normally the narrowest part in the outflow tract, has the same characteristics as a pulmonary valvular stenosis: local flow acceleration with a decrease in lateral pressure, due to the Bernoulli effect. It takes the form of an early systolic dip in the pulmonary artery pressure curve, registered just above the valve. It disappears further down the artery. To obtain the real mean pressure, it must be measured distal to the region where it is disturbed by the dip (Fig. 1).

The pulmonary branches at birth are narrow, and a systolic pressure loss of 10–15 mm Hg at the inflow may be the result. This is a physiological phenomenon which may cause a systolic ejection murmur and which disappears within 3–9 months. In VSD with large pulmonary flow the gradient may even be larger. Sometimes a real stenosis with a concomitant pressure gradient persists after normalization of the pulmonary flow.

A.C.G. Wenink et al. (eds.) The Ventricular Septum of the Heart, *75–86. All rights reserved.*
Copyright ©1981 by Martinus Nijhoff Publishers, The Hague/Boston/London.

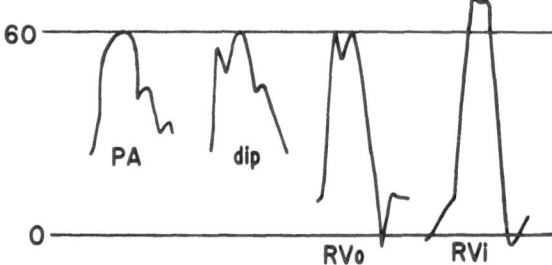

Fig. 1. Pressure curve in mm Hg in an infant of two months of age with isolated VSD: in the pulmonary artery, idem just above the pulmonary valve, in right ventricular outflow and inflow tract.

Needless to say the mean arterial pressure measured beyond these regions of stenosis-related reductions but in nonwedge position gives the best information on the peripheral arterial resistance. With increasing pulmonary vascular resistance and diminishing pulmonary flow, all proximal gradients decrease in magnitude, and may even disappear.

Aortic pressure. In order to maintain a reasonable aortic pressure in VSD with small systemic flow, the systemic peripheral resistance is increased. The pulmonary resistance, calculated from its relation to an assumed normal value of systemic resistance, will thus in reality be higher than estimated.

If, in case of a VSD, there is a slight difference in systolic pressure between the body of the left ventricle (LV) and the aorta, this is probably caused either by an anomalous subvalvular muscle or by a band of fibrotic tissue. Closure of the VSD with concomitant increase in aortic flow to normal values will enhance the pressure gradient. It is thus important to be on the lookout for even slight LV-LV or LV-aortic pressure gradients before operation.

Considerations of oxygen levels

Certain influences decrease the reliability of the information, based on oxygen saturation.

Large pulmonary flow. As we all know, in infants with VSD and large pulmonary flow the pulmonary arteriovenous difference in oxygen saturation is so small that variations of a few percent may considerably influence the calculation of the pulmonary flow. For practical purposes this is of little importance as the pulmonary resistance in these cases cannot be very high.

Small systemic flow. In these infants, the concomitant small systemic flow finds its expression in a large aortovenous difference in oxygen saturation. A slight aortic oxygen desaturation is not unusual. It is caused by pulmonary hypoventilation and possibly, in cases of pulmonary hypertension with equal pressures in both ventricles, by a right-to-left shunt at the ventricular level. In the latter case, knowledge of pulmonary venous oxygen saturation is essential for the calculation of flows.

The systemic mixed venous oxygen saturation is low. However, a relatively high oxygen level does not always indicate a large effective systemic flow. In septic shock, for instance, the oxygen use at the cellular level is depressed by metabolic insufficiency. To calculate the real systemic flow, measurement of the decreased total pulmonary oxygen uptake is indispensable. This is often impossible under life-threatening conditions. In hypoxic acidosis, on the other hand, small arteries may contract, and short-circuiting arteriovenous shunts may open up, thus decreasing local oxygen supply. The systemic flow is only partially effective. This, for instance, happens in the skin circulation in order to safeguard cardiac and cerebral oxygen supply.

Pulmonary resistance. In cases of VSD with pulmonary hypertension and a pulmonary vascular resistance of at least one-third of the systemic resistance, the risk of surgery is markedly increased. One of the methods to evaluate the reversibility of an elevated peripheral pulmonary vascular resistance is the administration of oxygen by inhalation. Pulmonary arterial pressure may decrease while pulmonary flow may increase in relation to systemic flow. To determine the influence of oxygen respiration on pulmonary flow, it is preferable to use the indicator dilution method for measuring flows during respiration of successively room air and pure oxygen, especially in left-to-right shunts. If the Fick method is used, one has to realize that the amount of oxygen dissolved in plasma, though negligible during room air respiration, plays a definite and easily underestimated role in the oxygen transport during respiration of oxygen. Without shunt (Table 1) the plasma provides 2.7%, and during the respiration of pure oxygen 16%, of the oxygen transport. In a medium-sized VSD (Table 2) respectively 3.2% and 33% is carried by plasma. According to Rudolph [1], even 50% of the oxygen may be transported by plasma. The real pulmonary flow in such a case would be half that calculated from the Fick method. Correction is indispensable. Endrys et al. [2] compared the apparent change in flows by using Fick and dye dilution methods. In the latter they found very little indication of increased flow whereas the uncorrected Fick measurements suggested a significant increase in pulmonary to systemic flow ratio during oxygen respiration. After correction the Fick method appeared to give data in close correlation with the dye dilution method.

Table 1. Pulmonary oxygen uptake in normal cases

	Room air				Pure oxygen			
	Oxygen				Oxygen			
		Erythrocytes				Erythrocytes		
Blood	Part. press.[a] mm Hg	sat.[b] %	cont.[c] vol%	Plasma cont.[d] vol%	Part. press.[a] mm Hg	sat.[b] %	cont.[c] vol%	Plasma cont.[d] vol%
Pulmonary vein	100	100	20	0.24	500	100	20	1.2
Pulmonary artery	40	75	15	0.1	40	75	15	0.1
Difference			5+	0.14			5+	1.1

[a] Partial pressure, [b] saturation, [c] content in case of normal hemoglobin, [d] content in normal hematocrit.

Table 2. Pulmonary oxygen uptake in cases of VSD

	Room air				Pure oxygen			
	Oxygen				Oxygen			
		Erythrocytes				Erythrocytes		
Blood	Part. press. mm Hg	sat. %	cont. vol%	Plasma cont. vol%	Part. press. mm Hg	sat. %	cont. vol%	Plasma cont. vol%
Pulmonary vein	100	100	20	0.24	500	100	20	1.2
Pulmonary artery	55	85	17	0.14	70	90	18	0.2
Difference			3+	0.1			2+	1

Considerations of blood velocity

In the near future the blood velocity curves obtained by the Doppler method will undoubtedly deepen our insight in cardiovascular hemodynamics, especially at the inflow side of the heart.

Inflow in the left heart. Rajagopalan et al. [3] recently published their findings on pulmonary and left atrial blood velocity both in experimental setups and in man. As we all know, the pressure curves are not alike in right atrium (RA) and left atrium (LA). The RA pressure has a dominant a wave; in the LA the mean pressure is a few mm Hg higher and the v wave is at least equal to the a wave. A large atrial septal defect (ASD) is the main cause of equal atrial pressures. In Figure 2, the RA and LA curves are also very similar; they are from a five-year-old girl without ASD but with VSD, pulmonary resistance at the systemic level, and a slightly decreased pulmonary flow. The a wave is

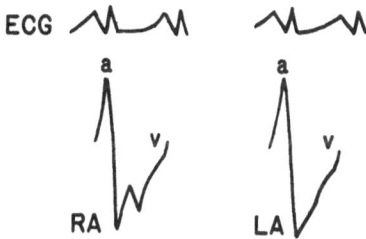

Fig. 2. Electrocardiogram and pressure curve in right and left atrium in a five-year-old girl with pulmonary arterial resistance at systemic level and a heart rate of 90/min.

superimposed on the v wave at a heart rate of 90/min. The v wave in the LA may be dominant in cases with increased pulmonary flow as in VSD without pulmonary resistance hypertension, but also in mitral incompetence. Figure 3 is a good example of v wave dominance in the LA of a three-month-old infant with a 4/1 ratio of pulmonary to systemic flow and a flow hypertension at a heart rate of 80/min.

The velocity curve in the large pulmonary veins is the mirror image of the LA pressure curve (Fig. 4).

The mechanism is probably as follows: The large pulmonary veins are wide enough to contain a stroke volume, but, not being supported by lung tissue, they are also collapsible. One might suppose that collapsed veins are obstructive to pulmonary flow, but the opposite appears to be true. Pulmonary venous forward flow is minimal during "high" LA pressure: early in diastole (v wave) and during auricular contraction (a wave), the veins are widely

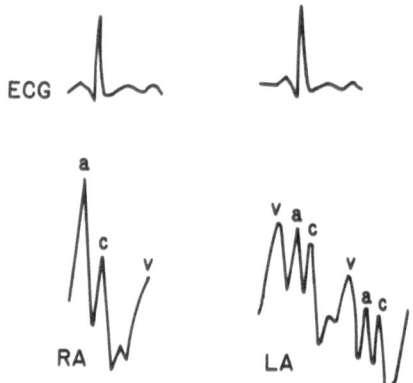

Fig. 3. Electrocardiogram and pressure curve in right and left atrium in a three-month-old infant with a pulmonary to systemic flow ratio of 4/1, a pulmonary flow hypertension, and a heart rate of 80/min.

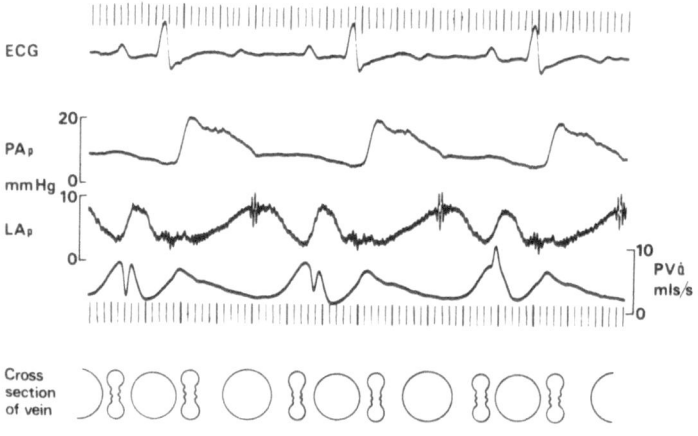

Fig. 4. Registration of electrocardiogram, pressure curves in pulmonary artery and left atrium, and a velocity curve of the pulmonary venous flow, with a summary of changes in cross-sectional area in extraparenchymal veins. From Rajagopalan et al. [3].

patent. With the drop in atrial pressure there is a rapid filling caused by venous collapse, comparable to a kind of passive peristalsis. The mechanism is much more instantaneous than capillary flow could be even though that is also pulsatile. Subsequently, the veins are reexpanded by forward flow. Whereas the above explanation is very plausible, it must be borne in mind that Rajagopalan's data give velocity rather than flow.

Since the latter is also determined by vascular cross section, additional information is still required for full understanding. On the other hand, flow and structural dimensions have been measured in man at all ages. In a normal newborn baby, the stroke volume may, under room temperature conditions, acutely increase from 4 to 7–8 ml, and that at least twice per second. As the LA volume at that moment is but 4 ml, the importance of the large storing capacity of the pulmonary veins is clear, and the more so in neonates with VSD and rapidly increasing pulmonary flow.

Inflow in the right heart. Kalmanson and Veyrat [4] investigated the right heart and its tributary veins. They demonstrated that in the jugular vein the velocity curve is the mirror image of the pressure curve. There is a backward flow during atrial contraction and a maximal forward flow during the x depression (systolic descent of the tricuspid valve) and the y depression (early diastolic rapid filling wave of the RV). The RA is large enough at birth to contain one stroke volume. They also registered the velocities in the RA, RV, and pulmonary artery (Fig. 5). The inflow part of the RA has a similar velocity characteristic to the caval veins and their tributaries: a negative or backward flow during atrial contraction. The RA outflow part shows a pattern identical to that in the RV inflow part: a positive flow during the a wave, a slight forward flow during ventricular systole, and a peak flow during RV diastole. The RV inflow part contributes little to the ejection, but much

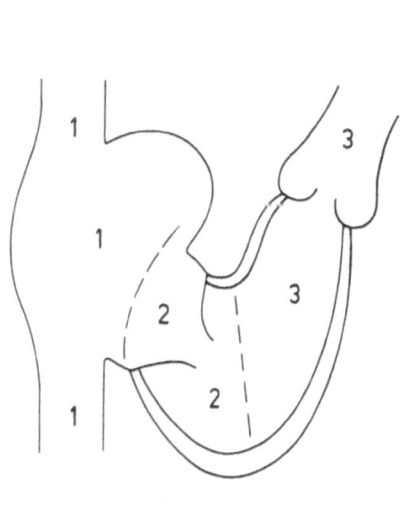

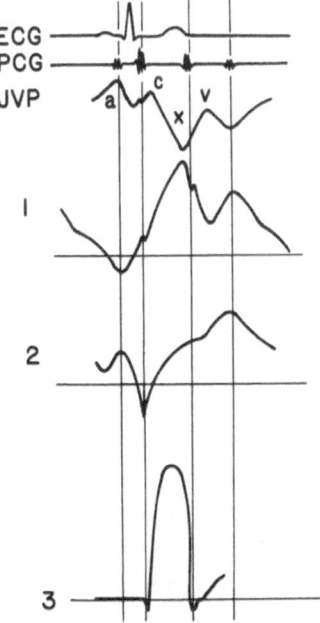

Fig. 5a. Diagrammatic cross section of caval veins, right atrium inflow (*1*), right atrium outflow and right ventricular inflow (*2*), and right ventricular outflow portion with pulmonary artery (*3*).

Fig. 5b. Electrocardiogram, phonocardiogram, and pressure curve in the jugular vein with a compilation of velocity curves in respectively the regions *1, 2,* and *3* of Figure 5a.

82

more to the diastolic filling. The systolic peak flows in the RV outflow part and the pulmonary artery are very similar. All this suggests that the hemodynamic influence of a VSD, at least after birth, depends not only on its size but also on its localization in the inflow or outflow part of the RV. It also indicates that the outflow portion is the important functional part of the RV as far as the pulmonary pressure is concerned.

FLOW AND STRUCTURE

Elevated pulmonary arterial resistance

Pulmonary hypertension with high vascular resistance is normal before, and especially during, birth. The resistance diminishes with the first breath of air and continues to decrease up to the age of at least two years. First the capillaries expand after a maximal compression of the thorax during birth, then the arteries widen and the amount of muscle in the wall of small arteries decreases, while the lungs continue to grow with increasing amount of alveoli and vascularity.

In cases of VSD the expansion of the capillaries takes place in a normal way. With increasing pulmonary flow the pulmonary hypertension may persist as "flow hypertension". A normal or delayed initial decrease in arterial resistance may be followed by an increase after the first days or weeks of life. It consists of muscular contraction followed by hypertrophy in the wall of small arteries [5].

Muscular contraction may bridle the high flow, but in cases where the full ejectile force of the subaortic ventricle is propagated into the pulmonary system, a pulmonary flow of three times the systemic flow may persist in combination with a high pulmonary pressure gradient. The resulting high flow velocity with steep systolic flow acceleration in the contracted resistance arteries causes intimal injury and cicatrization. Usually, however, the impact on the vessels is less vicious; the progression of the "resistance disease" is slower and may take many years. In all those cases where the VSD decreases in importance, the duration of abnormal flow impact is limited. This, as well as any kind of proximal stenosis, protects the lung vessels against progressive changes. However, after a given degree of pulmonary "resistance disease" is reached, the course will be progressive, independent of the original cause [6].

Another complication of large pulmonary flow in the infant may be the influence on pulmonary ventilatory function. There is a susceptibility to pulmonary edema and pneumonia. Partial hyperinflation may exist beside partial atelectasis. In the long run, permanent pulmonary damage may be the result, and it may even impede normal pulmonary growth.

Lung growth perturbance is one of the characteristics of Down's syndrome. With a large VSD it probably enhances irreversible pulmonary resistance disease at a young age.

Underdeveloped preductal aorta

When in the sixth embryonic week a VSD persists and there is a preferential flow through the pulmonary artery, the preductal aorta may become hypoplastic or even atretic, dependent on the structure of the LV outflow tract. If the VSD decreases or even closes spontaneously, before or after birth, and the anomaly of the left heart at that stage permits a normalization of aortic flow, enhanced growth of the ascending aorta occurs. However, some hypoplasia of the preductal aorta may persist, and coarctation at its entrance into the ductus arteriosus–descending aorta may develop [7]. Decrease in the size of the VSD, preventing the pulmonary "resistance disease", may even occur in the rare case of aortic preductal atresia.

Localization of the VSD

Localization and size of the VSD, together with ventricular and septal structure, determine the natural history of the pulmonary "resistance disease". In the following outline the VSDs are divided into those localized in the inflow portion, in the central part, and in the outflow tract of the RV. The nomenclature of the muscular defect is as described by Wenink et al. [8].

VSDs in RV inflow tract. Perimembranous VSDs may extend into the inflow part of the RV. They are very frequent and may initially cause a large pulmonary flow with moderate or no pulmonary resistance hypertension. They may decrease in size by ingrowing fibrous tissue, or they may close spontaneously by apposition or ingrowth of tricuspid tissue from the septal leaflet, even if initially large [9].

Posterior muscular VSDs are located between septal and posteromedial muscle. They are rare in isolated VSD, but frequent in transposition. Up till now, no signs of spontaneous closure have been found in the specimens of isolated VSD, but aortic hypoplasia or atresia had occurred in three of five patients, all of whom died in the first year of life. Those that had been catheterized had severe pulmonary hypertension.

The inflow VSD without muscular rim between VSD and tricuspid ring is usually part of the atrioventricular defect with anomalous inflow valves. The goose-neck-shaped LV outflow tract causes preferential flow through the pulmonary orifice, and pulmonary resistance hypertension is frequent. The defect does not close spontaneously.

VSDs in the central part of the RV. It is not quite clear whether these belong to the functional inflow or outflow portion of the RV. Perimembranous small VSDs often show ingrowth of fibrous tissue around the defect, making direct surgical closure a safe procedure. Small VSDs in the central muscular part may close spontaneously, but remain recognizable by a small dimple in the septum. The large central muscular VSD may give the appearance of Swiss cheese, caused by traversing trabecular structures on the right side. Spontaneous decrease or closure does not occur, and pulmonary resistance disease may be slow in its progression.

Marginal muscular VSDs. Isolated marginal defects are rare. They are often small, and may be rather tortuous channels. Even when multiple and situated in the outflow portion of the RV, they rarely or never cause pulmonary hypertension. We find them sometimes in combination with VSDs in any other localization.

VSDs in the outflow tract of the RV. The perimembranous VSD with smaller or larger extension in the RV outflow tract is usually subaortic: there is no tissue between aortic ring and VSD. The surgeon, looking through the VSD from an opened RV, sees the right aortic cusp. The localization in the RV is to the right, under the "crista" or even higher in the RV outflow tract, and also in or above the "crista" in direct subpulmonary position. The extreme subpulmonary position causes the most aggressive kind of pulmonary hypertension.

In some cases the defect is not only adjacent to the aortic valve ring, but the aortic valve is also malformed, being bicuspid or having cusps of unequal size or nonoptimal apposition in the commissures. The right coronary cusp, not supported by any septum, may prolapse. This usually occurs in the extreme subpulmonary VSD position, but may happen in any position of the subaortic VSD (Fig. 6). The primary result is aortic insufficiency. The prolapsed cusp may gradually obstruct the defect, causing a decrease in left-to-right shunt. As aneurysm of the sinus of Valsalva, it may cause a subpulmonary stenosis. The end result of this development is a rupture of the sinus with a large diastolic aorta-RV flow and with aortic insufficiency also into the LV [10]. Slight malalignment of ventricular and infundibular septum is found in the tetralogy of Fallot, the Eisenmenger complex, and the anomalies with elements of both these complexes. The accessibility of the pulmonary artery determines the result in functional respect. More complicated forms include the double-outlet ventricle and the Taussig–Bing complex. They have in common with truncus arteriosus communis persistens that the full ejectile force of the subaortic ventricle is propagated into the pulmonary artery to produce the most aggressive kind of pulmonary hypertension.

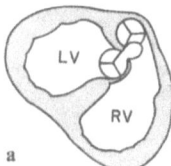 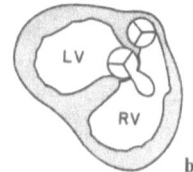

Fig. 6. Diagram of a cross section of the heart perpendicular to the longitudinal axis at outflow valvular level. Extreme positions of the subaortic VSD with aneurysm of the right coronary sinus of Valsalva with aortic cusp, (*a*) in subpulmonary and (*b*) in RV body position. From Sakakibara and Konno [10].

CONCLUSIONS

We may tend to forget that heart catheterization data in young infants have to be taken with a few grains of salt. The high v wave in the left atrium in cases of mitral incompetence is a reflection of the large pulmonary venous forward flow, rather than of mitral movement. Irreversible pulmonary arterial "resistance disease" at an early age is caused by anomalies with the same systolic pressure in aorta and pulmonary artery. The ventricular septal defect in the outflow tract of the right ventricle, especially in the absence of subpulmonary muscular protection, belongs to this category. The localization of the isolated VSD, whether in the functional inflow or outflow portion of the right ventricle, may well influence the natural history of the pulmonary resistance.

REFERENCES

1. Rudolph AM: Congenital diseases of the heart. Chicago, Year Book Medical, 1974, pp 128–129.
2. Endrys J, Kral B, Stransky P: Limitation of oxygen saturation method for measurement of left to right shunt during oxygen breathing [abstr]. Eur J Cardiol 10:327, 1979.
3. Rajagopalan B, Friend JAR, de J Lee G: Interrelations between pulmonary arterial and venous systems and lung capillary blood flow: observations in man and anesthetized dog. In: Baan J, Noordergraaf A, Raines J (eds) Cardiovascular system dynamics. Cambridge, MIT Press, 1978, pp 318–323.
4. Kalmanson D, Veyrat C: Clinical aspects of venous return: a velocimetric approach to a new system dynamics concept. In: Baan J, Noordergraaf A, Raines J (eds) Cardiovascular system dynamics. Cambridge, MIT Press, 1978, pp 279–305.
5. Wagenvoort CA, Neufeld HM, Dushane JW, Edwards JE: The pulmonary arterial tree in ventricular septal defect: a quantitative study of anatomic features in fetuses, infants and children. Circulation 23:740–748, 1961.
6. Hislop A, Haworth SG, Shinebourne EA, Reid L: Quantitative structural analyses of pulmonary vessels in isolated ventricular septal defect in infancy. Br Heart J 37:1014–1021, 1975.
7. Bruins C: Competition between aortic isthmus and ductus arteriosus: reciprocal influence of structure and flow. Eur J Cardiol 8:87–97, 1978.

8. Wenink ACG, Oppenheimer-Dekker A, Moulaert AJ: Muscular ventricular septal defects: a reappraisal of the anatomy. Am J Cardiol 43:259–264, 1979.
9. Somerville J: Congenital heart disease – changes in form and function. Br Heart J 41:1–22, 1979.
10. Sakakibara S, Konno S: Congenital aneurysm of the sinus of Valsalva. Am Heart J 75:595–603, 1968.

8. PHONOCARDIOGRAPHIC FOLLOW-UP IN VENTRICULAR SEPTAL DEFECT

LUC G. VAN DER HAUWAERT AND M. DUMOULIN

INTRODUCTION

Since the early days of phonocardiography, good correlations have been found between the phonocardiographic and hemodynamic findings in ventricular septal defects [1–6]. It is surprising therefore that this noninvasive and sensitive tool has not been used more extensively in the follow-up of children with this cardiac anomaly. Particularly in infants such information is lacking. The clinical course and changing auscultatory findings in infants have been discussed by Hoffman and Rudolph [7] and Collins and co-workers [8] in their outstanding surveys of the natural history of ventricular septal defects. These studies, however, concentrate on the hemodynamic changes and do not include a phonocardiographic analysis.

The purpose of our study is to document the natural history of ventricular septal defects in the first years of life by sequential phonocardiographic examinations.

METHODS

The 75 patients who form the basis of this report were infants with ventricular septal defects, born in the local maternity hospital or referred to the department of Pediatric Cardiology during a four-year period (1966–1970). Only patients with an isolated ventricular septal defect, younger than six months of age at the time of the first assessment, who had at least three phonocardiographic examinations, were included. Patients who died or needed an operation in the first year of life were excluded. The age at the first examination averaged 11 weeks. The follow-up was discontinued after spontaneous or surgical closure. The latter was electively carried out between four and six years of age. In the remaining unoperated patients the follow-up varied between six and eight years. Intervals between phonocardiographic examinations, which were always carried out together with a clinical, electrocardiographic, and radiological assessment, ranged from three months (during the first year or life) to one year.

All phonocardiograms were taken by the authors, using a technique pre-

A.C.G. Wenink et al. (eds.) The Ventricular Septum of the Heart, 87–104. All rights reserved.
Copyright ©1981 by Martinus Nijhoff Publishers, The Hague/Boston/London.

viously described [9]. Only sequences of two or three cardiac cycles, free of respiratory noise and artifacts, were used for further analysis. Besides the site of maximum intensity, duration, and shape of systolic and diastolic murmurs, loudness and splitting of the second sound were analyzed. The intensity of systolic murmurs was estimated on auscultation, using six grades (1 the softest, 6 the loudest murmur).

The patients were divided into three groups according to their clinical condition at the time of the initial examination. Group I: 18 infants with a small defect, in whom a typical murmur was the only pathological finding. Group II: 32 infants with a moderate or large left-to-right shunt, as shown by definite electrocardiographic and radiological changes, but no signs of congestive heart failure. Group III: 25 infants with the picture of a large ventricular septum defect and congestive heart failure.

One or two cardiac catheterizations were performed in 51 patients: two in group I, 25 in group II, and 24 in group III. Most patients in group III were catheterized between two and six months of age and, if clinical progress was satisfactory, recatheterized between two and five years. At the time of their first catheterization, all patients in group III had a systolic pulmonary artery pressure between 60% and 100% of systemic pressure and a pulmonary to systemic flow ratio of at least 2:1. Patients in group II were candidates for elective surgery and were therefore catheterized between three and five years of age. At the time of this hemodynamic study the pulmonary artery pressure was normal or slightly elevated, whereas the left-to-right shunt varied from small to large. The diagnosis rests exclusively on clinical grounds in 16 patients in group I, seven in group II, and one in group III.

RESULTS

At the initial examination, basically three types of systolic murmur could be distinguished. Type A: a high-frequency murmur starting immediately with the first sound, reaching a crescendo in the first half of systole, and ending before the second sound. Type B: a pansystolic murmur commencing with the first sound and ending at the second sound, sometimes exhibiting a striking crescendo in the second half of systole. Type C: a medium-frequency murmur starting shortly after the first sound, reaching a maximum in early or midsystole, and ending well before the second sound. The type A and B murmurs were associated with an intermittently split second sound of normal intensity. The type C murmur was usually followed by a loud and single second sound. A third sound or a low-frequency diastolic murmur could be recorded at the mitral area in most patients with a type B or C systolic murmur. In infants with a large mitral flow and short diastole this mitral murmur often showed a presystolic accentuation.

During the observation period the phonocardiographic pattern of these murmurs and sounds often underwent pronounced changes. This evolution will be described for the three clinical groups.

Group 1

Of the 18 patients in this group, eight had a low-intensity high-frequency early or midsystolic murmur (type A). On auscultation this murmur had a characteristic blowing quality. In seven this murmur disappeared (Fig. 1). In one patient the murmur persisted unchanged over the years. In the remaining ten patients, the murmur was pansystolic (type B). In seven the murmur disappeared (Figs. 2–4), in one it became softer and decrescendo (type A) but persisted, and in two it remained equally loud and pansystolic. Thus, 14 out of 18 patients in this group lost their murmur: seven before one year of age, and seven between one and two years. In most patients a gradual shortening and

Key to illustrations. The ECG (lead II) is always on top. On the middle and bottom channel a medium- and high-frequency phonocardiogram are recorded. The site at which the microphone was placed is indicated by the number and side of the intercostal space, e.g., 4L = fourth left intercostal space. Paper speed is 50 mm/s unless otherwise stated.

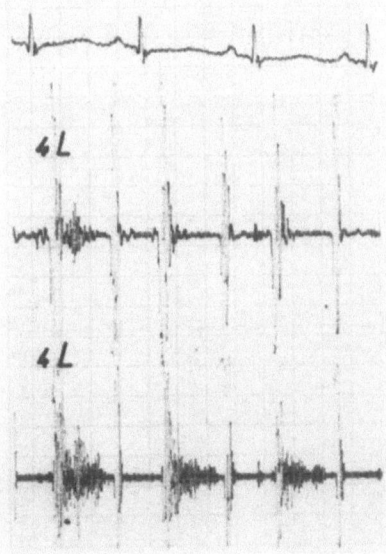

Fig. 1. Systolic murmur starting with the first sound and ending in the last third of systole (type A murmur), recorded in a seven-day-old otherwise healthy newborn. Because of its high-frequency vibrations it is better shown on the third than on the second channel. When this infant was reexamined at three months of age, the murmur had disappeared.

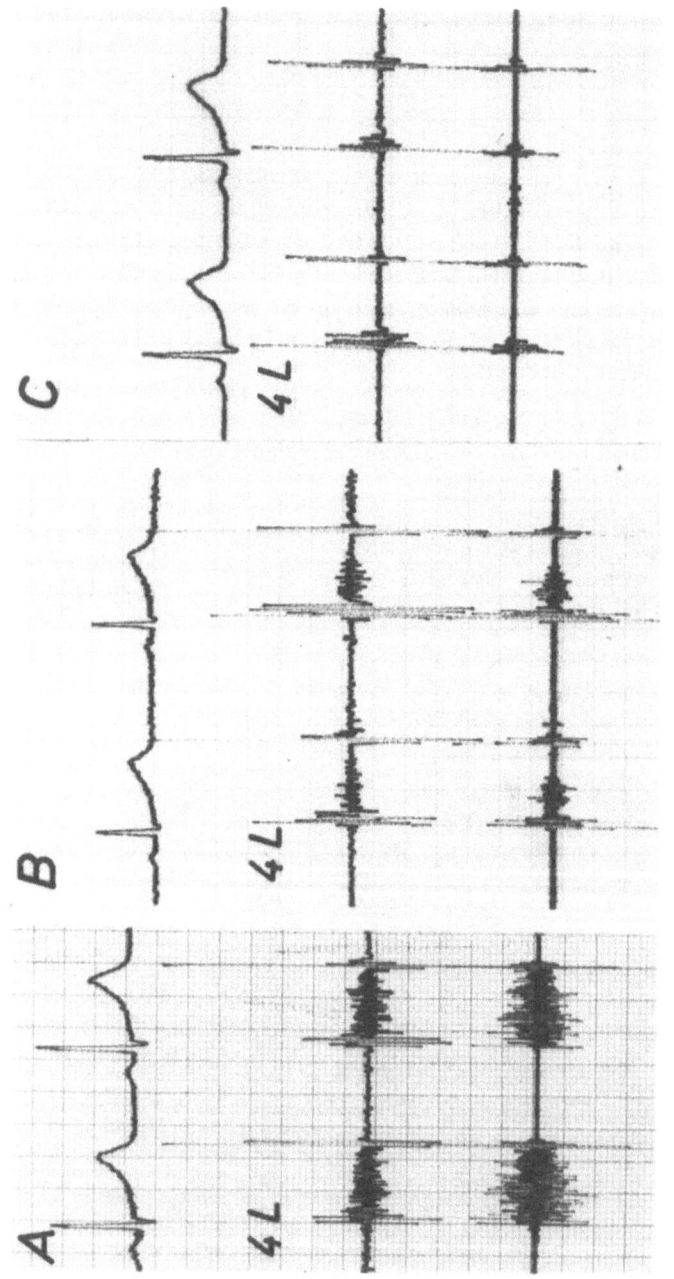

Fig. 2. Loud (on auscultation grade 4/6) pansystolic murmur in a three-month-old boy (*A*) with small ventricular septal defect. At nine months of age (*B*) the murmur was shorter and softer. Five months later (*C*) the murmur could no longer be heard or recorded.

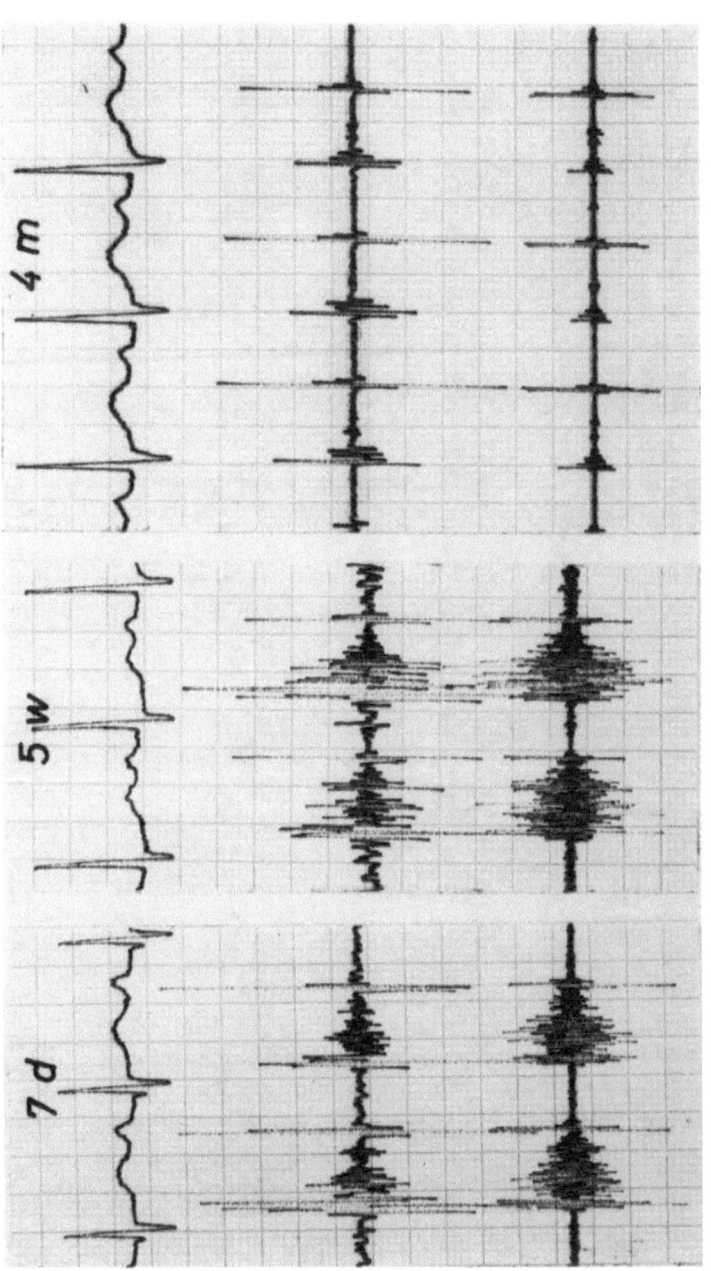

Fig. 3. Pansystolic murmur, softening in late systole, in an infant at seven days and five weeks of age. At five weeks the loudness of the murmur was clinically graded 4/6. By four months the murmur had disappeared.

92

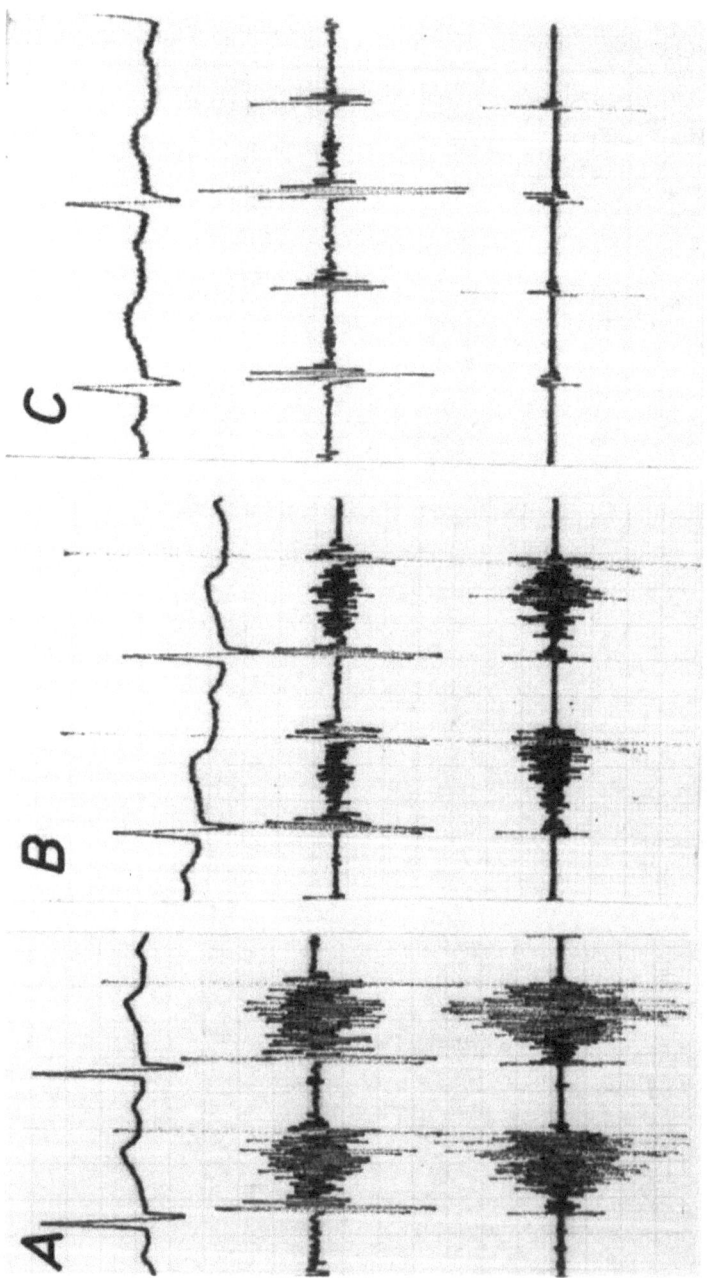

Fig. 4. This loud (grade 5/6) pansystolic murmur in a two-month-old child (*A*) exhibits a striking late systolic accentuation. At nine months (*B*) the murmur is less loud but shows the same unusual shape. When this boy was reexamined at age two (*C*) the murmur had disappeared.

softening of the murmur could be documented. In the final stage, before disappearance, the systolic murmur often occupied only the first half or third of systole (Fig. 2).

Group II

All 32 patients had, at some stage, a loud (grade 4–6/6) pansystolic murmur (type B). In the first days of life the murmur was sometimes faint and early systolic. However, when recorded a few weeks later, it usually had become louder and pansystolic. This evolution, illustrated in Figure 5, is probably related to changes in the hemodynamic condition: a fall in pulmonary vascular resistance and increase of the left-to-right shunt during the first weeks of life.

Of these 32 pansystolic murmurs, four disappeared (two before one year of age, two between three and five years), two became softer and shorter but persisted (type A), whereas 20 remained pansystolic throughout the first years of life. In six patients the phonocardiogram suggested the development of right ventricular outflow tract obstruction. In this subgroup the site of maximum intensity of the murmur shifted to the pulmonary area and the murmur itself became diamond-shaped. This evolution was always accompanied by a progressive widening of the splitting of the second sound and softening or disappearance of the pulmonary closure sound. Four of these six patients eventually became cyanotic and presented the clinical signs of tetralogy of Fallot. A representative example of this evolution is shown in Figure 6. In one of the patients with increasing right ventricular outflow obstruction, a murmer of aortic insufficiency was first recorded at two years of age.

Group III

By definition the 25 patients in this group had congestive heart failure. The initial phonocardiogram showed a pansystolic murmur (type B) in nine and a crescendo-decrescendo midsystolic murmur (type C) in the remaining 16 infants. A diastolic mitral murmur was recorded in nearly all.

In seven out of nine patients with a pansystolic murmur, the murmur remained pansystolic during the first years of life. In general its intensity increased when the signs of congestive heart failure subsided. In one patient the murmur became high-pitched and shorter (type A) between one and two years of age and disappeared between two and three years. Spontaneous closure of the ventricular septal defect in this patient was further substantiated by the regression of all clinical and electrocardiographic signs. In the remaining patient the murmur became very loud (grade 6/6) midsystolic and diamond-shaped. Concomitantly the splitting of the second sound widened,

94

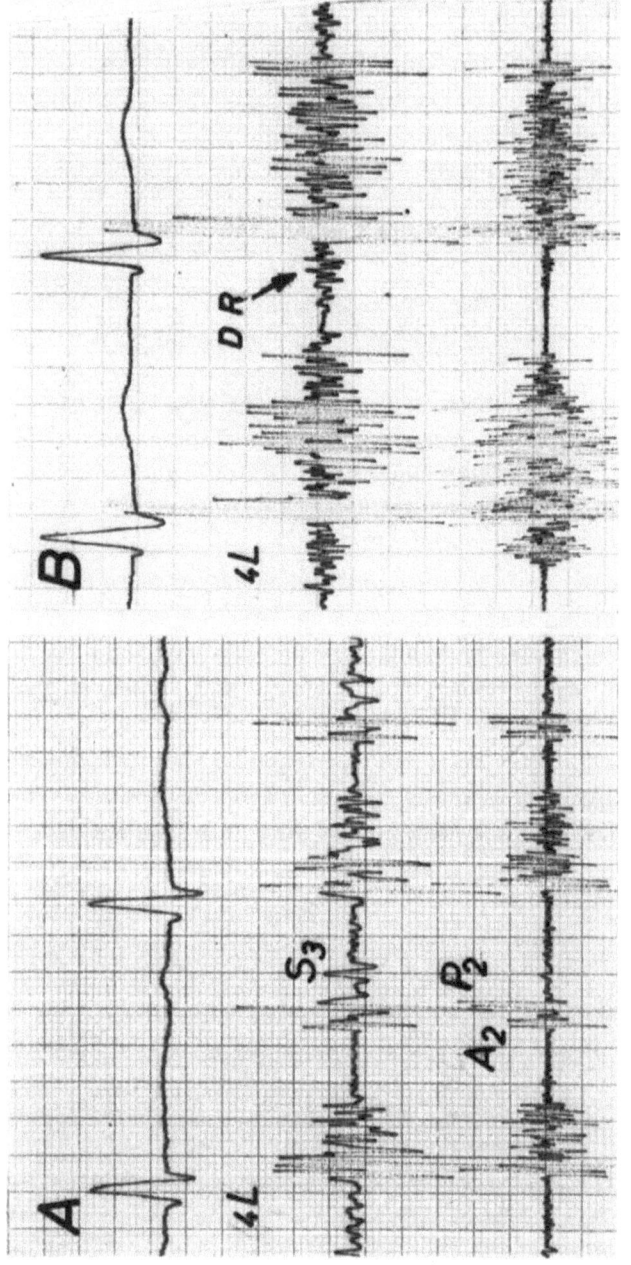

Fig. 5. The changing pattern of the murmur of ventricular septal defect in the neonate. Paper speed is 100 mm/s. At five days of age (*A*) the murmur is short, early systolic, and soft (on auscultation grade 2/6). The aortic (A_2) and pulmonary component (P_2) of the second sound and a prominent third sound (S_3) are distinctly visible. At two months of age (*B*) the murmur has become pansystolic and much louder (grade 5/6). The increase of the left-to-right shunt and mitral flow is also indicated by the prominent diastolic murmur (DR).

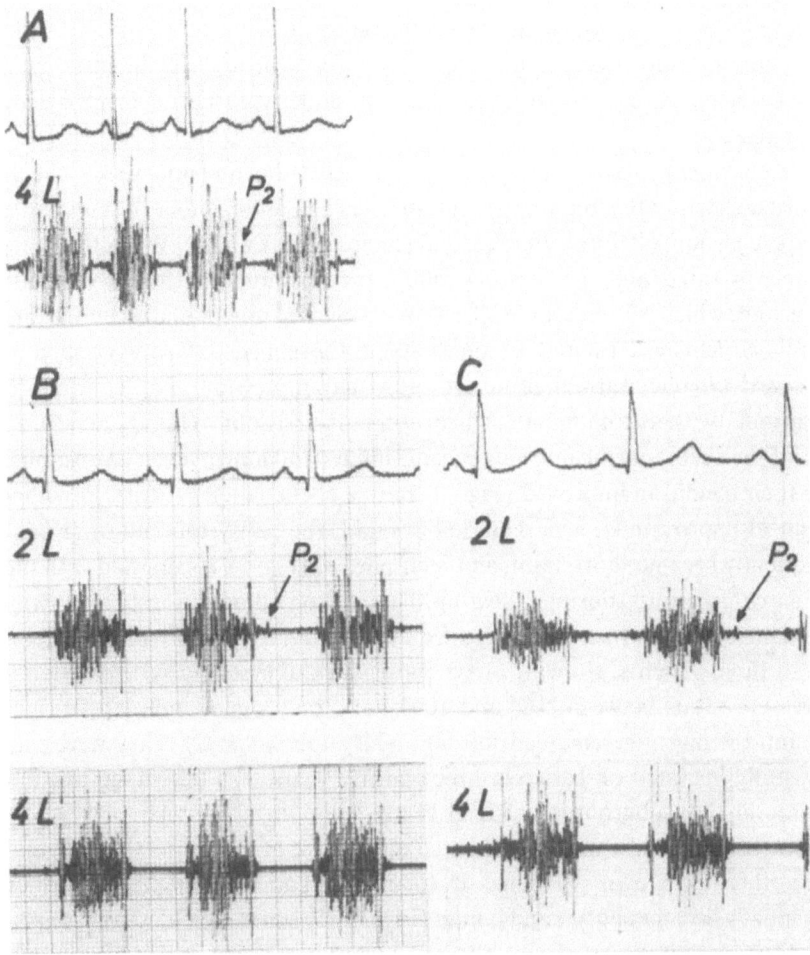

Fig. 6. In this four-month-old girl (*A*), belonging to the clinical group II, the murmur was pansystolic and the second sound narrowly split (30 ms). At 18 months of age (*B*), associated right ventricular outflow tract obstruction was suspected because of a late and soft pulmonary component of the second (P₂), 60 ms after the aortic component. At three years of age (*C*) the murmur, although pansystolic, was diamond-shaped and the splitting of the second sound had widened to 80 ms. By that time the patient had become slightly cyanosed. At cardiac catheterization, associated infundibular stenosis, right ventricular pressure at systemic level, and a small bidirectional shunt were found.

indicating the development of right ventricular outflow tract obstruction. In one of the seven patients with a persisting pansystolic murmur, a decrescendo diastolic murmur became audible at two years of age. Its intensity and duration increased over the years, as the underlying aortic insufficiency progressed.

In 16 patients the murmur was softer (graded 2–3/6) and not pansystolic. It started shortly after the first sound and reached a maximum in midsystole (type C), ending before a loud second sound (Figs. 7 and 8). When the heart rate was rapid and the diastolic filling period short, the mitral diastolic murmur, which was present in all, showed a marked presystolic accentuation, ending in a loud first sound. In some patients the sequence of a presystolic and an early systolic murmur produced the visual impression of a "continuous murmur" with maximum intensity around the first sound (Figs. 7 and 8). In 11 of the 16 infants the murmur became louder and longer, even pansystolic, as their condition improved (Fig. 7). In one of the latter patients, in whom clinical improvement was remarkably rapid, the pansystolic murmur subsequently became short, faint, and high-pitched (Fig. 9). It persisted with the same configuration during follow-up. The electrocardiogram and chest X-ray became normal, which also suggested nearly complete closure of the defect.

In three patients, shown to have pulmonary to systemic systolic arterial pressure ratios between 80% and 100%, and only a moderate left-to-right shunt, the murmur remained soft and midsystolic (type C). They were successfully operated on between three and five years. The remaining two patients in this subgroup developed severe pulmonary vascular obstructive disease. One patient was not operated on because of mental retardation and the other had Down syndrome. In the former patient the systolic murmur gradually became shorter and fainter (Fig. 10). When this child was examined at four and six years of age, the phonocardiogram showed a pulmonary ejection sound, a low-intensity murmur in early systole, a loud and single second sound, and a diastolic murmur of pulmonary insufficiency.

DISCUSSION

Our study confirms the well-established correlations between the phonocardiographic and hemodynamic findings in patients with ventricular septal defects [1–6]. The characteristics of the systolic murmur depend on the magnitude and duration of the pressure gradient between the ventricles and, indirectly, on the pulmonary arterial resistance and pressure. The murmur is therefore loud and pansystolic (type B) in small or moderate-sized defects, whereas it is usually softer and shorter, with an early or midsystolic accentuation (type C), in large defects with considerably raised pulmonary arterial

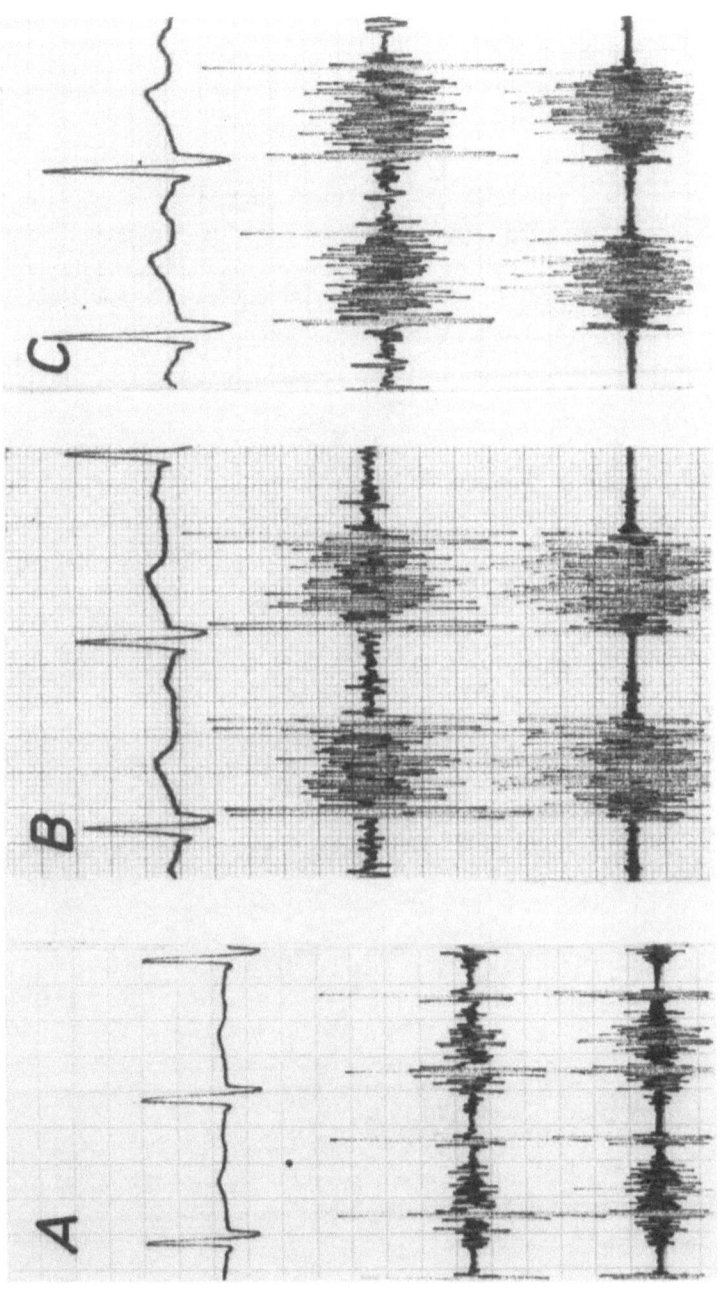

Fig. 7. Phonocardiogram at the fourth left intercostal space in a three-month-old baby (*A*) with large ventricular septal defect, pulmonary hypertension, and congestive heart failure. The systolic murmur (type C) has a crescendo in midsystole and ends well before a loud and single second sound. The diastolic murmur has a striking presystolic accentuation and ends with a loud first sound. The sequence of a presystolic and an early systolic murmur produces the visual impression of a "continuous murmur" with maximum intensity around the first sound. As the clinical condition improved, the systolic murmur became louder and pansystolic. It remained pansystolic as shown in panels *B* (at one year) and *C*, the last preoperative phonocardiogram taken at four years of age.

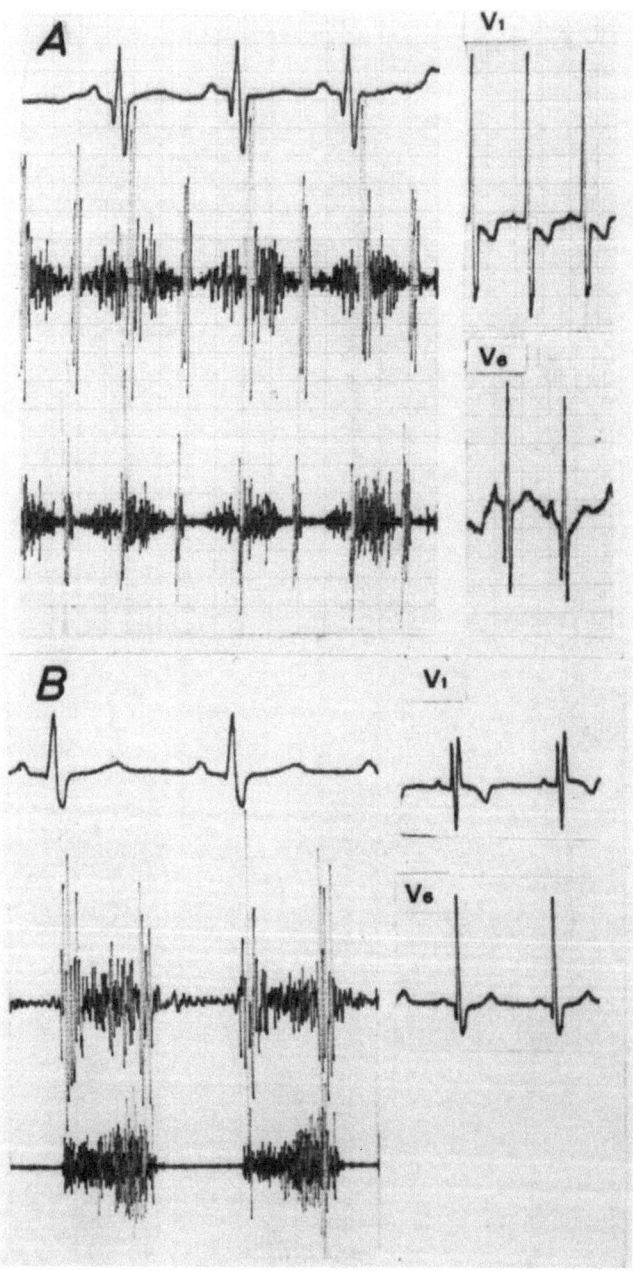

Fig. 8. At four months of age (*A*), when this child was in severe congestive heart failure, a characteristic sequence of a presystolic murmur, loud first sound, and midsystolic murmur (type C) is recorded. The ECG shows marked biventricular hypertrophy. The right ventricular pressure was at systemic level and the pulmonary to systemic flow ratio 2:1. At four years (*B*) the murmur was pansystolic with late systolic accentuation. The ECG showed an RSR pattern in V_1, but was otherwise within normal limits. At recatheterization, normal pulmonary artery pressure and a pulmonary to systemic flow ratio of 1.3:1 were found.

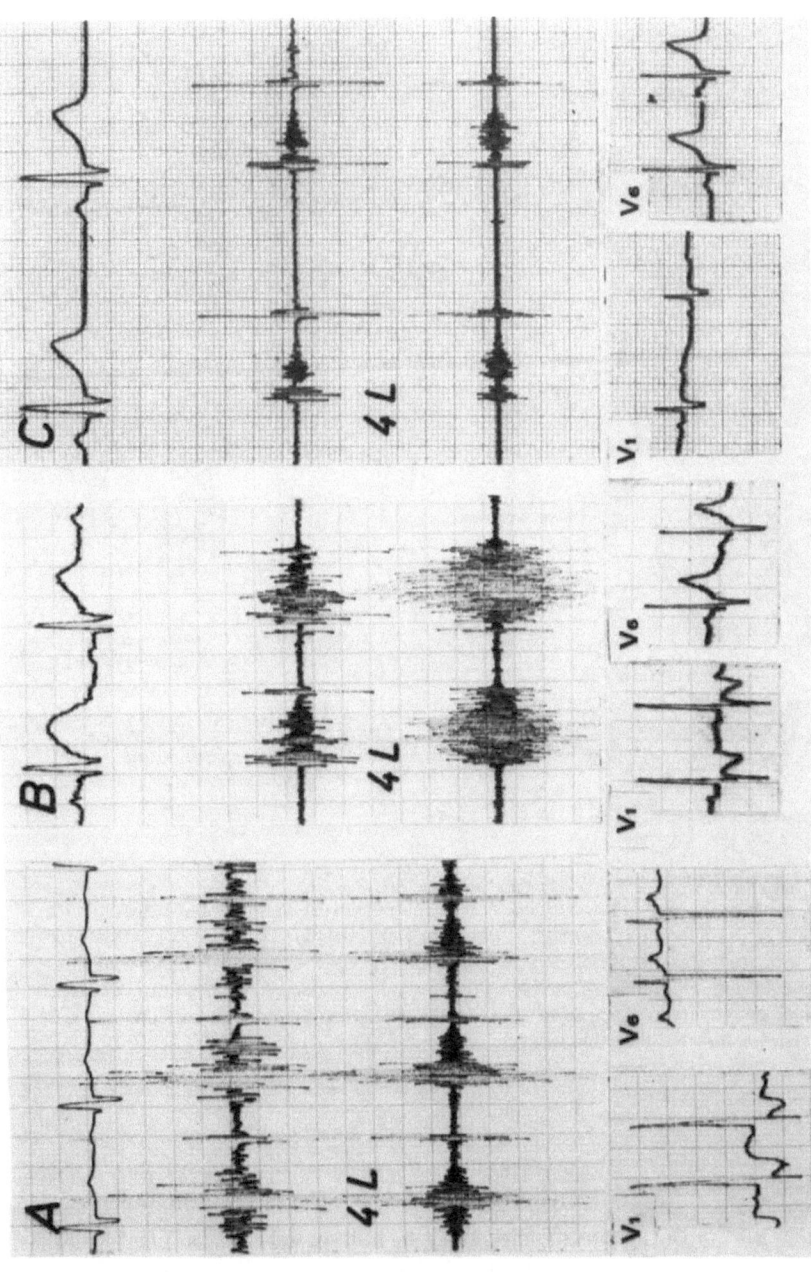

Fig. 9. At two months of age (*A*) this baby was in congestive heart failure. A presystolic mitral flow murmur, loud first sound, and early systolic murmur (type C) are recorded. The ECG shows marked right ventricular hypertrophy. Clinical improvement is accompanied by an increase of the length and loudness of the systolic murmur and disappearance of the diastolic murmur (panel *B*, recorded at six months). At age two years (*C*) a faint and short high-frequency murmur and a normal ECG were recorded. This observation shows that even in infants with congestive heart failure spontaneous closure may occasionally occur.

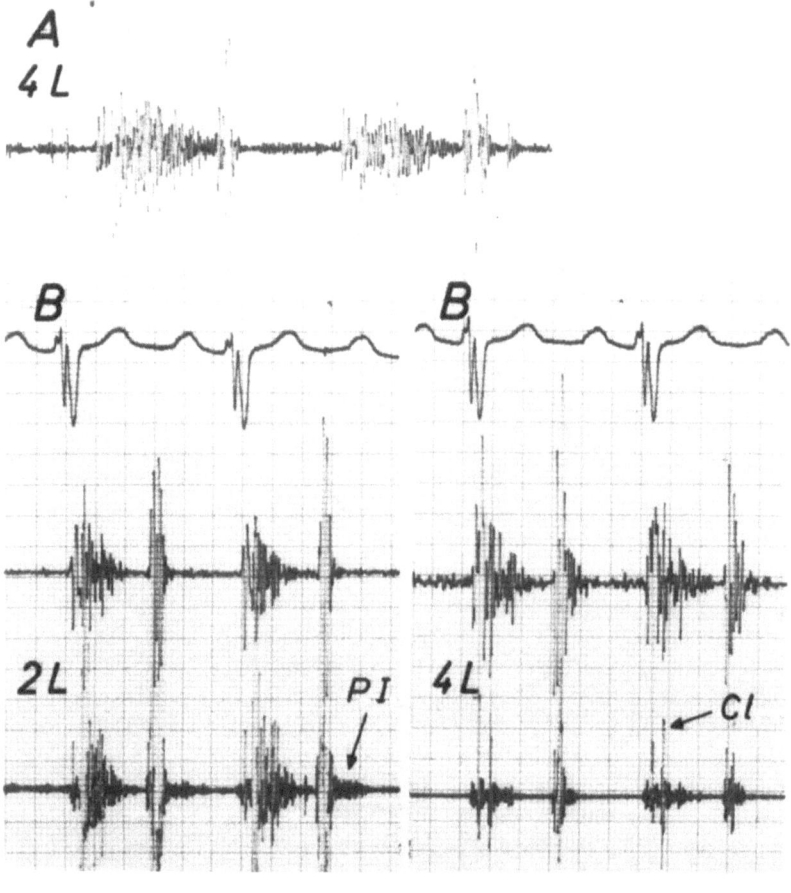

Fig. 10. Moderately loud (grade 3/6) midsystolic murmur in a two-month-old baby (*A*) with ventricular septal defect and congestive heart failure. Pulmonary artery pressure was at systemic level and the pulmonary to systemic flow ratio 3.2:1. At age four years (*B*) the murmur has become fainter (grade 2/6) and shorter. Note the loud ejection sound (Cl) and the early diastolic murmur of pulmonary insufficiency (PI). At recatheterization, pulmonary artery pressure was still at systemic level but the shunt was small and bidirectional.

pressure. In patients with severe pulmonary vascular disease, systemic right ventricular pressure, and minimal shunting, the defect may become silent. At the other end of the spectrum, very small or minute defects also produce an atypical murmur. On auscultation this murmur may be recognized by its site of maximum intensity, usually a small area in the third or fourth left intercostal space, and its blowing quality [10]. On the phonocardiogram [6, 10, 11] it starts with the first sound, reaches a crescendo in early or midsystole and softens rapidly before a normally split second sound (type A murmur).

Diastolic events also correlated well with the hemodynamic findings: large left-to-right shunts were always associated with a middiastolic mitral murmur. In infants with tachycardia and a short diastolic filling period, this murmur usually showed a striking presystolic accentuation. Finally, the intensity and splitting of the second sound were specifically influenced by two factors with opposite effect: high pulmonary artery pressure was generally associated with a loud and single second sound, whereas the development of right ventricular outflow tract obstruction produced widening of the splitting of the second sound and softening of its pulmonary component.

As can be anticipated from the rapid changes in cardiac growth, pulmonary vascular resistance, and left-to-right shunting in infants with ventricular septal defect, heart sounds and murmurs in these patients undergo equally pronounced changes during the first months of life. They have been commented on in studies dealing with the natural history of ventricular septal defect in infancy [7, 8, 12]. This evolution, however, has to the best of our knowledge not been documented by serial phonocardiographic studies. The main reason, presumably, is that the recording of phonocardiograms in infants is generally considered to be difficult or impossible. From personal experience we know that most technical difficulties can be overcome by patience and the use of a direct-writing recorder [9]. The overall results of our study are shown in a schematic diagram (Fig. 11).

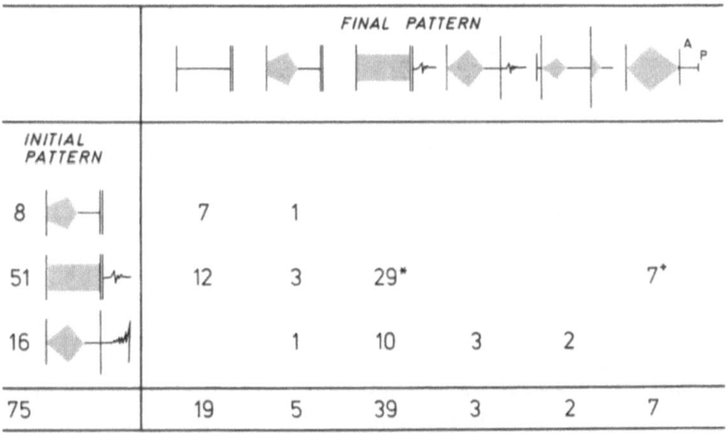

INITIAL PATTERN	FINAL PATTERN					
8	7	1				
51	12	3	29*			7*
16		1	10	3	2	
75	19	5	39	3	2	7

Fig. 11. Diagram showing the changes in the phonocardiographic pattern of heart sounds and murmurs in 75 patients with ventricular septal defect. At the first examination (average age 11 weeks) the murmurs were divided into three basic groups (types A, B, and C). The phonocardiographic findings at the last examination (3–8 years later, unless spontaneous closure had occurred at an earlier age) are represented in six columns: (1) spontaneous closure, (2) type A murmur, (3) type B murmur, (4) type C murmur, (5) severe pulmonary hypertension, (6) right ventricular outflow tract obstruction. (*⁺One patient in this group developed aortic insufficiency.)

Spontaneous closure was a frequent finding in infants with small or moderate-sized ventricular septal defects. Particularly the low-intensity high-frequency early or midsystolic murmur (type A) tended to disappear. This murmur is a fairly common finding in newborns [7, 18], but has also been described in older children [9, 10]. Of the 51 infants with a pansystolic murmur, 12 lost their murmur, simultaneously with other clinical evidence of heart disease. In the combined series of the eight patients with a nonpansystolic high-frequency murmur (type A) and the 51 patients with pansystolic murmur (type B), disappearance of the murmur and spontaneous closure occurred in 32%. This incidence is higher than that reported in most previous studies. It is, however, in accordance with the findings of Hoffman and Rudolph [7], who demonstrated complete closure in 36% of the infants with ventricular septal defect in their own local series. They consider this high percentage to reflect the true frequency of spontaneous closure if children are followed-up from birth, and expect it to be even higher if older patients are included. Spontaneous closure has indeed been reported in late childhood and, exceptionally, in adult life [13, 14].

With a few exceptions [12] little attention has been paid to the characteristics of murmurs and sounds in infants with large ventricular septal defects and congestive heart failure. In one-third only of our patients was the murmur pansystolic and loud, immediately suggesting the presence of the underlying anomaly. In two-thirds the murmur was "atypical", being midsystolic and relatively faint. In these infants the combination of a presystolic mitral flow murmur, ending in a loud first sound and a midsystolic murmur, often produced a characteristic phonocardiographic sequence (Figs. 7 and 8). It should be noted that this sequence may also be found in other conditions characterized by a large left-to-right shunt, increased mitral flow, and pulmonary hypertension, e.g., patent ductus arteriosus and truncus arteriosus. In the majority of patients the systolic murmur became louder and pansystolic as their condition improved and the signs of congestive heart failure subsided.

The presence or development of a pansystolic murmur in infants who had congestive heart failure usually indicated a favorable prognosis. Indeed, none of these patients developed severe pulmonary hypertension, whereas in many of them a significant reduction in left-to-right shunt and pulmonary artery pressure was observed. If surgery was required it could be carried out electively between three and six years of age. Conversely, the persistence of a midsystolic murmur was often associated with progressive pulmonary vascular disease. This was found to be the case in five out of 16 patients with this type of systolic murmur, two of whom eventually developed the full-blown picture of the Eisenmenger complex. We therefore consider the persistence of this type of murmur an important reason to follow infants closely and recatheterize them within six months, even if their symptoms are well controlled on medical treatment. Early surgery may be indicated if the pulmonary vascular resistance tends to increase.

A remarkable evolution was observed in seven patients (six in group II and one in group III) who initially had a pansystolic murmur. Their murmur tended to increase in intensity and become diamond-shaped over the years. Concomitant widening of the splitting of the second sound and softening of its pulmonary component made us suspect the development of right ventricular outflow tract obstruction, which was confirmed by cardiac catheterization in all. In four out of seven patients the infundibular pulmonary stenosis became so severe that their condition evolved into tetralogy of Fallot. This phenomenon was not observed in the study of Hoffman and Rudolph [7] which covered the age group from birth to approximately 2–3 years. It has, however, been reported in most studies based on a longer follow-up. Lynfield and co-workers [15] found evidence of progressive infundibular stenosis in four out of 32 patients who originally had the findings of uncomplicated ventricular septal defect. This observation corroborates the impression that, in patients with ventricular septal defect, the murmur of aortic insufficiency is rarely audible before four years of age [14].

Finally, two of our patients developed aortic insufficiency and a decrescendo-diastolic murmur. Both patients were two years of age when this murmur was first heard and recorded. In one patient, who also had infundibular stenosis, the insufficiency was slight, but in the other it was severe and progressive and required surgical correction at the time of the closure of the ventricular septal defect. This observation corroborates the impression that, in patients with ventricular septal defect, the murmur of aortic insufficiency is rarely audible before four years of age [14].

REFERENCES

1. Benchimol A, Dimond EG: Phonocardiography in ventricular septal defect. Correlation between hemodynamics and phonocardiographic findings. Am J Med 28:347–356, 1960.
2. Craige E: Phonocardiography in interventricular septal defects. Am Heart J 60:51–60, 1960.
3. Leatham A, Segal B: Auscultatory and phonocardiograph signs of ventricular septal defect with left-to-right shunt. Circulation 25:318–327, 1962.
4. Mannheimer E, Ikos D, Jonsson B: Prognosis of isolated ventricular septal defects. Br Heart J 19:333–344, 1957.
5. Schrire V, Vogelpoel L, Beck W, Nellen M, Swanepoel A: Ventricular septal defect: the clinical spectrum. Br Heart J 27:813–825, 1965.
6. Van der Hauwaert L, Nadas AS: Auscultatory findings in patients with a small ventricular septal defect. Circulation 23:886–891, 1961.
7. Hoffman JI, Rudolph AM: The natural history of ventricular septal defects in infancy. Am J Cardiol 16:634–653, 1965.
8. Collins G, Calder L, Rose V, Langford K, Keith J: Ventricular septal defect: clinical and

hemodynamic changes in the first five years of life. Am Heart J 84:695–705, 1972.

9. Van der Hauwaert LG: Phonocardiography. In: Watson H (ed) Paediatric cardiology. London, Lloyd-Luke, 1968, pp 89–114.

10. Evans JR, Rowe RD, Keith JD: Spontaneous closure of ventricular septal defects. Circulation 22:1044–1054, 1960.

11. Vogelpoel L, Schrire V, Beck W, Nellen M, Swanepoel A: The atypical systolic murmur of minute ventricular septal defects and its recognition by amylnitrite and phenylephrine. Am Heart J 62:101–118, 1961.

12. Fyler DC, Rudolph AM, Wittenborg MH, Nadas AS: Ventricular septal defect in infants and children. A correlation of clinical, physiologic and autopsy data. Circulation 18:833–851, 1958.

13. Bloomfield DK: Natural history of ventricular septal defect in patients surviving infancy. Circulation 29:914–955, 1964.

14. Corone P, Doyon F, Gaudeau S, Guérin F, Vernant P, Ducam H, Rumeau-Rouquette C, Gaudeul P: Natural history of ventricular septal defect. A study involving 790 cases. Circulation 55:908–915, 1977.

15. Lynfield J, Gasul BM, Arcilla R, Luan LL: The natural history of ventricular septal defects in infancy and childhood. Am J Med 30:357–371, 1961.

9. SPONTANEOUS CLOSURE OR CRITICAL DECREASE IN SIZE OF THE VENTRICULAR SEPTAL DEFECT IN TRICUSPID ATRESIA WITH NORMALLY CONNECTED GREAT ARTERIES: SURGICAL IMPLICATIONS

URSULA SAUER AND D. HALL

INTRODUCTION

The natural history of tricuspid atresia, absence of the right atrioventricular connection, is essentially dependent on the status of the ventricular septal defect (VSD). Complete closure of the VSD, otherwise referred to as bulbo-ventricular foramen or outlet foramen, apprears to be a major cause of the high mortality rate observed in the first year of life [1–9]. Incomplete closure of the VSD causes progressive subpulmonary or subaortic stenosis in the presence of normally connected or transposed great arteries, respectively [8, 10–17]. In this study the natural history of the VSD in tricuspid atresia with normally connected and related great arteries (ventriculoarterial concordance) (NCGA) and the effects of surgical interventions were assessed.

PATIENTS

The study group consisted of 25 patients seen between October 1973 and April 1979 who had tricuspid atresia and NCGA, 11 of whom had been investigated five months to 12 years previously. Follow-up period ranged accordingly up to 18 years. In addition to repeated physical examinations, electrocardiograms, and chest X-rays, standard cardiac catheterization was performed in all patients and cineangiocardiograms were obtained. Subsequent morphological assessment was enabled in seven patients at the time of surgery and in five from autopsy findings.

RESULTS (Table 1)

Spontaneous closure or reduction in size of the VSD was found to have occurred in 11 of the 25 patients (six female and five male), or 44%. Of these, three were found to have complete closure and eight demonstrated a reduction in size to less than 5 mm. The median age at documentation of the closure was 8.9 years, with a range from 124 days to 19.7 years. There were seven survivors and four nonsurvivors. The diagnosis of closure was estab-

Table 1. Documentation of closure of the "ventricular septal defect"

No.	Sex	Outcome	Type at 1st cath.	VSD closure	Documentation	Age at documentation	VSD size	Shunt present at documentation
1 PJ	M	Died	Ib	Complete	Angio/autopsy	1.5 y	Closed	Waterston + AAO-RVOC anastomosis (Goretex)
2 GH	M	Died	Ib	Complete	Angio/autopsy	15.8 y	Pinpoint	Blalock–Taussig left, stenosed + Glenn
3 AR	F	Died	Ic	Partial	Fontan op./autopsy	1.0 y	0.4 cm Diameter	Blalock–Taussig left, obliterated
4 BB	F	Died	Ic	Partial	Autopsy	134 d	0.5 cm Diameter	—
5 GC	F	Alive	Ic	Partial	Fontan op.	10.4 y	Small	—
6 KJ	F	Alive	Ib	Partial	Fontan op.	19.7 y	0.5 cm Diameter	Blalock–Taussig left, obliterated
7 JJ	F	Alive	Ib	Partial	Angio/Fontan op.	17.6 y	0.3 cm Diameter	Blalock–Taussig left + right
8 MT	M	Alive	Ib	Partial	Angio	8.9 y	Very small	Blalock–Taussig left, obliterated + Waterston
9 AU	M	Alive	Ib	Partial	Angio	9.8 y	Very small	Blalock–Taussig left
10 SC	M	Alive	Ib	Partial	Angio	4.3 y	Very small	Blalock–Taussig left, stenosed
11 UA	F	Alive	Ib	Complete	Clinically/phono	1.8 y	Closed	Blalock–Taussig left

M, male; F, female; VSD, "ventricular septal defect" (bulboventricular or outlet foramen); y, years; AAO, ascending aorta; RVOC, right ventricular outlet chamber.

lished clinically in one case (Fig. 1), angiocardiographically only in three, at surgery for Fontan procedure [18, 19] in three, and at autopsy in four patients. On classification according to pulmonary perfusion at the initial investigation, eight had type Ib (diminished flow) and three had type Ic (increased flow) [20, 21].

Cardiac catheterization (Table 2), initially indicated on the basis of hypoxia and increasing cyanosis in eight of the patients (type Ib) and congestive heart failure in three (type Ic), was first performed at a median age of five

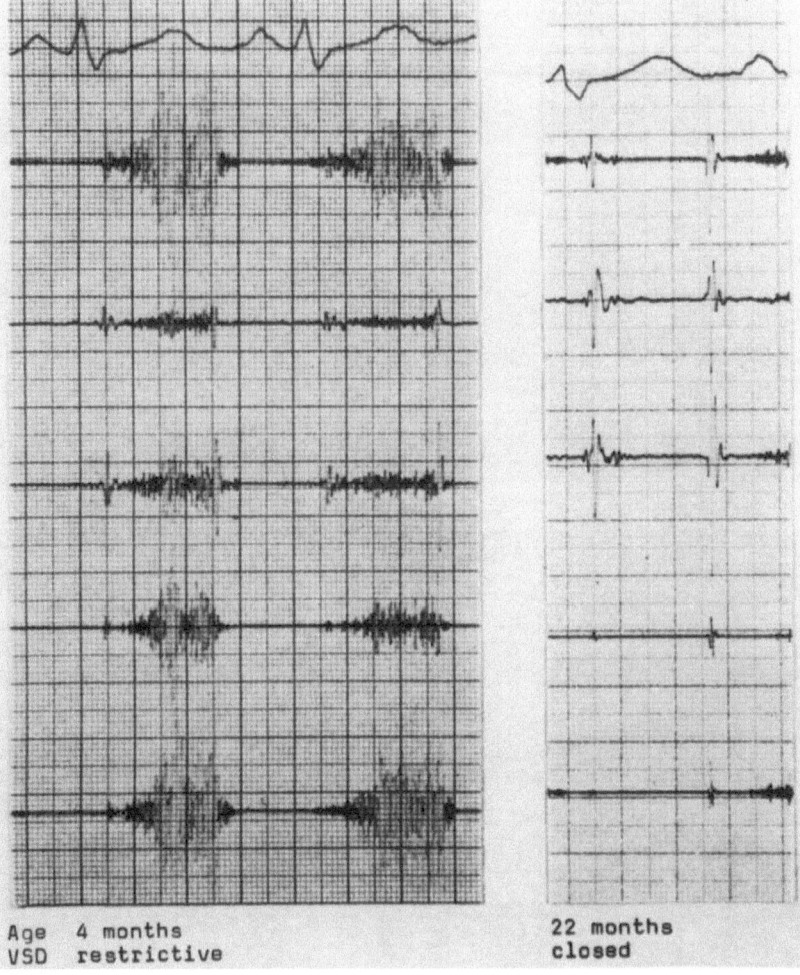

Age 4 months
VSD restrictive

22 months
closed

Fig. 1. Case no. 11. Patient with tricuspid atresia and normally connected great arteries (type Ib). Phonocardiograms at four and 22 months of age. During the interval the VSD murmur had disappeared, suggesting that the VSD had closed spontaneously. At $5\frac{1}{2}$ months of age a left Blalock–Taussig anastomosis was performed. ECG lead II, PCG 4th left ICS, 100 mm/s.

Table 2. Cardiac catheterization data

No.	Sex	1st Cardiac catheterization									2nd Cardiac catheterization					3rd Cardiac catheterization				
		Type	Age	BAS	Hct %	SAO_2 (LV) %	Q_p/Q_s	LV/RVOC mm Hg	Shunt	Age	Age	Hct %	SAO_2 (LV) %	Q_p/Q_s	LV/RVOC mm Hg	Age	Hct %	SAO_2	Q_p/Q_s	LV/RVOC mm Hg
1 PJ	M	Ib	42 d	+	46	(35)	—	—	Waterston	42 d	1.3 y	40	67	0.8	—					
2 GH	M	Ib	4.9 y	—	82	(30)	—	—	Bl-T left	4.9 y	12.8 y	63	77	0.6	80	15.4 y	60	75	1.0	
3 AR	F	Ic	36 d	+	46	(78)	3.3	42	Bl-T left	6 mo	—									
4 BB	F	Ic	43 d	—	39	67	1.9	15	—	—										
5 GC	F	Ic	5 mo	—	43	(85)	—	—	—	—	3.3 y	60	68	—	—	9.8 y	68	68	0.4	88
6 KJ	F	Ib	6.1 y	—	—	—	—	—	Bl-T left obliterated	10.3 y	16.9 y	59	78	1.1	83					
7 JJ	F	Ib	4.2 y	—	—	(46)	—	—	Bl-T left / right obliterated	4.2 y / 10.3 y	14.9 y	55	77	0.8	84	17.3 y	56	74	0.7	
8 MT	M	Ib	5 mo	+	63	(72)	1.2	—	Bl-T left obliterated / Waterston	1.2 y / 2.8 y	8.9 y	44	85	1.2	—					
9 AU	M	Ib	1.3 y	—	—	(55)	—	—	Bl-T left	1.4 y	9.8 y	63	58	0.3	—					
10 SC	M	Ib	29 d	—	39	(72)	—	—	Bl-T left stenosed	1.3 y	4.3 y	66	55	0.2	—					
11 UA	F	Ib	4.5 mo	—	47	66	0.7	—	Bl-T left	6 mo	—									
Mean values			5 mo (median)		51	61	1.8				9.8 y (median)	56	71	0.7	82		61	72	0.7	

	2nd Cardiac catheterization	3rd Cardiac catheterization
With functioning shunt	$n = 6$	$n = 1$
Without shunt	$n = 2$	$n = 2$

M, male; F, female; d, day(s); mo, month(s); y, year(s); Bl-T, Blalock–Taussig anastomosis; BAS, balloon atrial septostomy; Hct, hematocrit; SAO_2, systemic arterial oxygen saturation; SAO_2 (LV), oxygen saturation in the left ventricle; LV/ROC, systolic gradient between left ventricle and right ventricular outlet chamber across the "VSD".

months, range 29 days to 6.1 years. The mean systemic arterial oxygen saturation of 53% in type Ib indicated decreased pulmonary blood flow, whereas in type Ic it measured 77%. The mean Qp/Qs ratio was 1.8, but was obtained from only four of the children, including two with increased pulmonary blood flow (type Ic). The mean peak systolic pressure gradient across the VSD was 29 mm Hg (indicative of unrestrictive flow) in the latter two patients.

In the ten patients in whom right atrial (RA) and left atrial (LA) pressures were recorded, the a wave in the RA was higher than in the LA in nine and equal in one. The a-wave gradients ranged between 2 and 10 mm Hg. The highest a-wave gradients of 6, 9, and 10 mm Hg, respectively, were demonstrated in three infants with a patent foramen ovale which was associated with an aneurysm of the atrial septum in two. A balloon atrial septostomy was performed in three infants with a-wave gradients of 4.5, 10, and 9 mm Hg, respectively, the latter with a large aneurysm of the atrial septum.

At a mean interval of 6.8 years, a second cardiac catheterization was performed in eight patients with a median age of 9.8 years, range 15 months to 16.9 years. At this time a mean gradient of 82 mm Hg across the VSD, indicative of restricted flow (calculated mean Qp/Qs ratio 0.9), was found in three patients. The increase in oxygen saturation with a mean of 71% was mainly due to intercurrent shunt procedures in six of the patients, excluding one with a nonfunctioning Blalock–Taussig anastomosis.

A third cardiac catheterization was performed in three patients with a median age of 15.4 years at an interval of 2.4, 2.6, and 6.4 years, respectively. Except for the tendency toward increasing hematocrit values (mean 61%), the oxygen saturation (mean 72%), Qp/Qs ratio (mean 0.7), and a pressure gradient across the defect of 88 mm Hg in a single patient, remained essentially unaltered.

Cineangiocardiographic findings (Table 3) were obtained from injections into the left ventricular main chamber in the left anterior oblique projection, biplane right atrial injections, and from additional injections into the outlet chamber in five patients. At the initial investigation a large VSD was demonstrated in three infants (type Ic). A small or barely detectable defect was found in seven and occlusion of the defect in two patients at repeat cineangiocardiography. An aneurysm-like bulge with a small orifice at the site of the VSD was documented in seven patients (Figs. 2 and 3). An infundibular stenosis in the outlet chamber was present in eight children. It was severe in one and had progressed in most of the remaining patients from a contractile or functional to a fixed stenosis which was associated with a further decrease in pulmonary blood flow. Pulmonary valve stenosis was found in three patients, but was marked in only one. The outlet chamber, which was located anteriorly and to the right of the ventricle in all patients was small in six, moderately large in

Table 3. Summary of findings on repeat cineangiocardiography

No.	Sex	Type	VSD	RV infundibular stenosis	RV outlet chamber	PaV/AoV lat. view	"Aneurysm" at site of VSD	Other findings
1 PJ	M	Ib	Small – closed	Moderate	Small	0.7 – 0.6	+	Waterston with kinking of RPA and underperfusion of left lung; aneurysm of the atrial septum (BAS)
2 GH	M	Ib	Small – closed	Minimal	Moderately large	0.5 – 0.5	–	Blalock–Taussig left, stenosed
3 AR	F	Ic	Large	—	Large	1.0	–	—
4 BB	F	Ic	Large	—	Large	1.0	–	Aneurysm of the atrial septum
5 GC	F	Ic	Large – small	Moderate	Large – moderately large	1.2 – 0.8	+	—
6 KJ	F	Ib	Small – very small	—	Moderately large	– 0.9	–	Blalock–Taussig left, obliterated
7 JJ	F	Ib	Small – very small	—	Moderately large – small	0.5 – 0.6	+ Calcifications	Blalock–Taussig left + right
8 MT	M	Ib	Small – very small	Moderate – moderate to severe	Moderately large – very small	0.7 – 0.3	+	Blalock–Taussig left, obliterated, Waterston with kinking of RPA and underperfusion of left lung
9 AU	M	Ib	Small – very small	Moderate	Small	– 0.5	+	Blalock–Taussig left, pulmonary valve stenosis
10 SC	M	Ib	Small – very small	Moderate	Moderately large – small	– 0.5	+	Blalock–Taussig left stenosed, pulmonary valve stenosis
11 UA	F	Ib	Small	Moderate	Small	0.7	+	Pulmonary valve thickened

M, male; F, female; RV, right ventricle; PaV/AoV, ratio of pulmonary valve ring and aortic valve ring diameter; RPA, right pulmonary artery.

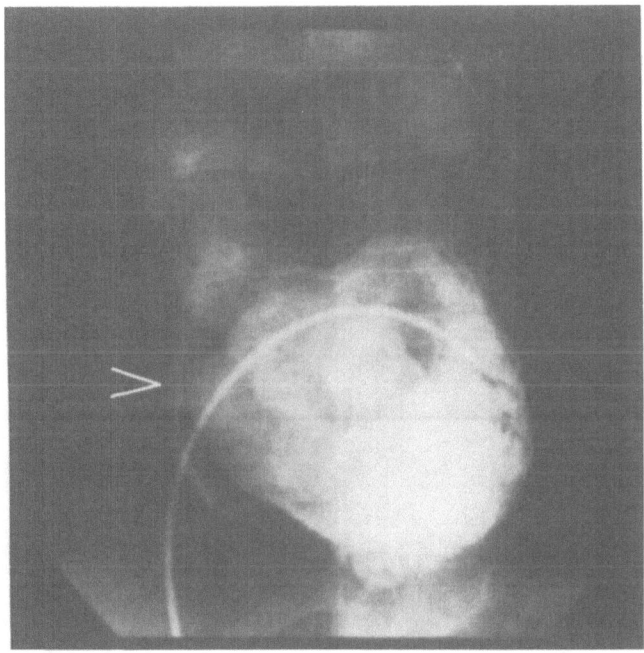

Fig. 2. Case no. 9. Patient aged 9.8 years with tricuspid atresia, normally connected great arteries (type Ib) and left Blalock–Taussig shunt which was performed at 1.4 years. Left ventricular cineangiocardiogram in the left anterior oblique position showing an aneurysmal bulge at the site of the VSD (arrow). The right ventricular outlet chamber is opacified through the very small VSD. At the height of the VSD there is an infundibular stenosis which separates the outlet chamber into a very inferior part and in a wider upper part.

three, and large in two patients. The size of the pulmonary valve, expressed as the ratio between the pulmonary valve ring and the aortic valve ring diameter on the lateral view, was one-half to three-quarters of the aortic valve in seven of the eight patients with type Ib, all with small VSD, moderately large or small outlet chamber, and associated infundibular stenosis. The pulmonary and the aortic valve were of equal size in the four remaining patients; three had type Ic with a large VSD as well as a large outlet chamber, but with a moderately severe infundibular stenosis in this outlet chamber in only one. The fourth patient had type Ib with a small VSD and a moderately large outlet chamber.

A posterosuperiorly directed stream of contrast medium on right atrial cineangiocardiograms in the posteroanterior and lateral views, present in all cases, was thought to be due to opacification through a patent foramen ovale or secundum type atrial septal defect [22, 23]. In two infants (cases no. 1 and 4), 42 days and three months of age, an aneurysm of the atrial septum was

112

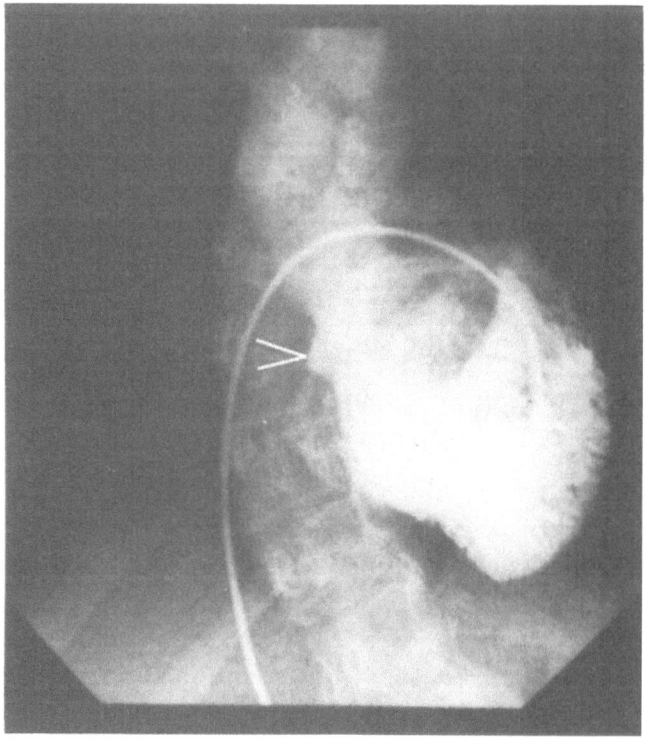

Fig. 3. Case no. 7. Patient aged 17.3 years with tricuspid atresia, normally connected great arteries (type Ib), and left and right Blalock–Taussig shunts which were performed at 4.2 and 10.3 years, respectively. Left ventricular cineangiocardiogram in the left anterior oblique position. Through a very small opening at the top of an aneurysmal bulge at the site of the VSD (arrow), only the narrow inferior part of the outlet chamber is opacified. A very tight fibrous infundibular stenosis and a small VSD, 0.3 cm in diameter, showing signs of closing, were found at subsequent Fontan operation.

demonstrated (Fig. 4a–c). Restriction of the interatrial defect, reflected by an a-wave gradient of 9 and 6 mm Hg and a mean pressure gradient of 2 and 5 mm Hg, respectively, necessitated a balloon atrial septostomy in the younger infant. Nevertheless, at repeat cineangiocardiography 14 months later, the aneurysm was essentially unchanged.

Aortograms in the seven patients with aortopulmonary shunts showed obliteration of the left Blalock–Taussig shunt in two and significant stenosis in a further two patients. Kinking and stenosis of the right pulmonary artery with preferential flow to the right lung was documented in both children with a Waterston anastomosis (cases no. 1 and 8) [8].

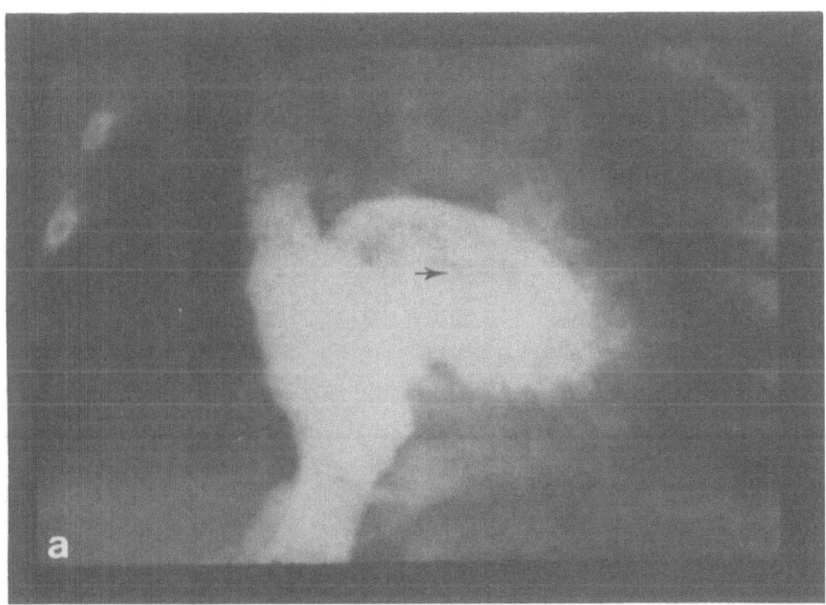

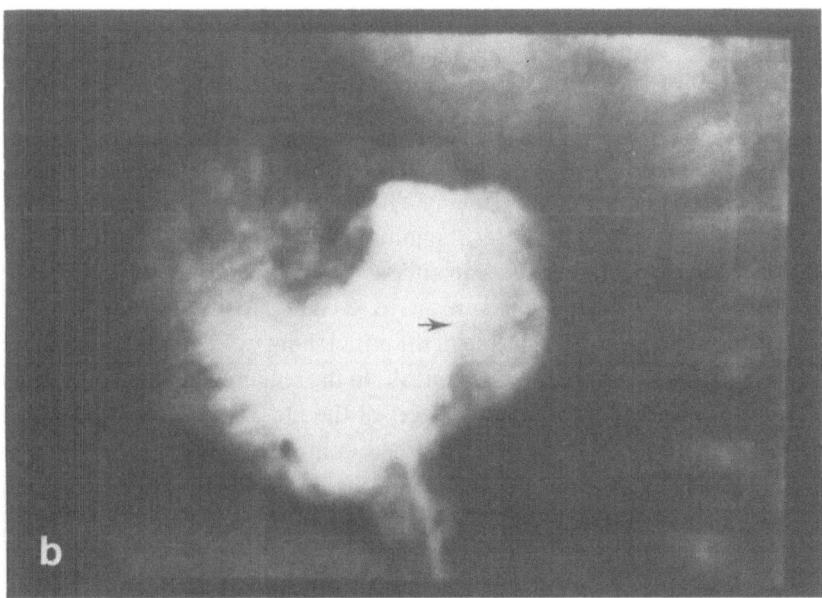

Fig. 4a and b. Case no. 1. Right atrial cineangiocardiogram of a 42-day-old infant, (*a*) posteroanterior and (*b*) lateral views. The posterosuperiorly directed stream of contrast medium is passing through the foramen ovale. There is also a large aneurysm of the atrial septum (arrow).

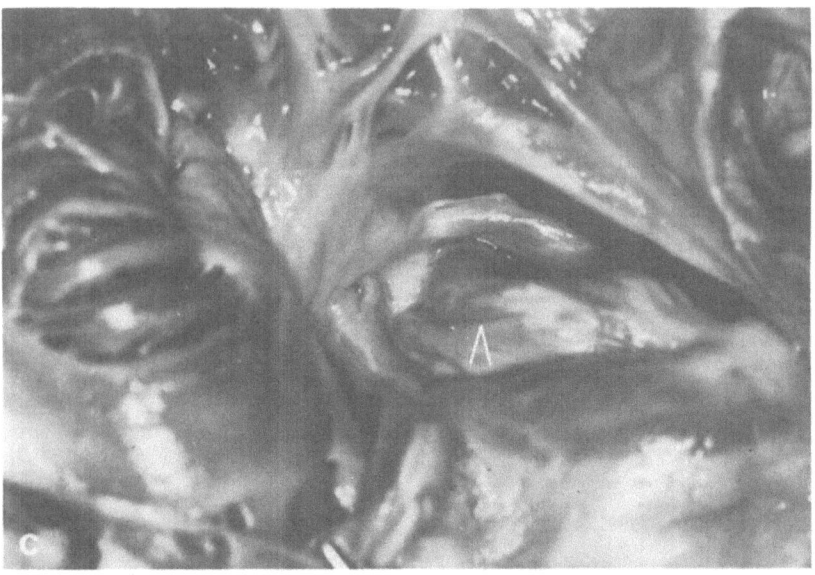

Fig. 4c. Autopsy specimen of the same patient as in Figure 4a and b at 18 months. Right atrial aspect of the fossa ovalis showing the aneurysm of the atrial septum (arrow) and the atrial septal defect at the site of the foramen ovale. A balloon atrial septostomy (BAS) was performed at the age of 42 days.

Surgery (Table 4)

Ten of the 11 patients underwent surgery. Nine with hypoxic symptoms required an aortopulmonary shunt at a median age of 1.3 years, range 42 days to 10.3 years. A left Blalock–Taussig shunt was performed in eight and a Waterston anastomosis in one as the initial operation. All nine patients required a second operation at a mean interval of 4.8 years, range six months to 10.8 years. Cyanosis and hypoxia recurred in eight patients. In four, significant stenosis or complete occlusion of the initial shunt was demonstrated, and the VSD size had diminished further in all. In the remaining patient (case no. 1), kinking of the right pulmonary artery at the site of the Waterston anastomosis had developed and the VSD had completely closed. The second surgical procedure was as follows: right Blalock–Taussig shunt in three; Waterston anastomosis, Goretex aortopulmonary anastomosis, and Glenn shunt in one patient each; reconstruction of the right pulmonary artery and Goretex anastomosis between the ascending aorta and the outlet chamber in one further child (case no. 1); and Fontan operation in the remaining two (cases no. 3 and 6). Seven years after the second Blalock–Taussig shunt, a Fontan operation was performed in one patient, age 17.6 years (case no. 7). In the tenth patient, a 10.4-year-old girl (case no. 5) who was markedly cyanosed

Table 4. Surgery in ten patients

No.	Sex	Type	BAS	1st Shunt	Age	Interval	2nd Shunt	Age	Interval	Modification of Fontan's operation	Age	Outcome
1 PJ	M	Ib	+	Waterston, kinking of RPA	42 d	1.4 y	AAO-RVOC Goretex anastomosis	1.5 y	—	—	—	Died
2 GH	M	Ib	—	Blalock–Taussig left	4.9 y	10.8 y	Glenn	15.7 y	—	—	—	Died
3 AR	F	Ic	+	Blalock–Taussig left	6 mo	—	—	—	6 mo	RAA-RVOC-direct anastomosis	12 mo	Died
5 GC	F	Ic	—	—	—	—	—	—	—	RAA-RVOC conduit	10.4 y	Alive
6 KJ	F	Ib	—	Blalock–Taussig left	10.3 y	—	—	—	9.4 y	RAA-RVOC conduit	19.7 y	Alive
7 JJ	F	Ib	—	Blalock–Taussig left	4.2 y	6.1 y	Blalock–Taussig right	10.3 y	7.3 y	RAA-RVOC conduit	17.6 y	Alive
8 MT	M	Ib	+	Blalock–Taussig left	1.2 y	1.5 y	Waterston kinking of RPA	2.7 y	—	—	—	Alive
9 AU	M	Ib	—	Blalock–Taussig left	1.4 y	8.9 y	Blalock–Taussig right	10.3 y	—	—	—	Alive
10 SC	M	Ib	—	Blalock–Taussig left	1.3 y	3.0 y	Goretex-AAO-PA anastomosis 0.6 – 0.4 cm	4.3 y	—	—	—	Alive
11 UA	F	Ib	—	Blalock–Taussig left	6 mo	1.3 y	Blalock–Taussig right	1.8 y	—	—	—	Alive

M, male; F, female; BAS, balloon atrial septostomy; d, day(s); mo, month(s); y, year(s); AAO, ascending aorta; RVOC, right ventricular outlet chamber; PA, pulmonary artery; RAA, right atrial appendage.

and very limited in her exercise tolerance, the Fontan operation was carried out as a primary corrective procedure.

Anatomical pathological findings

The hearts of four children who died were available for postmortem study. The oldest (case no. 2), who lived 15.8 years, succumbed to congestive heart failure. A Blalock–Taussig shunt had been performed at the age of 4.9 years and a Glenn anastomosis at 15.7 years, subsequent to cineangiographic documentation of VSD closure. The left aspect of the septum between main and outlet chambers revealed the pinpoint VSD which was separated from the aortic valve by a muscle bar and surrounded by fibrous endocardial proliferation (Fig. 5a). As viewed from the outlet chamber the VSD can be seen to be located low and posteriorly in the muscular septum (Fig. 5b). Histologi-

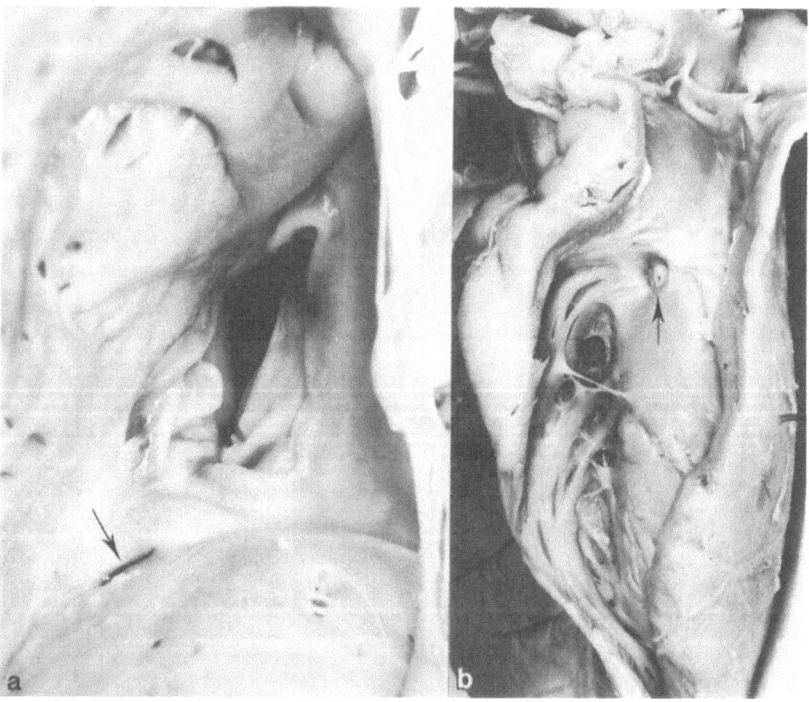

Fig. 5. (a) Case no. 2. Autopsy specimen of a 15.8-year-old patient with tricuspid atresia and normally connected great arteries (type Ib) with a left Blalock–Taussig shunt and a Glenn anastomosis performed at 4.9 and 15.7 years, respectively. Left ventricular aspect of the ventricular septum showing the pinpoint VSD (arrow) separated from the aortic valve by muscle and surrounded by fibrous endocardial proliferation. (*b*) Autopsy specimen from the same patient as in Figure 5a. Right ventricular outlet chamber. The pinpoint VSD (arrow) is located low and posterior in the muscular septum.

cally there was marked hypertrophy of the myocardial cells with patchy areas of interstitial fibrosis. The heart weighed 620 g.

The youngest infant lived for 134 days (case no. 4). The child underwent cardiac catheterization at the age of three months because of congestive heart failure. At this time the VSD was large and the Qp/Qs ratio was 1.9. At autopsy, 43 days later, the VSD had decreased in size to approximately 5 mm.

A further patient who lived one year (case no. 3) died perioperatively after a Fontan procedure required subsequent to occlusion of a left-sided Blalock–Taussig shunt performed at six months and spontaneous closure of the VSD. The cineangiocardiogram, at one month of age, revealed a nonrestrictive defect. At autopsy, the defect was found to be nearly obliterated by fibrous tissue [8].

A fourth patient (case no. 1) was acyanotic at birth, but underwent emergency catheterization at the age of 42 days because of severe hypoxia (Fig. 6a). A Waterston anastomosis was performed immediately. Follow-up catheterization at the age of 15 months showed kinking of the anastomosis leading to almost exclusive perfusion of the right lung (Fig. 6b). Antegrade perfusion of the left lung had apparently terminated with closure of the defect. When viewed from the main chamber, the septum showed the VSD to be closed completely (Fig. 6c). As viewed from the outlet chamber there is a dimple at the site of the VSD which is located low in the muscular septum at the junction between the upper, subpulmonary, and smooth portion (infundibular septum) and the trabeculated lower portion (Fig. 6d). This patient, too, died perioperatively, after an attempt to anastomose the outlet chamber with the ascending aorta and to reconstruct the pulmonary artery.

DISCUSSION

The 44% incidence (11 of 25 patients) of spontaneous closure or critical decrease in the size of the VSD in tricuspid atresia with NCGA in this study is comparable with that reported by Bharati et al. [24, 25] (27.5%), by Rao [15] (38%), and by Dische [26] (23%), and with the 20%–25% incidence of spontaneous closure in isolated ventricular septal defect [27–39].

As in previous reports [6, 40], the age at the initial investigation, median age five months, range 29 days to 6.1 years in this study, was representative of the onset of symptoms: three infants had congestive heart failure due to increased blood flow through a large VSD (type Ic). The remaining eight children suffered from hypoxia with increasing cyanosis and hematocrit values, decreasing pO_2, dyspnea on exertion, headache and dizziness in some instances, and hypoxic episodes and convulsions in one patient each. Spontaneous diminution in size of the VSD or functional and eventual anatomical closure

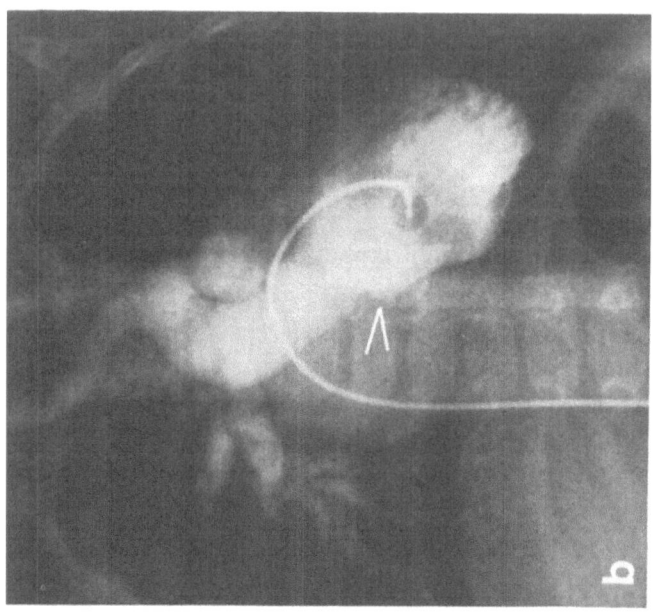

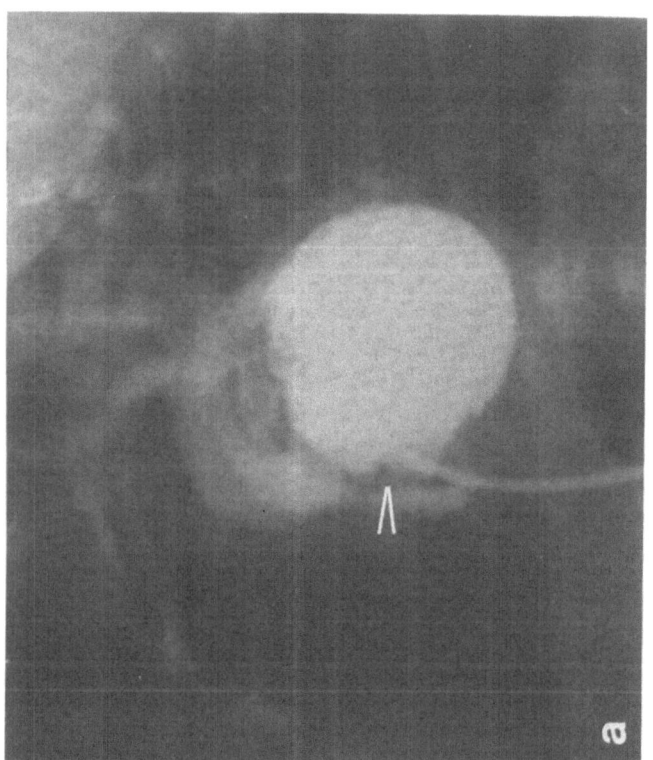

Fig. 6. (*a*) Case no. 1. Patient with tricuspid atresia, normally connected great arteries with decreased pulmonary blood flow (type Ib), who was acyanotic at birth. Left ventricular cineangiocardiogram in the left anterior oblique position at 42 days. The narrow right ventricular outlet chamber is opacified through a small VSD (arrow). (*b*) The same patient as in Figure 6a with a large Waterston anastomosis. Left ventricular cineangiocardiogram in the posteroanterior view at 15 months. The VSD has closed completely (arrow). Due to kinking of the right pulmonary artery there is preferential flow to the right lung with opacification of the main pulmonary artery and the large right pulmonary artery through the Waterston anastomosis while the left pulmonary artery can barely be visualized.

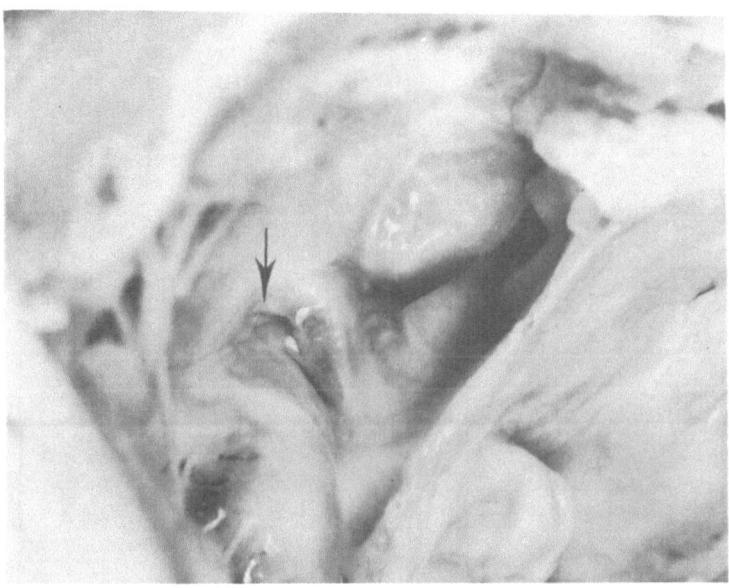

Fig. 6c. Autopsy specimen of the same patient as in Figure 6a and b, aged 1.5 years. Left ventricular aspect of the ventricular septum showing the VSD (arrow) to be closed completely.

of the defect, in several patients associated with the development of an infundibular stenosis in the outlet chamber, was generally attested to by the decreasing intensity or disappearance of the VSD murmur as also reported previously [6, 10, 13–15, 17, 41–43].

Although spontaneous closure of the VSD in tricuspid atresia with NCGA, similar to isolated VSDs [27, 28, 32, 36, 37, 44, 45], occurs most frequently in infancy [15] and accounts for the early onset of hypoxia and for the high mortality in the first year of life, it may occur at a later age, even up to the third decade [46].

The age at which spontaneous closure or critical decrease in the size of the VSD was documented in the present study ranged from 134 days to 19.7 years, median age 8.9 years: in four children the defect had closed completely or partially before two years of age, in six after eight years of age, and in one by 4.3 years. Survival was enabled by intercurrent shunt procedures. The median age at first shunt in nine of the 11 patients of 1.3 years, range 42 days to 10.3 years, is comparable with that in previously reported studies [6, 40, 47].

In patients with a functioning shunt, however, spontaneous VSD closure may first be documented at reinvestigation prior to an elective Fontan procedure, during subsequent open-heart surgery, or at autopsy, since typical

120

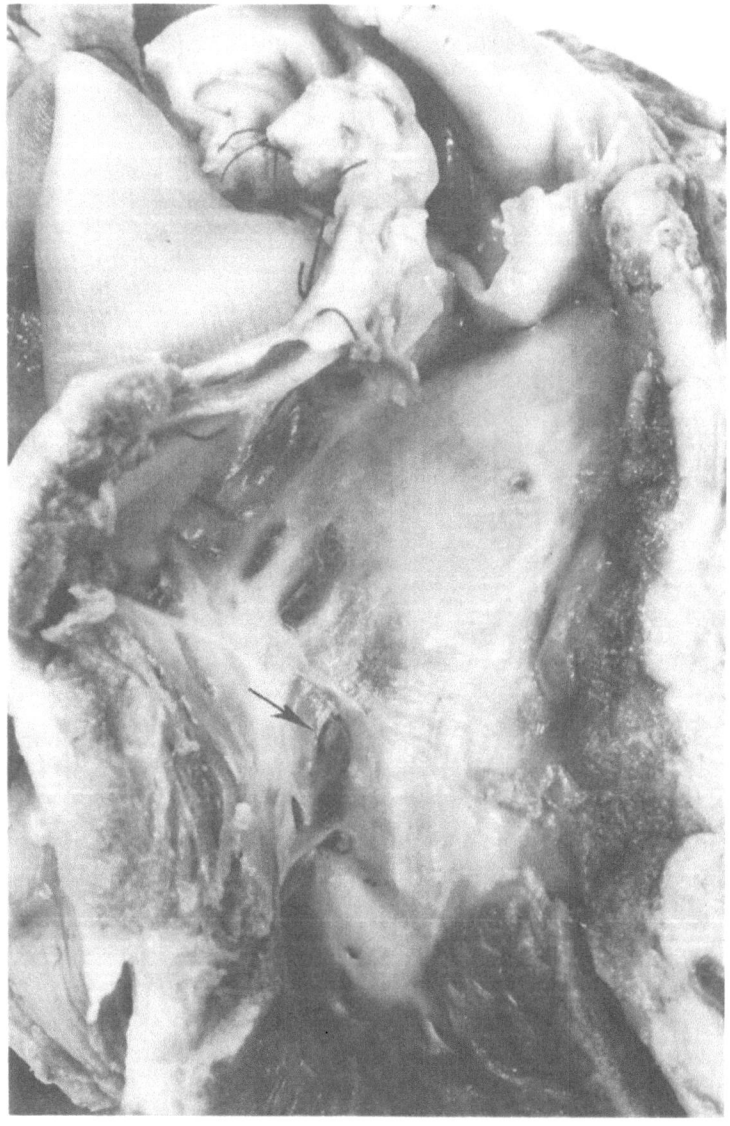

Fig. 6d. Autopsy specimen from the same patient as in Figure 6a–c. Right ventricular outlet chamber. There is only a dimple (arrow) at the site of the VSD which is located low in the muscular ventricular septum at the junction between the upper subpulmonary and smooth portion and the trabeculated lower portion. In the right anterior wall the Goretex anastomosis can be seen.

symptoms may not be readily apparent. Thus, the age at documentation of VSD closure may be representative of the actual age at closure only in patients without previous shunt procedures.

There is evidence that even large defects may occasionally close within a short period of time [15, 17]. This was documented to occur within 43 days in one infant in this series (case no. 4). Nevertheless, VSD closure in tricuspid atresia with NCGA, although reportedly related to age, is independent of the size of the defect at the initial investigation and uninfluenced by systemic-to-pulmonary artery shunts. It may, however, be related to the site or type of the VSD, as has been shown in isolated VSDs [17, 32, 38].

On "left ventricular" cineangiocardiogram in the left anterior oblique projection our findings demonstrated that the VSD was generally located in the anterior-superior border of the main chamber, below the infundibular septum and separated from the aortic valve cusps by a radiolucency. The angiocardiographic appearance resembled that of a defect in the anterior apical muscular septum described by Soto et al. [48]. Injection into the outlet chamber revealed the VSD to be inferior to the infundibular septum.

Correlation of the cineangiocardiographic findings with the findings at autopsy was possible in three cases (nos. 1, 2, and 3). Viewed from the ventricular aspect of the septum, the VSD was situated in the muscular septum below the right coronary aortic cusp and the commissure between the right coronary and the posterior acoronary aortic valve cusp. It was separated from the aortic valve by a muscular bar and surrounded or covered by thickened fibrous endocardial tissue. From the outlet chamber the defect was much smaller than on the left ventricular aspect, being positioned beneath the infundibular septum, posterior to the superior-anterior portion of the trabecula septomarginalis. A defect in this location is considered to be consistent with a foramen bulboventriculare [1–4]. According to Anderson et al. [1] the separation of the bulboventricular foramen from the aortic valve is the result of direct fusion of the infundibular septum with the bulboventricular septum, which may also explain the general absence of the membranous septum [49]. In this type of VSD, which can be assumed to have been present in the majority of cases with tricuspid atresia and NCGA, studied morphologically, the spontaneous closure rate was 20%–40% [1, 15, 24, 26, 42, 49, 50]. In only six of 91 cases reported by Bharati et al. [24], the defect varied in its location being more anterior, directly beneath the right coronary aortic cusp rather than below the acoronary cusp and entering the outlet chamber either beneath the arch of the septal and parietal bands or more anteriorly closer to the pulmonary trunk. This latter position is distinct from that of the common type VSD with its location inferior to the infundibular septum and posterior in the outlet chamber. Based on an anatomical study of 60 cases with tricuspid atresia and NCGA by L. Becú, 1976, Somerville [17] also distinguished two types of VSD as viewed from the ventricle: a rarer "low" muscular defect and a more common cephalad defect, which was separated from the aortic valve by a muscular band. Hypertrophy of this muscular band had resulted in subaortic stenosis in two cases with a closing cephalad type of defect. In both types of VSD, complete spontaneous closure was demonstrated, the probability of closure being even greater in the "low" muscular defect. It can also be assumed that the defect in the cephalad subaortic position is consistent with the typical VSD in tricuspid atresia with NCGA, while the "low" muscular defect is exceptional. A further variation is the presence of either one (in four of 91 cases reported by Bharati et al. [24]) or multiple additional defects [26]. It can be assumed that these additional defects, which are located without exception in the muscular septum, also behave like isolated muscular VSDs and thus will close spontaneously in 20%–50%. In an occasional case there may be a situation, as has been documented in a patient with tricuspid atresia associated, however, with transposition of the great arteries [51], in which the typical VSD is completely occluded while the additional muscular defect has remained patent.

Since the VSD in tricuspid atresia and NCGA is located in the muscular septum, the mechanisms of diminution and spontaneous closure should be the same as has been described previously for the isolated muscular septal defect [38]: (1) relative reduction in size of the VSD with growth [52], (2) apposition of the margins of the VSD [53], (3) encroachment of the VSD by muscular hypertrophy [54], (4) septal hypertrophy [55], and (5) closure by endocardial fibrous proliferation and thrombus formation [42, 43]. The relation of the conduction tissue to the VSD in tricuspid atresia with NCGA was studied by serial histological sectioning by Guller et al. [56], Bharati and Lev [57], and Becker et al. [58]. They have demonstrated a posterior short atrioventricular node situated adjacent to the central fibrous body which then pierced it to become the bundle. This was short and penetrated the myocardium beneath the mitral valve to reach a subendocardial position on the left side of the septum below the posterior aortic valve cusp. The left bundle branch originated close to the nodal-bundle junction and was situated posterior to the VSD. The right bundle branch traversed the posteroinferior and distal wall of the defect to become located in a nearly subendocardial position in the outlet chamber to the right and just inferior to the VSD as illustrated in Figure 7.

In contradiction to the report of Anderson et al. [1], who found a good-sized outlet chamber even when secondary constriction of the VSD had occurred, our results together with the experience of others [17, 24, 49, 59–61] suggest that the size of the VSD is the primary determinate for the size of the outlet chamber, the pulmonary valve and pulmonary artery. Once the VSD decreases in size and limits flow, the initially adequately large outlet chamber

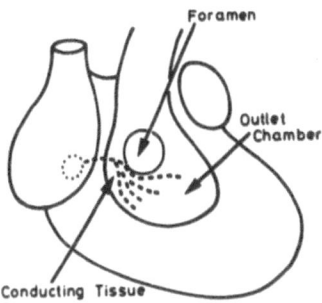

Fig. 7. Diagram of the heart with tricuspid atresia and normally connected great arteries, as viewed from the front, showing the conduction tissue to be to the right and inferior to the VSD (outlet foramen). Courtesy of Dr. Anton Becker.

and pulmonary arteries will not grow normally and thus become less suitable for a Fontan procedure [62]. The results of this study show that the natural history of tricuspid atresia with NCGA generally includes spontaneous diminution in size or complete closure of the VSD, reported to occur preferentially in infancy and early childhood, and that survival until the patients attain the age and size suitable for a Fontan operation is dependent on intercurrent palliative shunt procedures. Thus, in view of this natural history of the VSD, pulmonary artery banding is generally contraindicated in infants with tricuspid atresia, NCGA but with an unrestrictive VSD and increased pulmonary blood flow, who initially have congestive heart failure [6, 17, 47, 63]. The possibility of the patients eventually undergoing a Fontan operation also mitigates against a balloon atrial septostomy [64, 65] or a Blalock–Hanlon atrial septectomy [66], unless the mean pressure gradient between right and left atria exceeds 5 mm Hg, associated in some instances with an aneurysm of the atrial septum [67, 68], and the patient has signs of systemic venous obstruction [6, 68, 69].

The initial procedure has usually been an attempt to reestablish adequate pulmonary blood flow [6, 8, 11, 40, 47, 70–77], in our patients generally with a left Blalock–Taussig shunt. The Waterston anastomosis [40, 76] appears to be less suitable for patients with tricuspid atresia and NCGA (type Ib) since it may be associated with a number of complications. In the early postoperative course the shunt may prove inadequate or excessive. Pulmonary hypertension and pulmonary vascular obstructive disease may intervene in the late course [6, 40, 47]. While these complications may also occur in other types of central aortopulmonary shunts, the Waterston anastomosis, in particular, may lead to kinking of the right pulmonary artery and preferential flow to the right lung with subsequent pulmonary hypertension and hypoperfusion of the left lung [61]. Should the VSD in these patients close spontaneously, as has been documented in two of our patients (cases no. 1 and 8), the antegrade flow into the left lung would terminate. Similarly, in patients with tricuspid atresia and NCGA (type 1b), and a Glenn anastomosis [74], VSD closure dictates cessation of the blood flow to the left lung [15]. Consequently, the Blalock–Taussig shunt remains the palliative procedure of choice in patients with tricuspid atresia and NCGA (type Ib) [15, 40, 75]. Since, however, surgical shunts generally are outgrown, in our experience and that of others [47], after a mean duration of approximately five years, most of these patients will require a further palliative procedure before a physiological correction can be performed. While a second shunt operation, such as a Blalock–Taussig anastomosis on the contralateral side [15] or a Glenn anastomosis in children of over two years of age [47], may allow more adequate growth of the pulmonary arteries, the size of the outlet chamber remains uninfluenced unless pulmonary valve insufficiency is present.

Thus, a more desirable outcome with respect to suitability for physiological correction or Fontan operation [8, 16–19, 62, 78–101] may be enabled by providing a hemodynamic situation which encourages enlargement of the outlet chamber and of the pulmonary artery. Since the variability of the localization of the VSD is negligible and since the anatomical relationship of the conduction tissues to the boundaries of the defect is well defined, a procedure to enlarge the VSD either as the initial operation in infants in whom the failure rate of the Blalock–Taussig shunt is considered to be increased, or as an alternative to a second shunt procedure in younger children, warrants consideration. The presence of a further defect, however, should be ruled out by careful inspection of the septum and a possibly associated infundibular stenosis should be properly delineated.

Enlargement of the VSD in patients with tricuspid atresia and NCGA (type Ib), as originally reported by Brock [59] (Fig. 8), has subsequently been

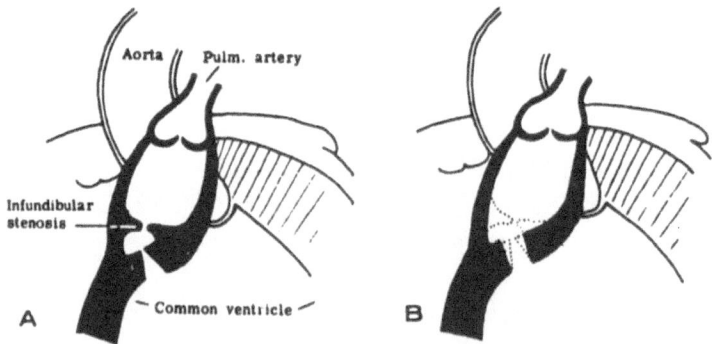

Fig. 8. Diagrams illustrating the intraoperative findings in a 12½-year-old girl with tricuspid atresia, normally connected great arteries, a very small VSD (0.4 × 0.2 cm) and severe infundibular stenosis (type Ib) before (*A*) and after (*B*) enlargement of the VSD. Resection of the infundibular stenosis was carried out by Sir Russel Brock in 1962 [17].

quantitatively delineated by Fontan [81, 102] to require an increase in the size of the VSD to a mean diameter of the pulmonary valve ring according to the patients weight, based on data of Lev et al. [103], plus 20%. In addition to a resection of the infundibular stenosis, closure of the incision in the outlet chamber with a patch [104] should be undertaken. Thus, to counteract the natural tendency to spontaneous closure or reduction in size of the VSD, the patency of which is critical in patients with tricuspid atresia, limited surgical enlargement of the VSD during infancy to afford adequate growth of the outlet chamber and augment pulmonary blood flow should be considered as an alternative to systemic-to-pulmonary artery shunts.

SUMMARY

Spontaneous closure or critical decrease in the size of the ventricular septal defect in tricuspid atresia with normally connected and related great arteries is relatively common. The 44% incidence (11 of 25 patients) is comparable with that reported in the literature and with the incidence of spontaneous closure in isolated ventricular septal defects. It is reported to occur preferentially in infancy and accounts for the early onset of hypoxia and for the high mortality rate of 79% observed in the first year of life. It is independent of the size of the ventricular septal defect at the initial investigation, and not accelerated by systemic-to-pulmonary artery shunts, but possibly related to the site of the ventricular septal defect.

The median age at documentation can be assumed to be generally representative of surgical palliation in infancy, the median age at first shunt being 1.3 years. Limited surgical enlargement of the ventricular septal defect during infancy to afford adequate growth of the outlet chamber and augment pulmonary blood flow warrants consideration as an alternative to systemic-to-pulmonary artery shunts.

Acknowledgments. We wish to thank Professor W. Gössner for allowing us to examine the autopsy specimens. We also thank Miss Yvonne Aeschbach for her help during the preparation of the manuscript. This study has been published previously in *Herz* 5:369–384, 1980.

REFERENCES

1. Anderson RH, Shinebourne EA, Becker AE, Macartney FJ, Quero-Jiménez M, Tynan MJ, Arnold R, Smith A, Wilkinson JL: Tricuspid atresia. J Thorac Cardiovasc Surg 74:325–327, 1977.
2. Anderson RH, Wilkinson JL, Gerlis LM, Smith A, Becker AE: Atresia of the right atrioventricular orifice. Br Heart J 39:414–428, 1977.

3. Anderson RH, Becker AE, Macartney FJ, Shinebourne EA, Wilkinson JL, Tynan MJ: Is "tricuspid atresia" a univentricular heart? Pediatr Cardiol 1:51–56, 1979.
4. Anderson RH, Shinebourne EA, Becker AE, Macartney FJ, Wilkinson JL, Tynan MJ: Tricuspid atresia and univentricular heart. Pediatr Cardiol 1:165–166, 1979/80.
5. Campbell M: Tricuspid atresia and its prognosis with and without surgical treatment. Br Heart J 23:699–710, 1961.
6. Dick M, Fyler DC, Nadas AS: Tricuspid atresia: clinical course in 101 patients. Am J Cardiol 36:327–337, 1975.
7. Kühne M: Über zwei Fälle kongenitaler Atresie des Ostium venosum dextrum. Jahrb Kinderheilkd 63:235–249, 1906.
8. Sauer U, Mocellin R: Angiocardiographic left ventricular volume determination in tricuspid atresia. Comparison of patients with and without palliative surgery. Herz 4:148–255, 1979.
9. Van Praagh R, Ando M, Dungan WT: Anatomic types of tricuspid atresia: clinical and developmental implication. Circulation [Suppl 2] 43 and 44:11–115, 1971.
10. Gallaher ME, Fyler DC: Observations on changing hemodynamics in tricuspid atresia without associated transposition of the great vessels. Circulation 35:381–388, 1967.
11. Kyger ER, Reul GJ Jr, Sandiford FM, Wukasch DC, Hallman GL, Cooley DA: Surgical palliation of tricuspid atresia. Circulation 52:685–690, 1975.
12. Neches WH, Park SC, Lenox CC, Zuberbuhler JR, Bahnson HT: Tricuspid atresia with transposition of the great arteries and closing ventricular septal defect. Successful palliation by banding of the pulmonary artery and creation of an aorticopulmonary window. J Thorac Cardiovasc Surg 65:538–542, 1973.
13. Rao PS, Sissman NJ: Spontaneous closure of physiologically advantageous ventricular septal defects. Circulation 43:83–90, 1971.
14. Rao PS, Linde LM, Liebman J, Perrin E: Functional closure of physiologically advantageous ventricular septal defects. Observations in three cases with tricuspid atresia. Am J Dis Child 127:36–40, 1974.
15. Rao PS: Natural history of the ventricular septal defect in tricuspid atresia and its surgical implications. Br Heart J 39:276–288, 1977.
16. Somerville J, Ross DN: Tricuspid atresia – new hope with radical palliative surgery. Br Heart J 37:782, 1975.
17. Somerville J: Congenital heart disease – changes in form and function. Br Heart J 41:1–22, 1979.
18. Fontan F, Baudet E: Surgical repair of tricuspid atresia. Thorax 26:240–248, 1971.
19. Fontan F, Mounicot FB, Baudet E, Simonneau J, Gordo J, Gouffrant JM: Correction de l'atrésie tricuspidienne: rapport de deux cas "corrigés" par l'utilisation d'une technique chirurgicale nouvelle. Ann Chir Thorac Cardiovasc 10:39–47, 1971.
20. Edwards JE, Burchell HB: Congenital tricuspid atresia: a classification. Med Clin North Am 33:1177–1196, 1949.
21. Keith JD, Rowe RD, Vlad P: Heart disease in infancy and childhood, 2nd edn. New York, Macmillan, 1967, p 647.
22. Tandon R, Edwards JE: Atrial septal defect in infancy. Circulation 49:1005–1010, 1974.
23. Williams HJ, Tandon R, Edwards JE: Persistent ostium primum coexisting with mitral or tricuspid atresia. Chest 66:39–43, 1974.
24. Bharati S, McAllister Hz, Tatooles CJ, Miller RA, Weinberg M, Bucheleres HG, Lev M: Anatomic variations in underdeveloped right ventricle related to tricuspid atresia and stenosis. J Thorac Cardiovasc Surg 72:383–400, 1976.
25. Bharati S, Lev M: The concept of tricuspid atresia complex as distinct from that of the single ventricle complex. Pediatr Cardiol 1:57–62, 1979.
26. Dische R: Personal communication, 1977.
27. Alpert BS, Mellits D, Rowe RD: Spontaneous closure of small ventricular septal defects. Probability rates in the first five years of life. Am J Dis Child 125:194–196, 1973.
28. Blackstone EH, Kirklin JW, Bradley EL, DuShane JW, Appelbaum A: Optimal age and results in repair of large ventricular septal defects. J Thorac Cardiovasc Surg 72:661–679, 1976.

29. Campbell M: The natural history of ventricular septal defect. Br Heart J 33:246, 1971.
30. Collins G, Calder L, Rose V, Kidd L, Keith J: Ventricular septal defect: clinical and hemodynamic changes in the first five years of life. Am Heart J 84:695–705, 1972.
31. Freedom RM, White RD, Pieroni DR, Varghese PJ, Krovetz LJ, Rowe RD: The natural history of the so-called aneurysm of the membranous ventricular septum in childhood. Circulation 49:375–384, 1974.
32. Hoffman JIE, Rudolph AM: Natural history of ventricular septal defect in infancy. Am J Cardiol 16:634, 1965.
33. Hoffman JIE: Natural history of congenital heart disease: problems in its assessment with special reference to ventricular septal defects. Circulation 37:97–125, 1968.
34. Hoffman JIE, Rudolph AM: The natural history of isolated ventricular septal defect with special reference to selection of patients for surgery. Adv Pediatr 17:57–78, 1970.
35. Hoffman JIE: Natural history of ventricular septal defect. Br Med J 1:571–572, 1971.
36. Keith JD, Rose V, Collins G, Kidd BSL: Ventricular septal defect: incidence, morbidity and mortality in various age groups. Br Heart J [Suppl 1] 33:81, 1971.
37. Li MD, Keith JD: Spontaneous closure of ventricular septal defects. Am Heart J 80:432–433, 1970.
38. Mesko ZG, Jones JE, Nadas AS: Diminution and closure of large ventricular septal defects after pulmonary artery banding. Circulation 48:847–855, 1973.
39. Varghese PJ, Rowe RD: Spontaneous closure of ventricular septal defects by aneurysmal formation of the membranous septum. J Pediatr 75:700–703, 1969.
40. Patel R, Fox K, Taylor JFN, Graham GR: Tricuspid atresia. Clinical course in 62 cases (1967–1974). Br Heart J 40:1408–1414, 1978.
41. Marcano BA, Riemenschneider TA, Ruttenberg HD, Goldberg SJ, Gyepes M: Tricuspid atresia with increased pulmonary blood flow. An analysis of 13 cases. Circulation 40:399–410, 1969.
42. Meng LCC: Spontaneous closure of ventricular septal defect in tricuspid atresia. J Pediatr 75:697–700, 1969.
43. Menner K, Rautenburg HW: Ungewöhnlicher Verlauf bei einem Kind mit einer Atresie der Tricuspidalklappe. Arch Kinderheilkd 183:171–175, 1971.
44. Clarkson PM, Frye RL, DuShane JW, Burchell HB, Wood EH, Weidman WH: Prognosis for patients with ventricular septal defect and severe pulmonary vascular obstructive disease. Circulation 38:129, 1968.
45. Weidman WH, Gersony WM, Nugent EW, DuShane JW, Rowe RD: Indirect assessment of severity in ventricular septal defect. Circulation [Suppl 1] 56:24–35, 1977.
46. Roberts WC, Morrow AG, Mason DT, Braunwald E: Spontaneous closure of ventricular septal defect. Anatomic proof in an adult with tricuspid atresia. Circulation 27:90–94, 1963.
47. Williams WG, Rubis L, Fowler RS, Rao MK, Trusler GA, Mustard WT: Tricuspid atresia: results of treatment in 160 children. Am J Cardiol 38:235–240, 1976.
48. Soto B, Coghlan CH, Bargeron LM Jr: Angiography of ventricular septal defects. In: Anderson RH, Shinebourne AE (eds) Paediatric cardiology 1977. Edinburgh, Livingstone, 1978, pp 125–137.
49. Guller B, Titus JL: Morphological studies in tricuspid atresia. Circulation 38:977–986, 1968.
50. Hoffman JIE: Natural history of congenital heart disease: problems in its assessment with special reference to ventricular septal defects. Circulation 37:97–125, 1968.
51. Fontan F: Personal communication, 1978.
52. French H: Possibility of a loud congenital heart murmur disappearing when a child grows up. Guys Hosp Gaz 32:87, 1918.
53. Edwards JE, Dry TJ, Parker RL, Burchell HD, Wood EH, Bulbulian AH: An atlas of congenital anomalies of the heart and great vessels. Springfield IL, Charles E Thomas, 1954, p 67.
54. Suzuki H, Lucas RV Jr: Spontaneous closure of ventricular septal defect. Arch Pathol 85:31, 1967.

55. Evans JR, Rowe RD, Keith JD: Spontaneous closure of ventricular septal defects. Circulation 22:1044–1054, 1960.

56. Guller B, DuShane JW, Titus JL: The atrioventricular conduction system in two cases of tricuspid atresia. Circulation 40:217–226, 1969.

57. Bharati S, Lev M: The conduction system in tricuspid atresia with regular d-transposition. Abstr Circ [Suppl 2] 53 and 54:170, 1976.

58. Becker A, Meyboom EJ, Wilkinson JL, Smith A: "Tricuspid atresia" is a form of uni-ventricular heart: a concept supported by the anatomy of the atrioventricular conduction tissue [abstr]. In: Association of European Paediatric Cardiologists, 16th annual general meeting, Budapest, 1978.

59. Brock R: Tricuspid atresia: a step toward corrective treatment. J Thorac Cardiovasc Surg 47:17–25, 1964.

60. Guller B, Kincaid OW, Ritter DG, Titus JL: Angiocardiographic findings in tricuspid atresia: correlation with hemodynamic and morphologic features. Radiology 93:531–540, 1969.

61. Somerville J, Barbosa R: Radical corrective surgery after Waterston shunts. In: Longmore DB (ed) The current status of cardiac surgery. Lancaster, England, MTP Medical and Technical, 1975, pp 78–83.

62. Choussat A, Fontan F, Besse P, Vallot F, Chauve A, Bricaud H: Selection criteria for Fontan's procedure. In: Anderson RH, Shinebourne AE (eds) Paediatric cardiology 1977. Edinburgh, Livingstone, 1978, pp 559–566.

63. Tingelstad JB, Lower RR, Howell TR, Eldrige WJ: Pulmonary artery banding in tricuspid atresia without transposed great arteries. Am J Dis Child 121:434–437, 1971.

64. Rashkind WJ, Miller WW: Creation of an atrial septal defect without thoracotomy: palliative approach to complete transposition of the great arteries. JAMA 196:991, 1966.

65. Rashkind WJ, Friedman S, Waldhausen JA, Miller WW: Management of tricuspid atresia in infancy: use of balloon-catheter atrial septostomy followed by ascending aorta to right pulmonary artery anastomosis [abstr]. Circulation [Suppl 2] 35 and 36:217, 1967.

66. Blalock A, Hanlon CR: The surgical treatment of complete transposition of the aorta and the pulmonary artery. Surg Gynecol Obstet 90:1, 1950.

67. Freedom RM, Rowe RD: Aneurysm of the atrial septum in tricuspid atresia. Diagnosis during life and therapy. Am J Cardiol 38:265–267, 1976.

68. Sauer U: Primitive ventricle – angiocardiography and haemodynamics with absent atrio-ventricular connexion. In: Anderson RH, Shinebourne AE (eds) Paediatric cardiology 1977. Edinburgh, Livingstone, 1978, pp 360–372.

69. Lenox CC, Zuberbuhler JR: Balloon septostomy in tricuspid atresia after infancy. Am J Cardiol 25:723–726, 1970.

70. Alvarez-Diaz F, Brito JM, Cordovilla G, Pérez de León J, Sanchez PA, Brodiú CM: Ascending aorta–right pulmonary artery anastomosis: Waterston's operation. Thorax 28:152–157, 1973.

71. Bargeron LM Jr, Karp LB, Barcia A: Late deterioration of patients after superior vena cava to right pulmonary artery anastomosis. Am J Cardiol 30:211–216, 1972.

72. Deverall PB, Lincoln JCR, Aberdeen E, Bonham-Carter RE, Waterston DJ: Surgical management of tricuspid atresia. Thorax 24:239, 1969.

73. Edwards WS, Bargeron LM Jr: The superiority of the Glenn operation for tricuspid atresia in infancy and childhood. J Thorac Cardiovasc Surg 55:60–69, 1968.

74. Glenn WWL, Brown M, Whittemore R: Circulatory bypass of the right side of the heart: cava-pulmonary artery shunt – indications and results. In: Cassels DE (ed) The heart and circulation in the newborn and infant. New York, Grune and Stratton, 1966, pp 345–357.

75. Taussig HB, Keinonen R, Momberger N, Kirk H: Long-term observations on the Blalock–Taussig operation. IV: Tricuspid atresia. Johns Hopkins Med J 132:135–145, 1973.

76. Waterston DJ: The treatment of Fallot's tetralogy in infants under the age of one year [in Czech]. Rozhl Chir 41:183, 1962.

77. Williams WG, Rubis L, Trusler GA, Mustard WT: Palliation of tricuspid atresia. Arch Surg 110:1383–1386, 1975.

78. Björk BO, Olin CL, Bjarke BB, Thorén CA: Right atrial–right ventricular anastomosis for correction of tricuspid atresia. J Thorac Cardiovasc Surg 77:452–458, 1979.

79. Bowman FO Jr, Malm JR, Hayes CJ, Gersony WM: Physiological approach to surgery for tricuspid atresia [abstr]. Circulation 62:91–96, 1980.

80. Fontan F, Choussat A, Brom AG, Chauve A, Deville C, Castro-Cels A: Repair of tricuspid atresia – surgical considerations and results. In: Anderson RH, Shinebourne EA (eds) Paediatric cardiology 1977. Edinburgh, Livingstone, 1978, pp 567–580.

81. Fontan F: Evolution of therapeutical concepts in tricuspid atresia. Edgar Mannheimer lecture. In: Association of European Paediatric Cardiologists, 16th annual meeting, Budapest, 1978.

82. Gago O, Salles CA, Stern AM, Spooner E, Brandt RL, Morris JD: A different approach for the total correction of tricuspid atresia. J Thorac Cardiovasc Surg 72:209–214, 1976.

83. Gale AW, Danielson GK, McGoon DC, Wallace RB, Mair DD: Fontan procedure for tricuspid atresia [abstr]. Circulation 62:91–96, 1980.

84. Henry JN, Danielson GK: Successful "correction" of tricuspid atresia: results of a detailed anatomical study. Surg Forum 25:163–165, 1974.

85. Henry JN, Devloo RAE, Ritter DG, Mair DD, Davis GD, Danielson GK: Tricuspid atresia – successful surgical "correction" in two patients using porcine xenograft valves. Mayo Clin Proc 49:803–810, 1974.

86. Hurwitt ES, Young D, Escher DJW: The rationale of anastomosis of the right auricular appendage to the pulmonary artery in the treatment of tricuspid atresia. Application of this procedure to a case of cor triloculare. J Thorac Cardiovasc Surg 30:503–512, 1955.

87. Just-Viera JO, Rivé-Mora E, Altieri PI, Girod CE: Tricuspid atresia and the hypoplastic right ventricular complex: complete correction for long term survival. Surg Forum 22:165–166, 1971.

88. Kreutzer G, Galindez E, Bono H, de Palma C, Laura JP: An operation for the correction of tricuspid atresia. J Thorac Cardiovasc Surg 66:613–621, 1973.

89. Lamberti JJ, Thilenius D, de la Fuente D, Lin CY, Arcilla R, Replogle RL: Right atrial partition and right ventricular exclusion. Another surgical approach for complex cyanotic congenital heart disease. J Thorac Cardiovasc Surg 71:386–391, 1976.

90. Miller RA, Pahlajani D, Serratto M, Tatooles C: Clinical studies after Fontan's operation for tricuspid atresia [abstr]. Am J Cardiol 33:157, 1974.

91. Robicsek F, Sanger PW, Taylor FH, Najib A, Tavana M: Complete bypass of the right heart. Am Heart J 66:792, 1963.

92. Robicsek F, Sanger PW, Golucci V: Long-term complete circulatory exclusion of the right side of the heart: hemodynamic observations. Am J Cardiol 18:867, 1966.

93. Robicsek F, Sanger PW, Golucci V, Daugherty HK: Long-term circulatory exclusion of the right heart. Surgery 59:431–437, 1966.

94. Ross DN, Somerville J: Surgical correction of tricuspid atresia. Lancet 1:845–849, 1973.

95. Sanger PW, Robicsek F, Taylor FH, Golucci V: Observations on partial and complete circulatory exclusion of the right heart. J Cardiovasc Surg (Torino) 6:30, 1965.

96. Seki S, Ohba O, Tanizaki M, Takahashi S, Teramoto S, Sunada T: Construction of a new right ventricle on the epicardium – a possible correction for underdevelopment of the right ventricle. J Cardiovasc Surg (Torino) 70:330, 1975.

97. Serratto M, Miller RA, Tatooles C, Ardekani R: Hemodynamic evaluation of Fontan operation in tricuspid atresia. Circulation [Suppl 3] 54:99–101, 1976.

98. Stanford W, Armstrong RG, Cline RE, King TD: Right atrium–pulmonary allograft for the correction of tricuspid atresia. J Thorac Cardiovasc Surg 66:105–111, 1973.

99. Tatooles CJ, Ardekani RG, Miller RA, Serratto M: Operative repair of tricuspid atresia. Ann Thorac Surg 21:499, 1976.

100. Tatooles CJ, Ardekani RG, Miller RA, Serratto M: Results following physiological repair for tricuspid atresia. Ann Thorac Surg 22:578–583, 1976.

101. Walker DR, Sbokos CG, Lennox SC: Correction of tricuspid atresia. Br Heart J 37:282–286, 1975.

102. Annecchino FP, Fontan F, Chauve A, Quaegebeur J: Palliative reconstruction of the right

ventricular outflow tract in tricuspid atresia: a report of 5 patients. Ann Thorac Surg 29:317–321, 1980.

103. Lev M, Rowlatt UF, Rimoldi HJA: Pathologic methods for study of congenitally malformed hearts. Methods for electrocardiographic and physiologic correlation. Arch Pathol 72:493, 1961.

104. Rittenhouse EA, Mohri H, Yates WG, Tenckhoff L, Reichenbach DD, Merendino KA: Ventricular enlargement for underdeveloped right ventricle and associated anomalies. J Thorac Cardiovasc Surg 68:229–236, 1974.

10. THE VENTRICULAR SEPTUM IN HEARTS WITH AN ATRIOVENTRICULAR DEFECT

ARNOLD C.G. WENINK

INTRODUCTION

A striking feature of hearts with an atrioventricular defect is the pathology of the atrioventricular valve or valves. All along has this pathology been a criterion for further classification of hearts within this group [1–9], which is of great surgical significance. Because most of this pathology has been attributed to faulty development of the atrioventricular endocardial cushions [3, 4, 10], these malformations have been called endocardial cushion defects.

An interatrial shunt is also a common feature. Although this "persistent ostium primum" was described as resulting from deficient atrial septation [11], many investigators have concluded that the atrial septum is not necessarily abnormal [1, 4, 10, 12–14].

The reason for including this malformation in a book on the ventricular septum is the scooped out appearance of this septum [15], which has been recognized in all forms of the anomaly [13, 14, 17–21]. The presence or absence of a ventricular septal defect "in the accepted sense" [16] depends solely on atrioventricular valve attachment [21, 22].

It will subsequently be shown that the abnormal position of the aortic orifice [14, 20, 21, 23] may also be explained by abnormal development of the ventricular septum.

PATHOLOGICAL ANATOMY OF THE VENTRICULAR SEPTUM

It is the deficiency of the posterior portion of the septum that characterizes all hearts with this malformation. The deficiency is present in so-called partial (Fig. 1) as well as complete (Fig. 2) forms. If one took the valve leaflets out, it would no longer be possible to tell the difference, although indeed the degree of septal deficiency may vary.

Evidently, the septal component that is deficient is the inlet septum. Although the defect may be very large (not in the sense of an interventricular communication, but in the sense of absent muscular tissue), it never extends beyond the trabecula septomarginalis. This means that the bulboventricular septum is principally normal (Fig. 3).

A.C.G. Wenink et al. (eds.) The Ventricular Septum of the Heart, *131–138. All rights reserved.*
Copyright ©1981 by Martinus Nijhoff Publishers, The Hague/Boston/London.

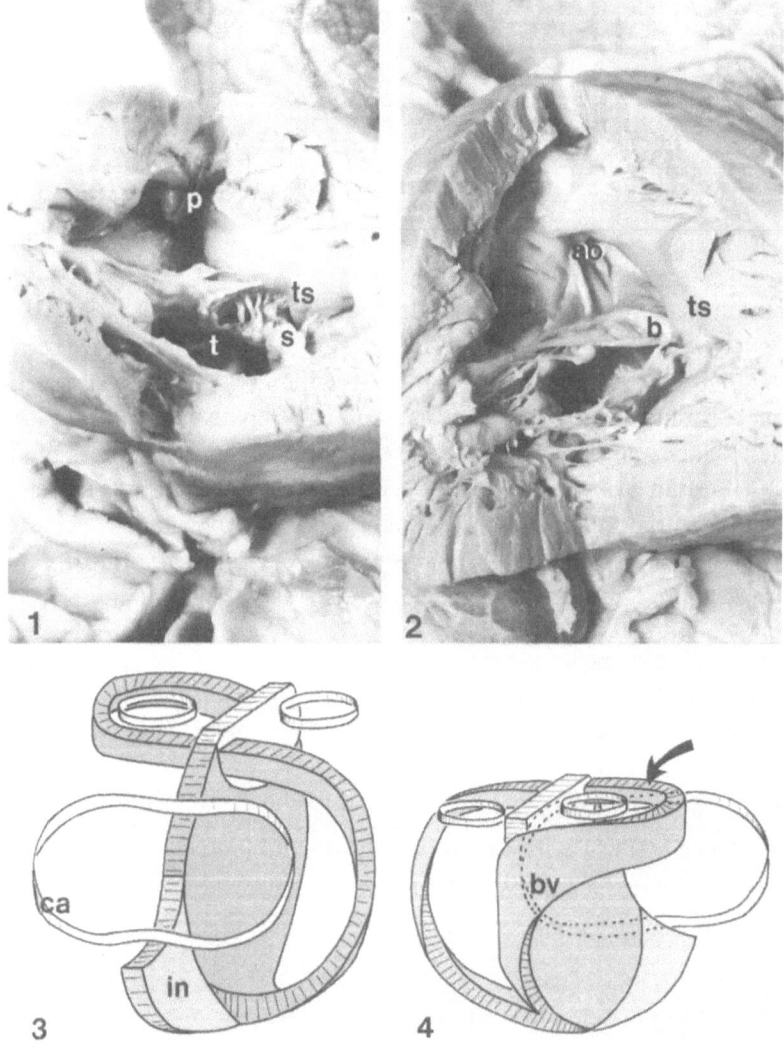

Figs. 1–4. (*1*) Atrioventricular defect with two atrioventricular annuli, i.e., partial form. Right ventricular view; t, tricuspid orifice; p, pulmonary orifice. Particularly the septal leaflet of the tricuspid valve (s) has come down toward the apex of the right ventricle, and is abnormally close to the trabecula septomarginalis (ts).

(*2*) Atrioventricular defect with one common atrioventricular annulus, i.e., complete form. The valve is abnormally close to the trabecula septomarginalis (ts). The inlet septum is not more deficient than in the case illustrated in Figure 1, but there is a floating anterior bridging leaflet (b). As a consequence, there is free access from this right ventricle to the aortic orifice (ao). Note the aortic-atrioventricular fibrous continuity.

(*3*) Septal components in an atrioventricular defect. Right-posterior view. The inlet septum (in) is deficient. Compare with Figure 7 in Chapter 3. Although a common annulus (ca) is illustrated, this does not influence septal anatomy.

(*4*) Septal components in an atrioventricular defect. Left-anterior view. If there is aortic-atrioventricular discontinuity (arrow), the interposing musculature is continuous with the deviating portion (bv) of the anterior septum.

However, the anatomy of the left ventricular outflow tract in these hearts (see Draulans-Noë et al., Chapter 11, this book) suggests coexistent anomalies of the bulboventricular fold. The basal portion of the ventricular septum that is anterior to the aortic orifice may show sizeable extensions toward the anterior ventricular wall. The anatomy presents itself as a leftward deviation of the septum [24, 25] and may seriously hinder the outflow into the aorta. In addition to this excess of myocardium, all these hearts exhibit an anterolateral muscle bundle [26, 27], which causes a clockwise displacement of the area of aortic-atrioventricular fibrous continuity (Draulans-Noë et al., Chapter 11, this book).

The excess of septal myocardium anterior to and below the aortic orifice often leads, in the presence of a free-floating anterior valve leaflet, to the anatomy of double-outlet right ventricle [28]. In the most extreme cases, with aortic-atrioventricular discontinuity, the myocardium between the aortic and atrioventricular valves can be traced without interruption into the deviating portion of the anterior septum (Figs. 4 and 5).

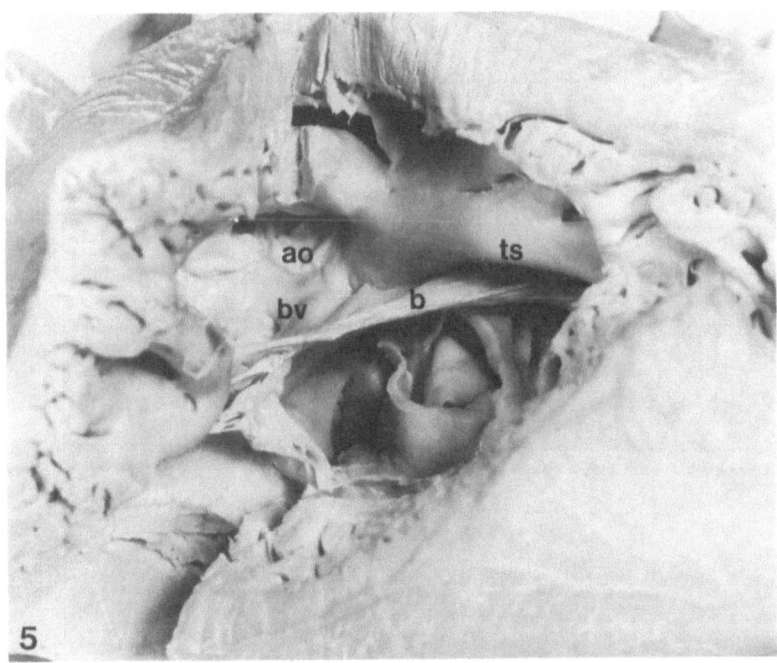

Fig. 5. Atrioventricular defect with double-outlet right ventricle. Right ventricular view. Note that the muscular bar (bv) between the aortic orifice (ao) and the anterior bridging leaflet (b) of the common valve is continuous with the anterior septum (ts). Together they constitute the bulboventricular fold.

DEVELOPMENTAL CONSIDERATIONS

Deficiency of the inlet septum as seen in these hearts can easily be explained on the basis of normal septation (Chapter 3, Fig. 5). The trabeculated myocardium on the posterior wall of the embryonic ventricle does probably give rise to an elevation, but this elevation remains inconspicuous. In particular the increase in size that takes place in the sixth week of development fails to occur (Fig. 6). The remnant of this inlet septum gains the normal contact with the anterior bulboventricular septum and the alignment of these components is correct. In other words, in atrioventricular defects the ventricular septum runs to the crux, the crux being defined as that point at which the atrial septum reaches the posterior atrioventricular junction. One may ask,

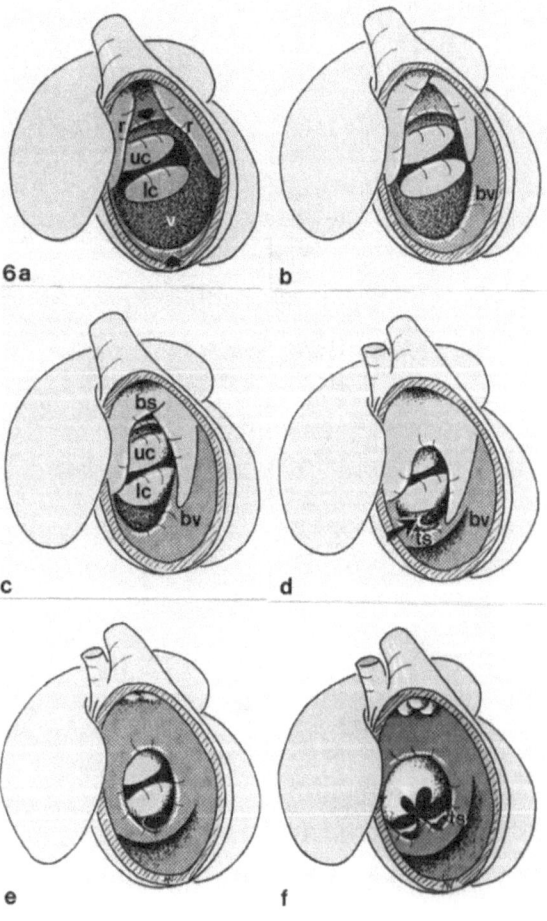

then, on what grounds a malalignment of atrial and ventricular septa could be reported [6, 29]. This may depend on the way in which the plane of the ventricular septum has to be determined. In the normal heart, the atrial septum is adjacent to the inlet septum and has no important relationships with the bulboventricular septum. Alignment of atrial and ventricular septa is obviously determined by considering the plane of the inlet septum. In atrioventricular defects, however, there is not much of an inlet septum. What is more, the entire inlet portions of the ventricles have failed to enlarge, which brings the atrioventricular annulus much closer to the apex than in normal hearts. If, in this situation, alignment of atrial and ventricular septa has to be determined, one is inclined to take the bulboventricular septum as a standard (Fig. 7). Being part of the bulboventricular fold, this septum is not in the same plane as the inlet septum. It has a tendency to reach to the right of the atrioventricular orifices.

Generally speaking, a ventricular septum that runs to the crux consists of both inlet and bulboventricular components, however small the inlet component may be. It is only the inlet component that has a constant relationship to the crux of the heart.

These developmental considerations are also pertinent with respect to the site of the conducting tissues. The atrioventricular bundle receives contributions from the atrioventricular and bulboventricular rings of specialized myocardium [30]. The atrioventricular ring tissue is related to the developing

---

Fig. 6. Diagrams to show abnormal ventricular septation as is thought to lead to an atrioventricular defect. Compare with Figure 5 in Chapter 3, p. 26. Right-lateral view. The right parietal wall of the bulbus has been removed.

(*a*) Preseptation stage. The bulboventricular fold (arrow) encircles the bulboventricular orifice, through which the ventricular cavity (v) is seen. Part of the fold is hidden by the endocardial bulbar ridges (r). The atrioventricular orifice is guarded by the upper (uc) and lower (lc) atrioventricular endocardial cushions.

(*b*) Outgrowth of the bulbar and ventricular cavities leads to accentuation of the bulboventricular fold (bv). There is no indication of a ridge on the posterior ventricular wall.

(*c*) The anterior portion of the bulboventricular fold has formed the bulboventricular septum (bv). The cranial portion of the bulboventricular fold is nearly completely hidden by the bulbar septum (bs), resulting from fusion of the bulbar ridges. The upper (uc) and lower (lc) endocardial cushions have not fused, and there is still a common atrioventricular orifice.

(*d*) Because of deficient development of the inlet septum (arrow), the interventricular communication persists. The right and apical portion of the bulboventricular fold has formed the trabecula septomarginalis (ts) and separates the deficient inlet septum from the bulboventricular septum (bv).

(*e*) Muscularization of the endocardial bulbar ridges makes further distinction between bulboventricular fold and bulbar (i.e., adult infundibular) septum impossible. Together they surround the ostium between inlet and outlet portions of the right ventricle.

(*f*) Mature right ventricle, after full development of a common atrioventricular valve. The small inlet part, containing the right half of the common valve, is separated from the outlet part, containing the pulmonary valve, by the trabecula septomarginalis (ts).

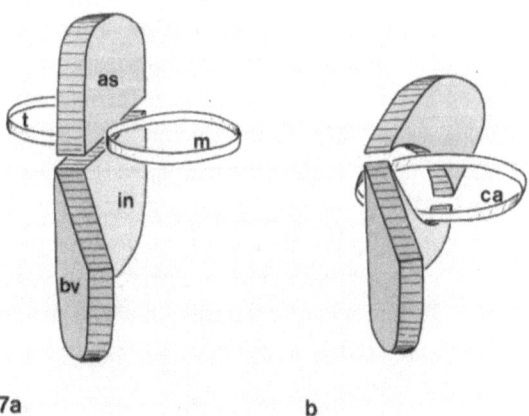

7a   b

Fig. 7. (a). Diagram to show the relationships of the atrial septum (as) with the inlet septum (in) and the bulboventricular septum (bv) in the normal heart. Anterior view; m, mitral annulus; t, tricuspid annulus. The atrial septum is in good alignment with the inlet septum, but not with the bulboventricular septum. The different planes of atrial and bulboventricular septa are not very obvious because of interposition of the well formed inlet septum. (*b*) The same in the case of an atrioventricular defect. A common annulus (ca) is illustrated. The (normal) angle between atrial and bulboventricular septa does strike because only a short inlet septum is interposed between the two.

inlet myocardium and thus the proximal portion of the bundle lies on the inlet septum. If the bulboventricular septum fuses properly with this inlet septum, that is, if the septum "runs to the crux" (and if there is a normal bulboventricular loop; see Chapter 16), the heart has a posterior connecting node and bundle. This is the case in atrioventricular defects, albeit that the node and the bundle are displaced posteriorly [31–33].

The other pathological feature of the septum pertains to the left ventricular outflow tract. It can be understood by realizing that the anterior septum develops as part of the bulboventricular fold. The basal portion of this fold, which lies in the inner curvature of the developing heart, does not normally contribute to the septum. It encloses the aortic orifice and contributes to the formation of the aortic leaflet of the mitral valve. The excess of myocardium seen in this area in atrioventricular defects must be explained as a more or less muscular bulboventricular fold (Fig. 5), which tends to push the aorta toward the right as in double-outlet right ventricle. When the bulboventricular fold is completely muscular, there is no aortic-atrioventricular fibrous continuity.

Some final remarks have to be made on the pathology of the atrioventricular valves. The surgical importance of this pathology is beyond doubt, but from a developmental point of view it is not very exciting. The essentials of atrioventricular defects have been explained above on the basis of derangement of early septational processes. These take place before there are any atrioventricular valve leaflets. The formation of the valves and tension apparatus is a relatively late occurrence [34]. It is therefore not surprising that the elaboration of myocardium, as is essential for valve formation, would lead to abnormal valves, if there is preexistent myocardial pathology.

The endocardial cushions have been carefully left out of the above considerations. They do not form any part of the septum nor do they contribute to the valves [34]. Atrioventricular defects are not "endocardial cushion defects".

REFERENCES

1. Wakai CS, Edwards, JC: Developmental and pathologic considerations in persistent common atrioventricular canal. Mayo Clin Proc 31:487–499, 1956.
2. Wakai CS, Edwards JC: Pathologic study of persistent common atrioventricular canal. Am Heart J 56:779–794, 1958.
3. Campbell M, Missen GAK: Endocardial cushion defects. Common atrioventricular canal and ostium primum. Br Heart J 19:403–418, 1957.
4. Van Mierop LHS, Alley RD, Kausel HW, Stranahan A: The anatomy and embryology of endocardial cushion defects. J Thorac Cardiovasc Surg 43:71–83, 1962.
5. Rastelli G, Kirklin JW, Titus JL: Anatomic observations on complete form of persistent common atrioventricular canal with special reference to atrioventricular valves. Mayo Clin Proc 41:296–308, 1966.
6. Tenckhoff L, Stamm SJ: Analysis of 35 cases of the complete form of persistent common atrioventricular canal. Circulation 48:416–427, 1973.
7. Ebert PA, Goor DA: Complete atrioventricular canal malformation: further clarification of the anatomy of the common leaflet and its relationship to the VSD in surgical correction. Ann Thorac Surg 25:134–143, 1978.
8. Hagler DJ, Tayik AJ, Seward JB, Mair DD, Ritter DG: Real time wide-angle sector echocardiography: atrioventricular canal defects. Circulation 59:140–150, 1979.
9. Piccoli GP, Wilkinson JL, Macartney FJ, Gerlis LM, Anderson RH: Morphology and classification of complete atrioventricular defects. Br Heart J 42:633–639, 1979.
10. Ugarte M, Enriques de Salamanca F, Quero M: Endocardial cushion defects. An anatomical study of 54 specimens. Br Heart J 38:674–682, 1976.
11. Patten BM: Persistent interatrial foramen primum. Am J Anat 107:271–280, 1960.
12. Baron MG, Wolf BS, Steinfeld L, Van Mierop LHS: Endocardial cushion defects. Specific diagnosis by angiocardiography. Am J Cardiol 13:162–175, 1964.
13. Frater RWM: Persistent common atrioventricular canal. Anatomy and function in relation to surgical repair. Circulation 32:120–129, 1965.
14. Van Mierop LHS: Embryology of the atrioventricular canal region and pathogenesis of endocardial cushion defects. In: Feldt RM (ed) Atrioventricular canal defects. Philadelphia–London–Toronto, WB Saunders, 1976, pp 1–12.
15. Sternberg C: Beiträge zur Herzpathologie. Centralbl Allg Pathol Pathol Anat 24 (Ergänzungsheft: Verh Dtsch Pathol Ges 16): 253–262, 1913.
16. Al Omeri M, Bishop M, Oakley C. Bentall HH, Cleland WP: The mitral valve in endocardial cushion defects. Br Heart J 27:161–176, 1965.
17. Goor D, Lillehei CW, Edwards JE: Further observations on the pathology of the atrioventricular canal malformation. Arch Surg 97:954–962, 1968.

138

18. Blieden LC, Randall PA, Castaneda AR, Lucas RV, Edwards JE: The "goose neck" of the endocardial cushion defect: anatomic basis. Chest 65:13–17, 1974.
19. Titus JL, Rastelli GC: Anatomic features of persistent common atrioventricular canal. In: Feldt RH (ed) Atrioventricular canal defects. Philadelphia–London–Toronto, WB Saunders, 1976, pp 13–35.
20. Van Mierop LHS: Pathology and pathogenesis of endocardial cushion defects: surgical implications. In: Davila JC (ed) 2nd Henry Ford Hospital International Symposium on Cardiac Surgery. New York, Appleton–Century–Crofts, 1977, pp 201–207.
21. Piccoli GP, Gerlis LM, Wilkinson JL, Loszadi K, Macartney FJ, Anderson RH: Morphology and classification of atrioventricular defects. Br Heart J 42:621–632, 1979.
22. Toussaint M, Planche CL, Ribierre M: Le canal atrio-ventriculaire complet. Etude anatomique de 31 cas de formes isolées. Coeur 9:1171–1175, 1978.
23. Shaner RF: Malformation of the atrioventricular endocardial cushions of the embryo pig, and its relation to defects of the conus and truncus arteriosus. Am J Anat 84:431–456, 1949.
24. Wenink ACG: Considerations pertinent to the embryogenesis of transposition. In: Van Mierop LHS, Oppenheimer-Dekker A, Bruins CLDC (eds) Embryology and teratology of the heart and the great arteries. The Haque, Leiden University Press, 1978, pp 129–135.
25. Moene RJ, Oppenheimer-Dekker A, Moulaert AJ, Wenink ACG, Gittenberger-de Groot AC, Roozendaal H: The concurrence of dimensional aortic arch anomalies and abnormal left ventricular muscle bundles. Pediatr Cardiol (in press).
26. Moulaert AJMC: Ventricular septal defects and anomalies of the aortic arch. Thesis, University of Leiden, 1974.
27. Moulaert AJ, Oppenheimer-Dekker A: Anterolateral muscle bundle of the left ventricle, bulboventricular flange and subaortic stenosis. Am J Cardiol 37:78–81, 1976.
28. Thiene G, Frescura C, DiDonato R, Galluci V: Complete atrioventricular canal associated with conotruncal malformations: anatomical observations in 13 specimens. Eur J Cardiol 9:199–213, 1979.
29. Yokoyama M, Ando M, Takao A, Sakakibara S: The location of the coronary sinus orifice in endocardial cushion defects. Am Heart J 85:302–307, 1973.
30. Wenink ACG: Development of the human cardiac conducting system. J Anat 121:617–631, 1976.
31. Lev M: The architecture of the conduction system in congenital heart disease. I. Common atrioventricular orifice. Arch Pathol 65:174–191, 1958.
32. Feldt RH, Titus JL: The conduction system in persistent common atrioventricular canal. In: Feldt RH (ed) Atrioventricular canal defects. Philadelphia–London–Toronto, WB Saunders, 1976, pp 36–43.
33. Wenink ACG, Anderson RH, Thiene G: The conducting system in hearts with atrioventricular canal malformations. In: Van Mierop LHS, Oppenheimer-Dekker A, Bruins CLDC (eds) Embryology and teratology of the heart and the great arteries. The Hague, Leiden University Press, 1978, pp 55–61.
34. Van Gils FAW: The development of the human atrioventricular heart valves. J Anat 128:427, 1979.

11. ECHOCARDIOGRAPHY AND ANGIOCARDIOGRAPHY IN ATRIOVENTRICULAR DEFECT

H.A. YVONNE DRAULANS-NOË, PAUL J. VOOGD, ARNOLD C.G. WENINK, AND
ELMA LIGTVOET-GUSSENHOVEN

INTRODUCTION

Echocardiography and angiocardiography are important methods in the *diagnosis* of atrioventricular defect (AVD), in the *estimation of the severity* of the anomaly, and in the evaluation of associated anomalies, such as *left ventricular outflow tract* (LVOT) obstruction.

Anatomical considerations

The diagnosis of AVD, and estimation of the severity of the anomaly and of LVOT narrowing, are based on the characteristic anatomical features of the anomaly: septal deficiency, mitral valve malformation, and malposition. In the normal heart the anterior mitral leaflet (AML) extends in a plane parallel to the ventricular septum from the anterolateral to the posteromedial commissure. Its line of attachment can be divided into three parts (Fig. 1):

1) A short *free-wall attachment*, running along the free wall of the left ventricle from the anterolateral commissure to the middle of the left coronary aortic cusp.
2) An *aortic attachment*, continuous with the root of the aorta, where the fibrous mitral-aortic transitional zone borders on the inferior half of the left coronary aortic cusp, and then continues along the left half of the posterior, noncoronary aortic cusp until the membranous atrioventricular septum is reached.
3) The *septal attachment*, which runs for a short distance along the border of the atrioventricular septum to the posteromedial commissure.

In our study on the anatomy of the LVOT in AVD, the free-wall and aortic (Fig. 1) attachment of the AML proved to differ from that in the normal heart due to the presence of an (usually broad) anterolateral muscle bundle in almost all our specimens. The ALM, first described by André Moulaert in 1976[1], is a horizontal muscle bundle in the LVOT, between the left coronary aortic semilunar valve and the anterior mitral leaflet, and separates the anterior mitral leaflet from the anterolateral wall of the left ventricle. It is present in approximately 40% of normal hearts, and is thought to be a

A.C.G. Wenink et al. (eds.) The Ventricular Septum of the Heart, 139–155. All rights reserved.
Copyright © 1981 by Martinus Nijhoff Publishers, The Hague/Boston/London.

140

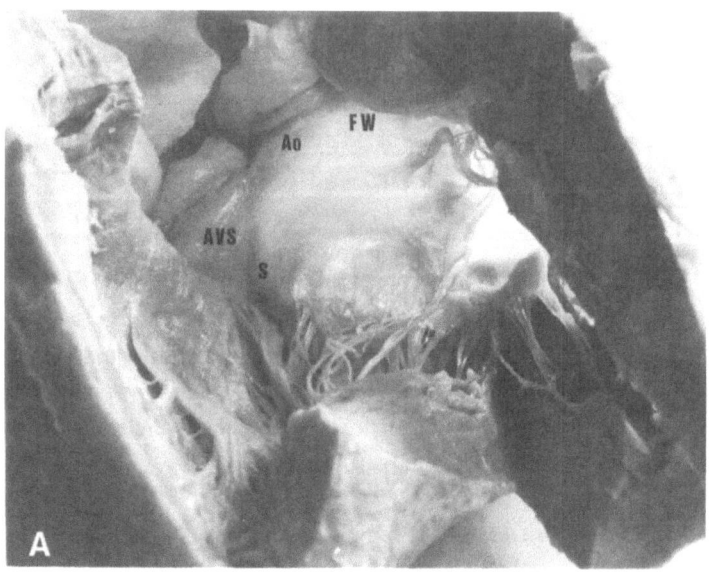

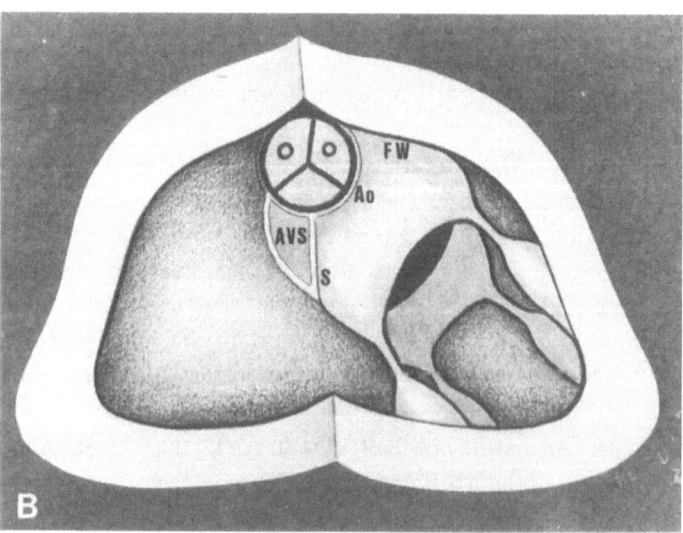

Fig. 1A and B. Left ventricular outflow tract and attachment of the anterior leaflet of the mitral valve in the normal heart: FW, free-wall attachment; Ao, aortic attachment; S, septal attachment; AVS, atrioventricular septum.

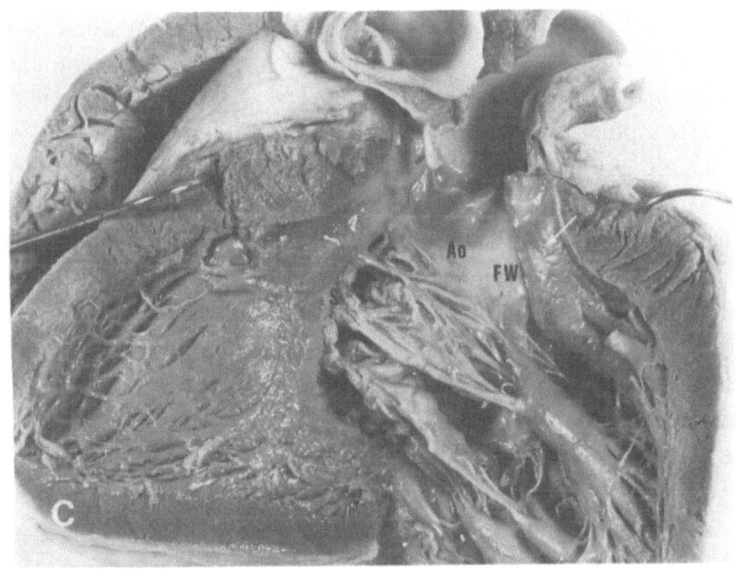

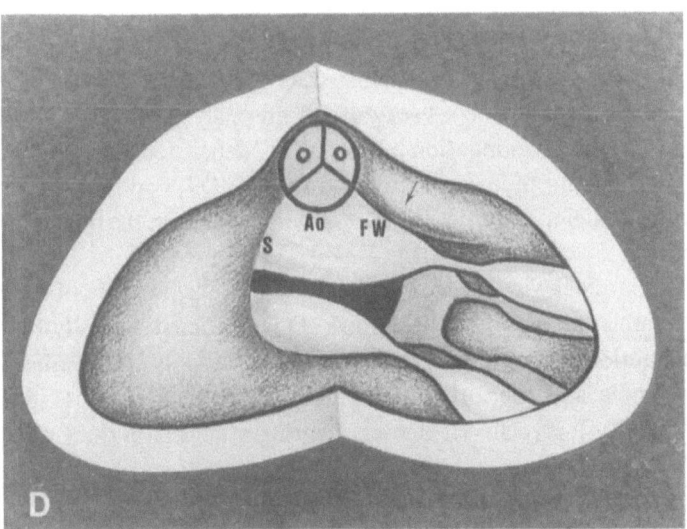

Fig. 1C and D. Left ventricular outflow tract and attachment of the anterior leaflet of the mitral valve in atrioventricular defect. Note the broad anterolateral muscle bundle (arrow), and the smooth, elongated free-wall attachment of the mitral valve to the bundle: Ao, aortic attachment; FW, free-wall attachment; S, septal attachment.

muscular remnant of the left extremity of the bulboatrioventricular flange.

Thus in AVD the *free-wall attachment* and the *aortic attachment* to the left coronary aortic cusp are *displaced* by the ALM. As the membranous atrioventricular septum is absent in AVD, the line of attachment of the AML continues along the noncoronary aortic cusp, until the membranous interventricular septum is reached at the level of the commissure with the right coronary aortic cusp. The *septal attachment* is anteriorly displaced and prolonged, as it continues along the rim of the defective muscular septum.

Summarizing, the displacement of the line of attachment results in a clockwise rotation of the AML, so that it now occupies a position perpendicular instead of parallel to the ventricular septum. In addition (Fig. 1) both the free-wall and septal attachment are considerably prolonged.

The presence of the anterolateral muscle bundle and the changed mitral valve position also influence the shape and boundaries of the LVOT. The outflow tract of the left ventricle (defined as the space anterior to the AML) is normally bordered medially by the septal wall and laterally by the AML and its papillary muscles, giving wide access to the aortic orifice. In AVD the LVOT is funnel-shaped, showing varying degrees of narrowing and elongation due to the anterior and apical displacement of the septal attachment of the AML. We refer to the decreased distance between this septal attachment and the anterior left ventricular wall as "deficiency of the anterior septum". The deficiency of the basal aspect of the ventricular septum (both inlet and anterior septum) was considered to be similar in the various forms of AVD, but it has recently been demonstrated [2] that the deficiency of the inlet septum increases with the severity of the anomaly. Deficiency of the inlet septum will result in elongation of the LVOT, deficiency of the anterior part of the ventricular septum in narrowing of the LVOT, and thus the degree of narrowing and elongation of the LVOT will depend on the degree of septal deficiency.

Due to the clockwise rotation of the AML and the presence of the anterolateral muscle bundle, the LVOT in AVD is bordered medially by the defective anterior part of the ventricular septum, laterally by the anterolateral muscle bundle, and inferiorly by the proximal part of the AML (Fig. 2). This part of the AML is relatively immobile, being attached on three sides.

DIAGNOSIS OF AVD

In 1964 Baron et al [3] first reported the angiocardiographic abnormalities which characterize AVD: the well-known goose-neck appearance on the left ventricular angiocardiograms. The goose-neck is formed by contrast trapped behind the mitral valve in diastole, thus outlining its attachment.

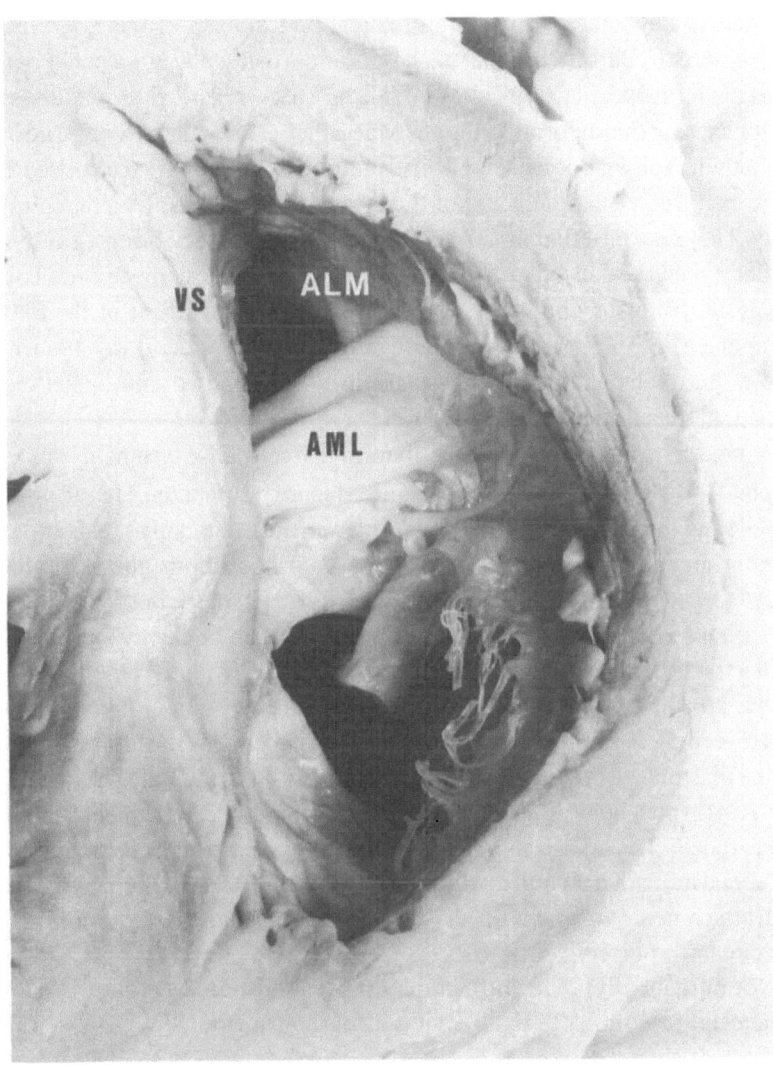

Fig. 2. Left ventricular outflow tract boundaries and mitral valve position in atrioventricular defect (apical view). The anterior mitral leaflet is rotated clockwise. The left ventricular outflow tract is bordered on the lateral side by the anterolateral muscle bundle, medially by the ventricular septum, and inferiorly by the proximal ("fixed") part of the anterior mitral leaflet.

There is still some discussion on the anatomical basis of this goose-neck appearance. In Baron's original paper, the abnormal septal attachment of the anterior mitral leaflet, typical of AVD, has been regarded as the decisive factor causing this deformity. Fergus Macartney et al. in their recent study on the angiographic appearance of atrioventricular defects [4] recognized the abnormal free-wall attachment of the bridging anterior leaflet angiographically. They reasoned that in common AVD with unattached bridging anterior leaflet (type C of Rastelli's classification) the radiological appearance could not result from the abnormally positioned septal attachment of the mitral component, as in the ostium primum defect, but was due to the abnormal free-wall attachment. The latter so far has been ignored and, when mentioned, has been specifically stated to be normal [3, 5].

A precise explanation for this abnormal free-wall attachment was not given. However, our anatomical studies identify the anterolateral muscle bundle and the resulting mitral valve displacement as the cause of this appearance. The diastolic goose-neck deformity with its smooth inferior border, seen as a wedge of contrast separating the left margin of the aortic valve from the nonopacified blood entering the left ventricle, can be clearly seen in cases with a free-floating anterior bridging leaflet. In AVD with the anterior mitral leaflet attached to the summit of the ventricular septum (ostium primum defect, complete AVD type A of Rastelli's classification) the inferior border of the diastolic goose-neck can either be caused by the septal attachment of the AML (puckered appearance) or by the free-wall attachment (smooth appearance). The inferior border of the systolic goose-neck will be caused by the septal attachment (Fig. 3). As stated by Fergus Macartney et al., the free-wall attachment can be identified by its localization immediately medial to the left circumflex artery.

Not infrequently, echocardiography proves to be an even more accurate diagnostic tool in AVD than angiocardiography, especially in those cases

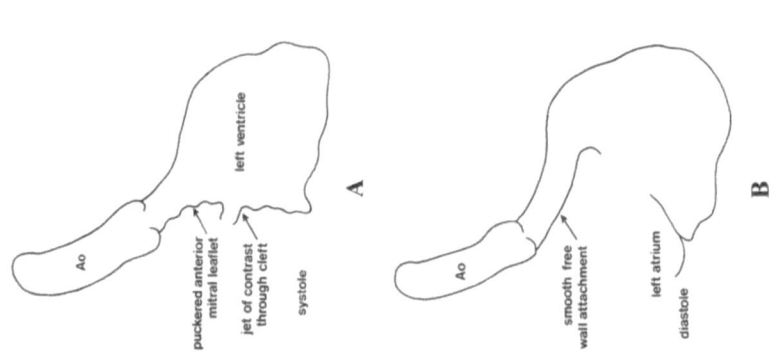

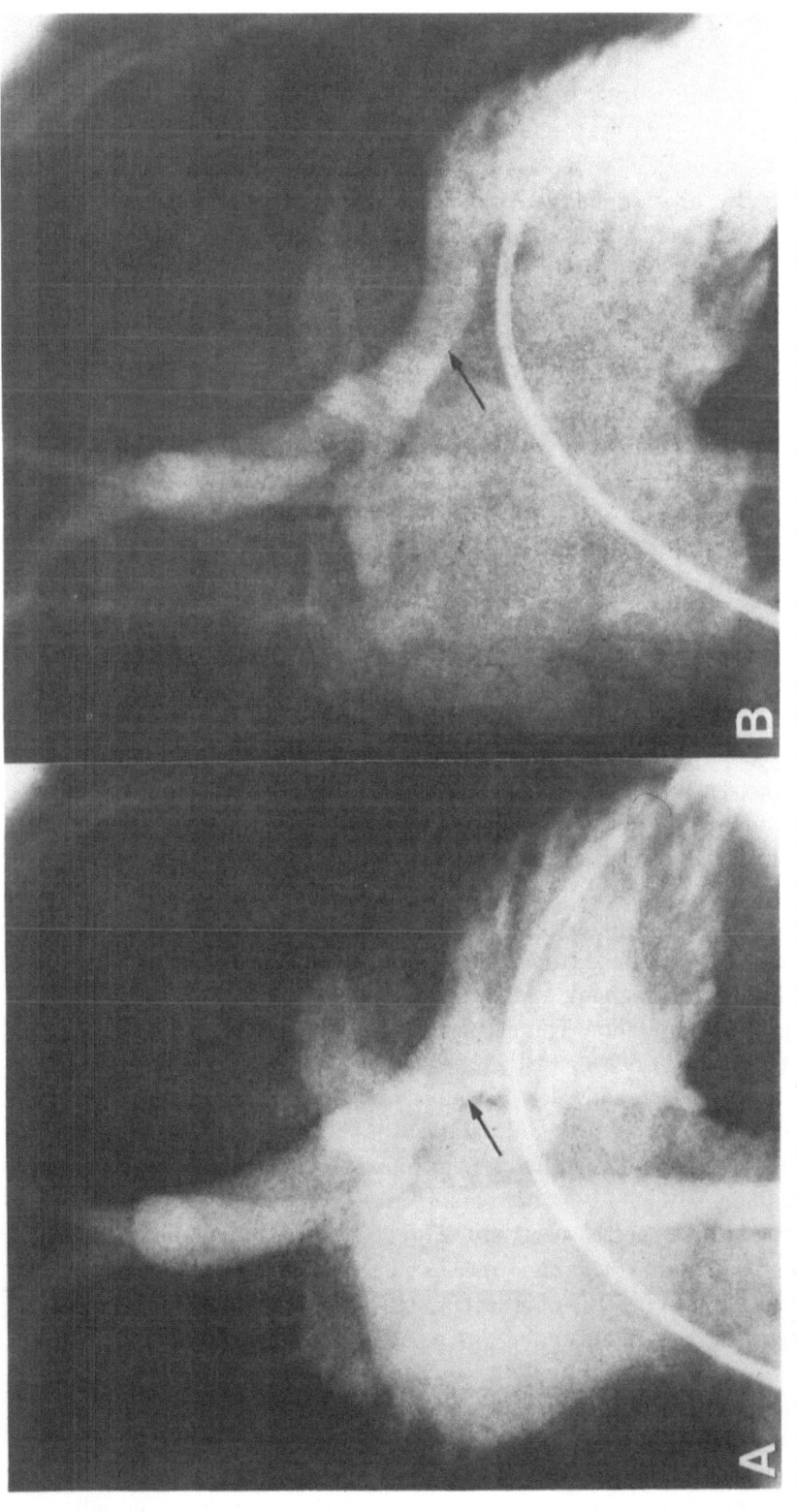

Fig. 3. Left ventricular angiogram in ostium primum atrial septal defect: (*A*) systole, (*B*) diastole. In systole the inferomedial border of the left ventricular outflow tract (arrow) is formed by the septal attachment of the anterior mitral leaflet (puckered appearance). In diastole it is formed by the smooth free-wall attachment (arrow).

where the left ventricular goose-neck is poorly visualized (for instance, in the presence of a large ventricular septal defect, obscuring the LVOT) or even absent, as in cases with isolated cleft mitral valve with little or no septal deficiency, or in complicated cases such as double-outlet right ventricle or transposition of the great arteries where the aorta does not arise from the left ventricle.

ESTIMATION OF SEVERITY

The severity of the AVD influences prognosis and results of surgical treatment. This depends particularly on the structure and function of the mitral valve. About half of the patients with AVD will have mild mitral valve dysfunction, one-third moderate, and one-sixth severe.

The objective of the preoperative evaluation must be to recognize the patient with severe mitral dysfunction, probably requiring mitral valve replacement. In the preoperative evaluation we try to distinguish those patients who are likely to do well with surgical correction mainly on the degree of mitral valve regurgitation assessed by auscultation and left ventricular angiography. However, such preoperative assessment of mitral valve dysfunction is typically inexact, and findings at operation correlate poorly with the interpretation of physical examination and left ventricular angiography. It still remains a difficult practical problem for the surgeon to determine at the time of operation which patients require valvular replacement. He must decide, at the time of exposure of the valves, on the degree of mitral valve regurgitation existing before repair (based primarily on clinical findings and the left ventriculogram), and on the probability of the repair reducing the degree of regurgitation. This means that the assessment at operation is based on the adequacy of leaflet tissue, which is again an imprecise judgment.

These considerations clearly demonstrate the necessity for additional information on the severity of the anomaly in the preoperative assessment.

In 1968 Somerville and Jefferson [5] found an association between severity of the anomaly and LVOT morphology. They compared the degree of mitral valve deformity, as seen at surgery, with changes in shape of the angiographic goose-neck during the cardiac cycle. A goose-neck with little or no change of the medial left ventricular border corresponded with a "bad" mitral valve at surgery, difficult to repair and with a poor surgical prognosis.

Angiocardiographically the severe forms of AVD with significant septal deficiency will show significant narrowing and elongation of the LVOT, with an immobile AML due the deficient cusp tissue, tethered by short chordae to the deficient ventricular septum.

We tried to estimate the severity of the AVD echocardiographically, by estimating elongation (2DE), mobility (2DE) and narrowing (2DE and M-mode scanning) of the LVOT. LVOT diameter was measured on M-mode scans and compared with normal values and with aortic diameter. The latter was expressed as a LVOT/aortic ratio. We had the impression that a long, rather immobile LVOT on 2DE and a reduced diameter with low LVOT/aortic ratio were suggestive of a severe anomaly with poor surgical prognosis.

LEFT VENTRICULAR OUTFLOW TRACT OBSTRUCTION

The majority of patients with AVD will have anatomical narrowing of the LVOT, because of the anterior displacement of the AML. LVOT obstruction, however, will occur only in the presence of additional obstructing factors: anterior septal hypertrophy and deviation, hypertrophy of the anterolateral muscle bundle, and/or large anomalous papillary muscle running into the LVOT (Fig. 4)

In 21 out of 41 specimens with AVD and narrow LVOT because of chordal attachment of the AML to a deficient VS, the LVOT was narrower than the aortic valve ring, with slight subvalvular AoS in ten cases, moderate in seven

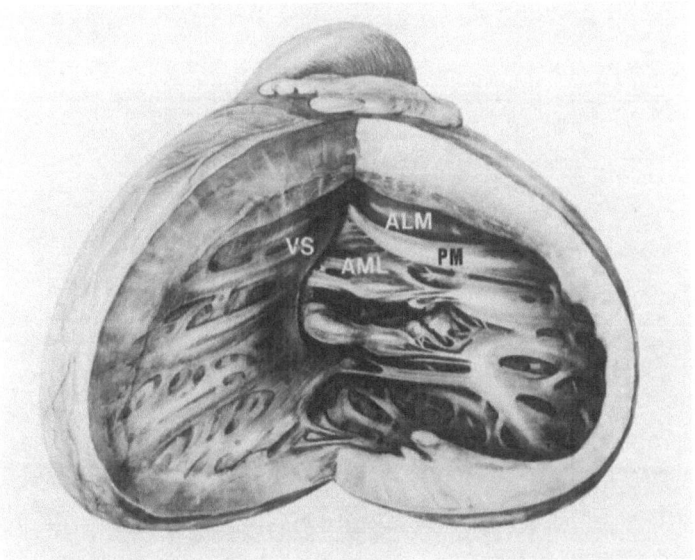

Fig. 4. Drawing of a hypothetical left ventricle with atrioventricular defect, and outflow tract narrowing. The causes of left ventricular outflow tract narrowing are shown; (1) anterior displacement of the anterior mitral leaflet (AML), due to septal deficiency; (2) focal septal hypertrophy (VS), usually with some leftward deviation; (3) hypertrophy of the anterolateral muscle bundle (ALM); (4) a large anomalous papillary muscle (PM).

148

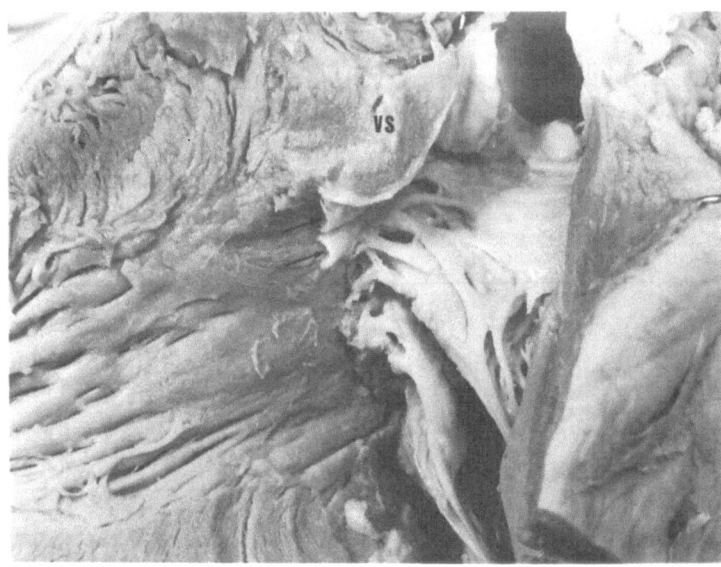

Fig. 5. Ostium primum defect, with severe subaortic stenosis, caused by hypertrophy of the anterior part of the ventricular septum (VS). Note the pouch-like endocardial masses (arrow) proximal to the obstruction, as can be observed in hypetrophic obstructive cardiomyopathy.

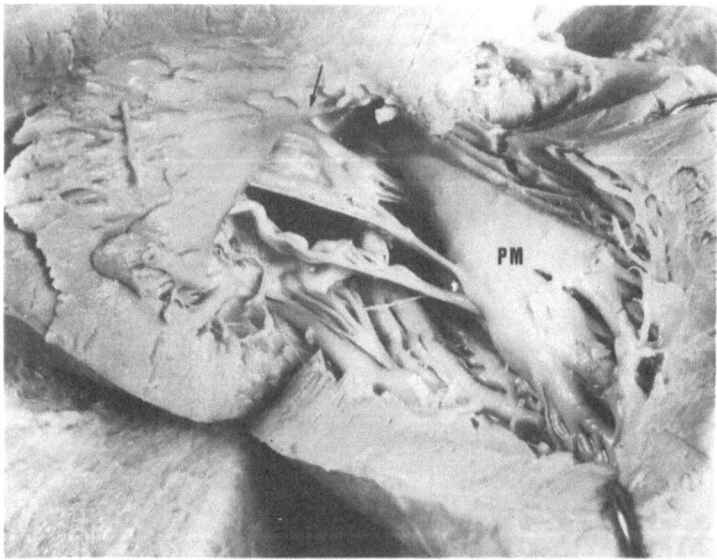

Fig. 6. Large anomalous papillary muscle (PM) causing further narrowing of the left ventricular outflow tract in complete atrioventricular defect with large ventricular septal defect and free-floating common anterior leaflet. Note the deficiency of the anterior part of the ventricular septum (arrow).

and severe in four cases. The obstruction was caused by septal hypertrophy and deviation, combined with hypertrophy of the anterolateral muscle bundle in three cases and/or large anomalous papillary muscle in three cases (Figs. 5 and 6).

This correlates well with our echocardiographic findings in 36 patients, where severe LVOT narrowing (LVOT/Ao ratio $\leq 50\%$) was found in four patients with significant LV/aortic pressure gradients (40 mm, 50 mm, 60 mm, and 110 mm Hg, respectively). In all four patients the diagnosis subvalvular aortic stenosis due to septal hypertrophy was confirmed at operation (Figs. 7 and 8). In one patient an anomalous papillary muscle running into the LVOT was described.

In the left ventricular angiocardiogram, septal hypertrophy and deviation can be recognized as a medial obstruction, and anterolateral muscle bundle hypertrophy will result in a lateral obstruction. A large papillary muscle can sometimes be seen as a filling defect on the frontal view.

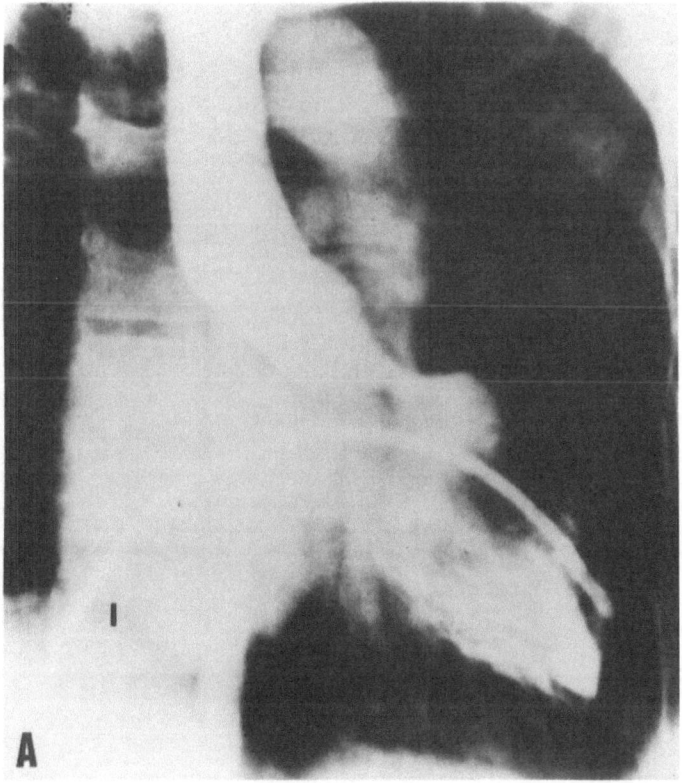

Fig. 7A. Ostium primum atrial septal defect with subvalvular aortic stenosis (gradient 60 mm Hg) caused by septal hypertrophy. Left ventricular angiogram showing the subvalvular obstruction.

150

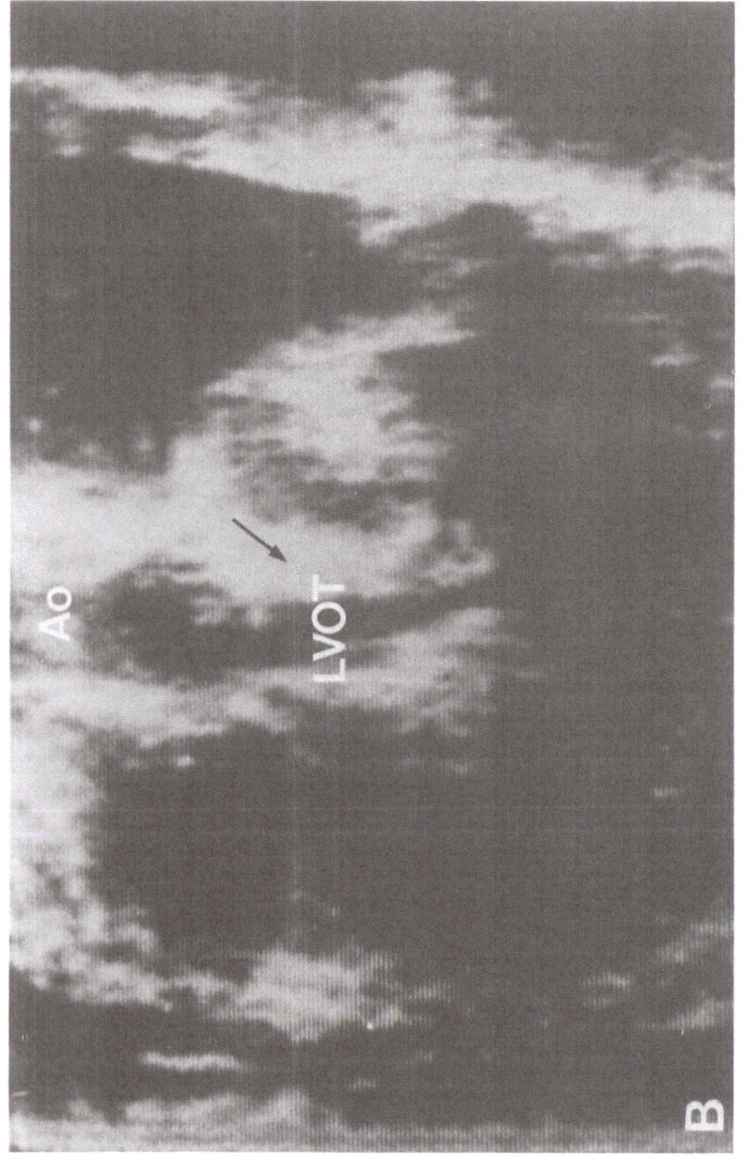

Fig. 7B. Two-dimensional echocardiography in the same patient as in *A* after correction with resection of the subaortic stenosis and mitral valve replacement (Hancock valve). The anterior part of the ventricular septum is still hypertrophied. The Hancock valve is anteriorly displaced (arrow), and the LVOT considerably narrowed; Ao, aorta.

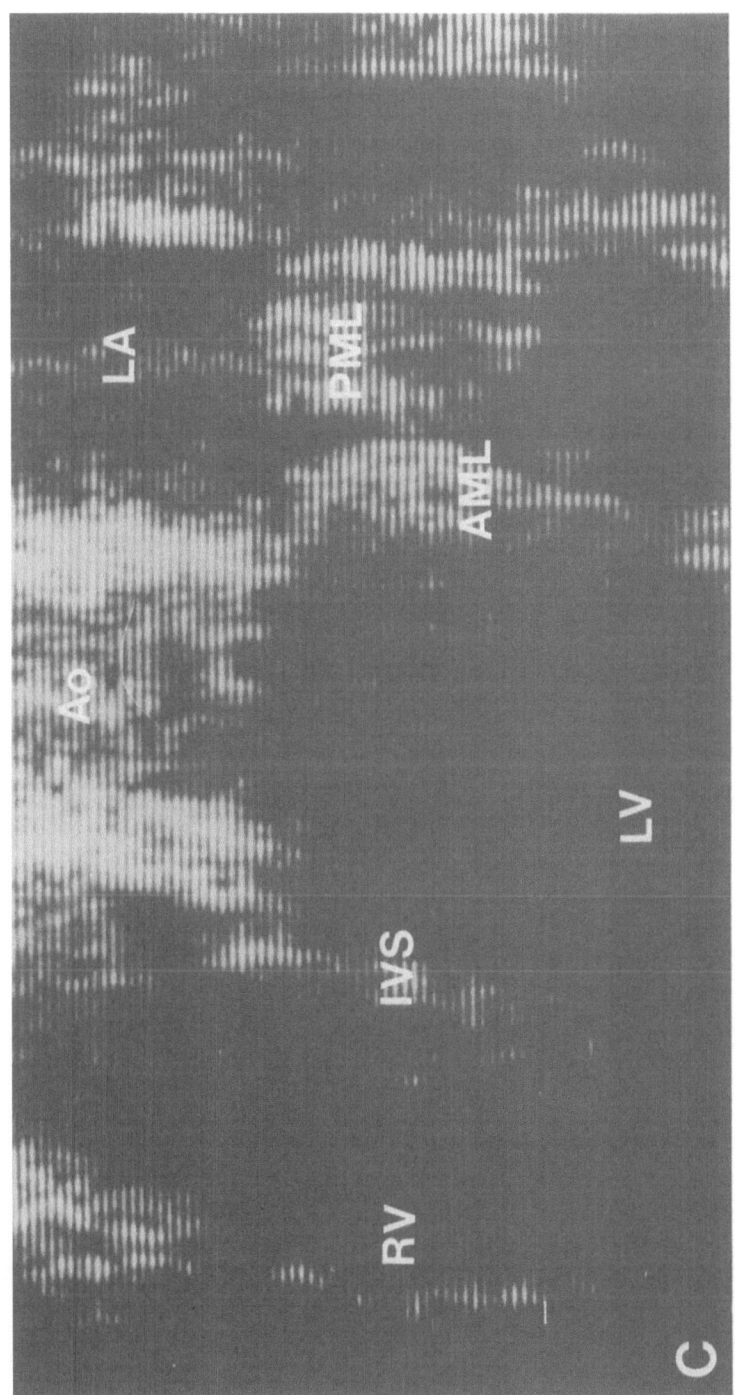

Fig. 7C. In comparison with *B*, a two-dimensional echocardiogram of the normal LVOT (end systole); Ao, aorta; LV, left ventricle; LA, left atrium; RV, right ventricle; AML, anterior mitral leaflet; PML, posterior mitral leaflet; IVS, ventricular septum.

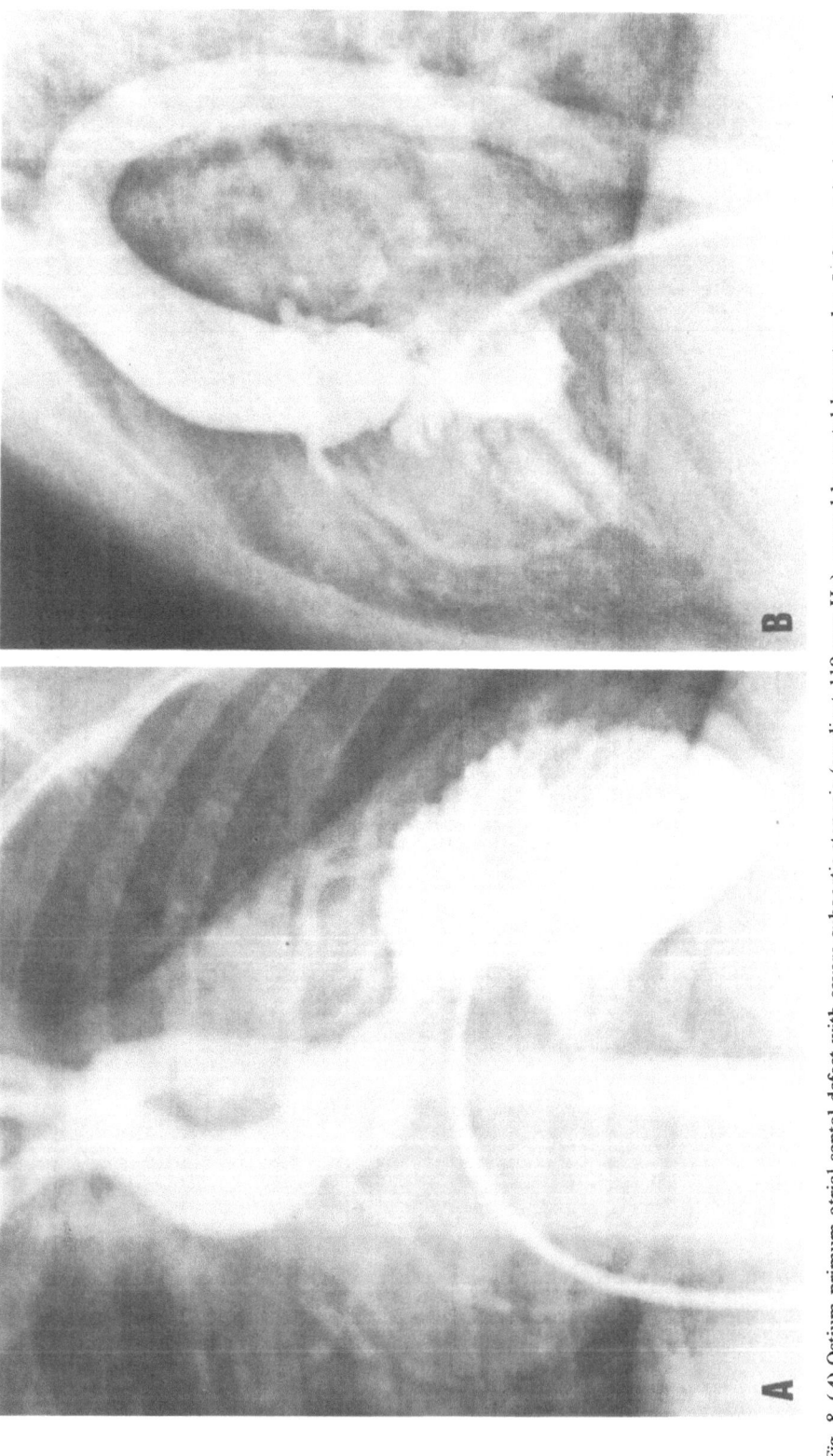

Fig. 8. (*A*) Ostium primum atrial septal defect with severe subaortic stenosis (gradient 110 mm Hg), caused by septal hypertrophy. Left ventricular angiocardiogram, frontal projection. (*B*) Lateral projection.

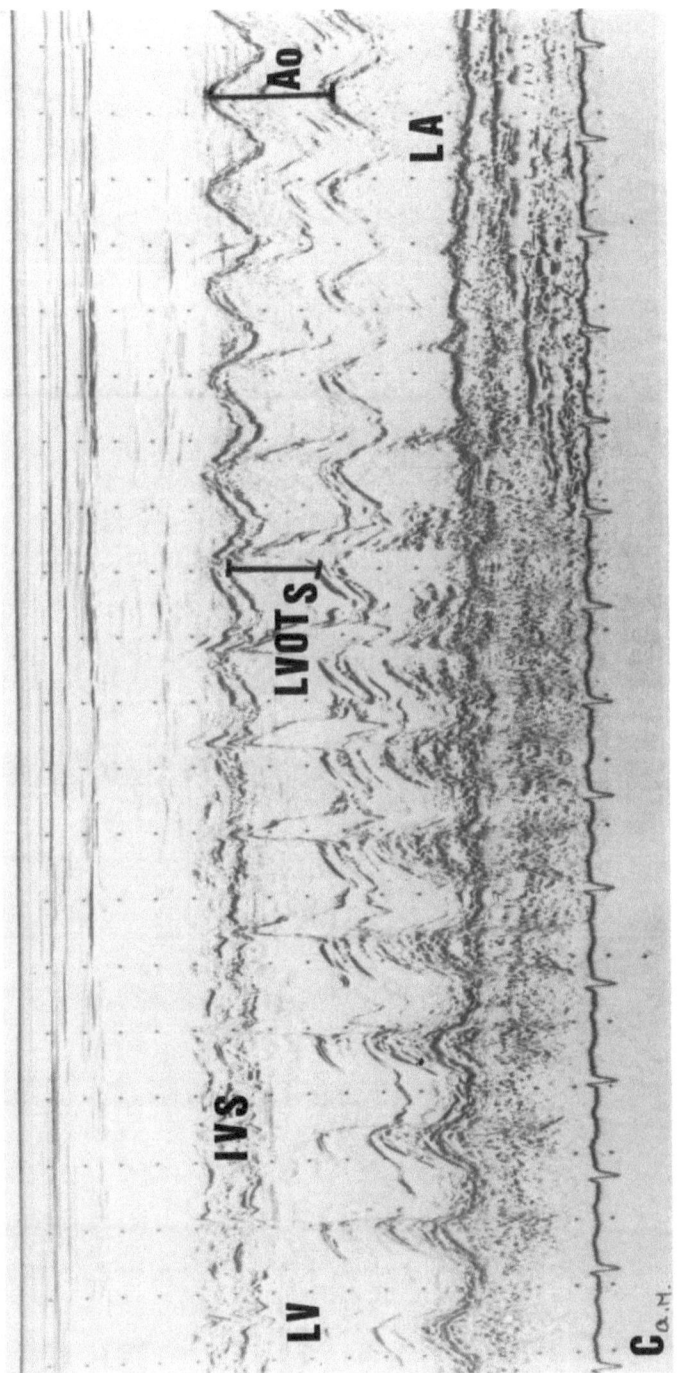

Fig. 8C. M-mode scan in ostium primum atrial septal defect. Abbreviations: see Figure 7.

154

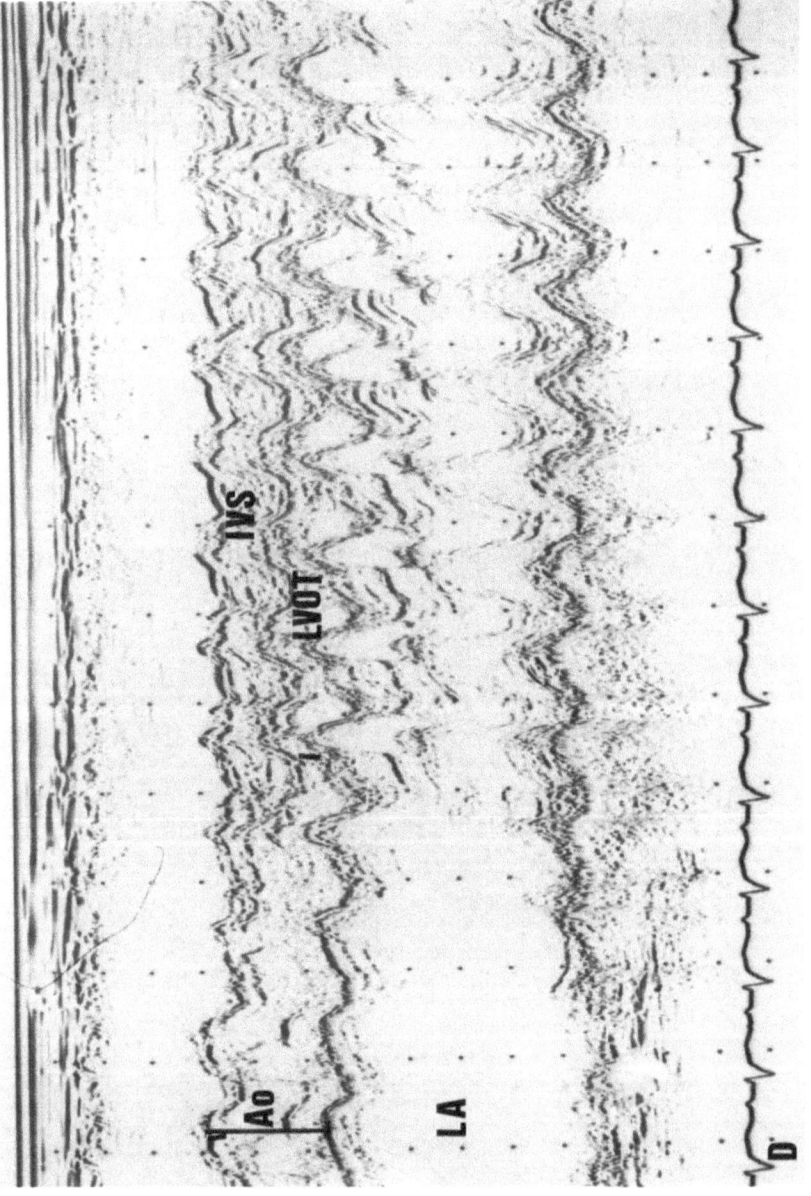

Fig. 8D. Same patient as in *A*. M-mode scan showing septal hypertrophy and LVOT narrowing. Abbreviations: see Figure 7.

SUMMARY AND CONCLUSIONS

The ventricular septal abnormalities, absence of the atrioventricular septum, deficiency of the interventricular septum, and hypertrophy and deviation of the anterior part of the muscular septum play a major part in AVD (Arnold Wenink, Chapter 10, this book).

Accurate knowledge of anatomical detail in AVD is necessary not only for the correct interpretation of angiocardiographic and echocardiographic findings, but also a prerequisite to the development of appropriate operative techniques.

As mitral valve dysfunction (especially in the severe cases frequently requiring mitral valve replacement) is caused not only by its malformation but also by the abnormal position due to the septal abnormality, it seems likely that attempts at surgical correction may have to include repair of the septal deficiency, even in those cases without interventricular communication.

The objective of the preoperative investigation must be to recognize the patient with severe mitral dysfunction and septal deficiency, probably requiring mitral valve replacement with ventricular septal extension. Little mobility of the mitral valve and a long and narrow left ventricular outflow tract are poor prognostic signs.

REFERENCES

1. Moulaert AJ, Oppenheimer-Dekker A: Anterolateral muscle bundle of the left ventricle, bulboventricular flange and subaortic stenosis. Am J Cardiol 37:78–80, 1976.
2. Piccoli GP, Gerlis LM, Wilkinson JL, Lozsadi K, Macartney FJ, Anderson RH: Morphology and classification of atrioventricular defects. Br Heart J 42:621–632, 1979.
3. Baron MG, Wolf BS, Steinfeld L, van Mierop LHS: Endocardial cushion defects. Am J Cardiol 13:162–175, 1964.
4. Macartney FJ, Rees PG, Daly K, Piccoli PG, Taylor JFN, de Leval MR, Stark J, Anderson RH: Angiocardiographic appearances of atrioventricular defects with particular reference to distinction of ostium primum atrial septal defect from common atrioventricular orifice. Br Heart J 42:640–656, 1979.
5. Somerville J, Jefferson J: Left ventricular angiocardiography in atrioventricular defects. Br Heart J 30:446–457, 1968.
6. Sahn DJ, Terry RW, O'Rourkem R, Leopold G, Friedman WF: Multiple crystal echocardiographic evaluation of endocardial cushion defect. Circulation 50:25–32, 1974.
7. Bom N, Lancee CT, van Zwieten G, Kloster EF, Roelandt J: Multiscan echocardiography. I. Technical description. Circulation 48:1066–1074, 1973.
8. Draulans-Noë HAY, Voogd PJ, Ligtvoet CM, Ridder J, Wenink ACG: Two-dimensional echocardiography in atrioventricular canal malformation: a diagnostic approach. Acta Med Scand [Suppl] 205/627:196–202, 1979.

12. STRADDLING AND OVERRIDING VALVES — SEGMENTAL MORPHOLOGY

ROBERT H. ANDERSON AND SIEW YEN HO

INTRODUCTION

Until relatively recently, hearts with straddling and overriding atrio-ventricular valves have tended to be considered an infrequent morphological curiosity. With the advent of more sophisticated surgical and diagnostic techniques it has been shown that the presence of such a lesion severely compromises the successful treatment of other anomalies such as ventricular septal defects, diagnosis now being possible by modern techniques such as echocardiography [1] or angiocardiography using views designed to profile the ventricular septum [2].

But, despite the increase in pre-operative recognition of hearts with straddling valves, correction of the lesion still carries a high mortality and morbidity [3, 4]. It is therefore advantageous to know the precise chamber combinations which can contain straddling and overriding valves, since this information not only aids their identification and repair, but also gives important clues to the disposition of the atrioventricular conduction tissues [5]. This latter point is of major significance since traumatic heart block was shown to be an important complication in their repair [4].

In this chapter, therefore, the basic features of an atrioventricular valve will be described and a distinction made between *overriding* of the valve annulus and *straddling* of the valve apparatus. Definitions will be given for the differentiation of a right valve or a left valve from a common valve. Finally the different chamber combinations permitting overriding or straddling will be described. It will be shown how knowledge of the chamber combinations and septal orientation permits the disposition of the conduction tissues to be predicted with a high degree of accuracy.

ATRIOVENTRICULAR VALVE MORPHOLOGY WITH REFERENCE TO STRADDLING AND OVERRIDING

Straddling versus overriding

In the "normal" heart the two atrioventricular valves are each committed in

158

their entirety to separate ventricular chambers. Both these atrioventricular valves have an annulus, leaflets and tension apparatus. In the congenital malformation known as "double inlet ventricle", both atrioventricular valves are connected to the same ventricular chamber in their entirety, all components of both atrioventricular valves being contained within the chamber. Hearts with either straddling or overriding atrioventricular valves are intermediates between these "normal" and "double inlet" situations. When describing the morphology and significance of these anomalous valves, we find it helpful to distinguish between the situation in which valve *annulus and leaflets* are committed to both of the ventricular chambers and that in which valve *tension apparatus* is committed to both ventricular chambers. This is because it is known that in some hearts the tension apparatus of a valve can be entirely contained within one chamber while the annulus and leaflets are positioned above a ventricular septal defect so that the valve orifice opens into both chambers. Following the lead of Tabry et al. [3], we describe this situation as *overriding* of the atrioventricular valve (Fig. 1a). In other hearts, in contrast, it is known that while the valve annulus and leaflets can be entirely committed to one ventricular chamber, part of the tension apparatus can extend through a ventricular septal defect to be tethered within the other ventricular chamber (Fig. 1b). It is this second situation which we distinguish as *straddling* of the atrioventricular valve, again following the convention of

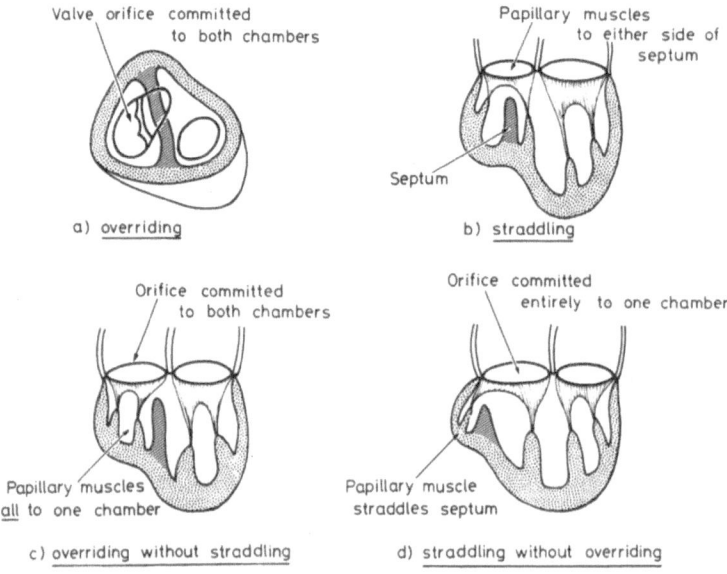

Fig. 1. Diagrams illustrating the difference between "straddling" and "overriding" as used in this chapter. Reproduced from reference 5 by permission of the *American Journal of Cardiology*.

Tabry et al. [3]. Most usually when an atrioventricular valve is connected to two chambers within the ventricular mass, there is both overriding and straddling; i.e. the valve annulus and leaflets and the tension apparatus are contained and tethered within both ventricular chambers. This is therefore termed overriding with straddling (Fig. 2) Bharati and her colleagues [6] have used the terms "annular straddling" to describe what we term overriding, and "peripheral straddling" to describe what we call straddling. The semantics are relatively unimportant. What is important is to appreciate the difference between connexion of the annulus and leaflets to two chambers and the tethering of the tension apparatus within two chambers (Fig. 2). This is because the commitment of the annulus and leaflets (the degree of override) determines the type of atrioventricular connexion present. Straddling in itself does not affect the type of atrioventricular connexion. As we will subsequently see, the determination of the type of connexion is of major importance when describing the chamber combinations of a heart with a straddling valve.

Nomenclature of chambers

We have already indicated how hearts with straddling and overriding valves are intermediate between "normal" hearts and hearts with "double inlet ventricle". The progression in this series is entirely dependent upon the degree of override of the valve annulus and leaflets. Thus in some hearts the entirety of annulus and leaflets are committed to the same chamber as receives the other atrioventricular valve. But in these hearts a small part of the tension apparatus of the valve can cross the septum to arise from a rudimentary ventricular chamber. There is little doubt that such a heart has a double inlet

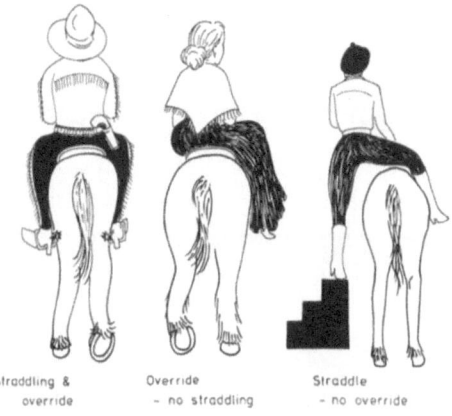

Straddling &   Override   Straddle
override   – no straddling   – no override

Fig. 2. Analogous situations which illustrate the difference between straddling and overriding.

atrioventricular connexion with a straddling atrioventricular valve (Fig. 3a). Conversely, in other hearts, one valve may be entirely committed to one ventricular chamber while the annulus and the leaflets of the other valve are entirely committed to the other ventricular chamber. In such a heart a small part of the tension apparatus can then pass through a ventricular septal defect. Again there is little doubt that in this heart there is a concordant, discordant or ambiguous atrioventricular connexion (depending on the nature of the atrial and ventricular chambers connected together by the valves) together with straddling of one valve (Fig. 3b). In these situations there is little difficulty in determining both the atrioventricular connexion present and the presence of a straddling atrioventricular valve. However, the names of the ventricular chambers in hearts with straddling valves but with these different types of atrioventricular connexion are controversial [5, 7, 8]. We believe [5] that it is best to name the ventricular chambers according to the atrioventricular connexion present. We take as our precedent for this the generally accepted concept that hearts with double inlet connexion are "single ventricles" [9, 10] and that single ventricles can possess rudimentary ventricular chambers [11]. Thus, hearts with straddling or overriding valves and double inlet connexion are treated as univentricular hearts. Their two chambers are respectively considered as a ventricle and a rudimentary chamber. Hearts with straddling or overriding valves and concordant, discordant or ambiguous connexion are treated as biventricular hearts and both chambers referred to as ventricles. The series of hearts between double inlet connexion on the one hand and concordant, discordant or ambiguous connexion on the other hand is split at its midpoint, following the concept suggested by Kirklin et al. [12] for overriding arterial valves. Only the choice of the midpoint as the division for this series is arbitrary. Everything else follows from the general

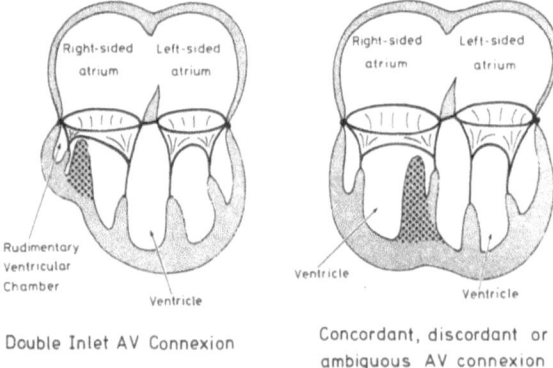

Fig. 3. Diagrams illustrating straddling right valve in the setting of double inlet versus one-to-one connexions.

agreement that hearts with double inlet connexion are univentricular [9, 10]. However, we would also state the degree of override we consider to be present. So, when considering the features of a straddling or overriding valve we determine first the nature of the chambers connected together by the valve, then the degree of override, which we state. From this we determine the type of atrioventricular connexion and then name the ventricular chambers accordingly.

Does a common valve straddle or override?

The convention thus far described for straddling or overriding valves has assumed that the affected valve is one of two valves (or rarely both valves). It is very evident that, within the definitions given, all hearts with a common atrioventricular orifice and an atrioventricular defect (complete atrioventricular canal malformation, complete endocardial cushion defect) also fulfill our criteria of straddling and overriding valves. This fact was recognised by Liberthson et al. [13], but these authors chose to exclude common valves from their category of straddling or overriding valves. We believe this to be an artificial exclusion. It is our opinion that if common valves are similarly treated with respect to overriding of their annulus and commitment of their tension apparatus to separate ventricular chambers, then they too should rightly be included within the category. Thus most frequently a common atrioventricular valve orifice will be more or less equally committed to right and left ventricular chambers, giving the balanced form of atrioventricular defect with straddling of its left anterior and posterior leaflets.

Rarer, but of major diagnostic and surgical significance, are the cases in which a common valve is unequally shared between right and left ventricles. These are the "dominant right" and the "dominant left" forms of atrioventricular defect described by Bharati and Lev [14]. But equally it must be remembered that a common valve can be entirely committed to a sole ventricular chamber as in the univentricular heart [8, 11]. Here then it must be remembered that hearts with a straddling common atrioventricular valve orifice can be intermediate between a univentricular heart and a biventricular heart just as can those with straddling right or left valves (Fig. 4). This is because hearts with common valves can show the same degrees of overriding of the common annulus as have been described with regard to the single right or left annulus in the setting of an overriding valve. Thus, there is a progression of commitment of the common annulus. This extends between exclusive commitment to one ventricular chamber with straddling of the tension apparatus to the situation where the annulus is equally committed between the two ventricular chambers. In this respect the determination of the atrioventricular connexion cannot be determined on a 50% rule since in the

162

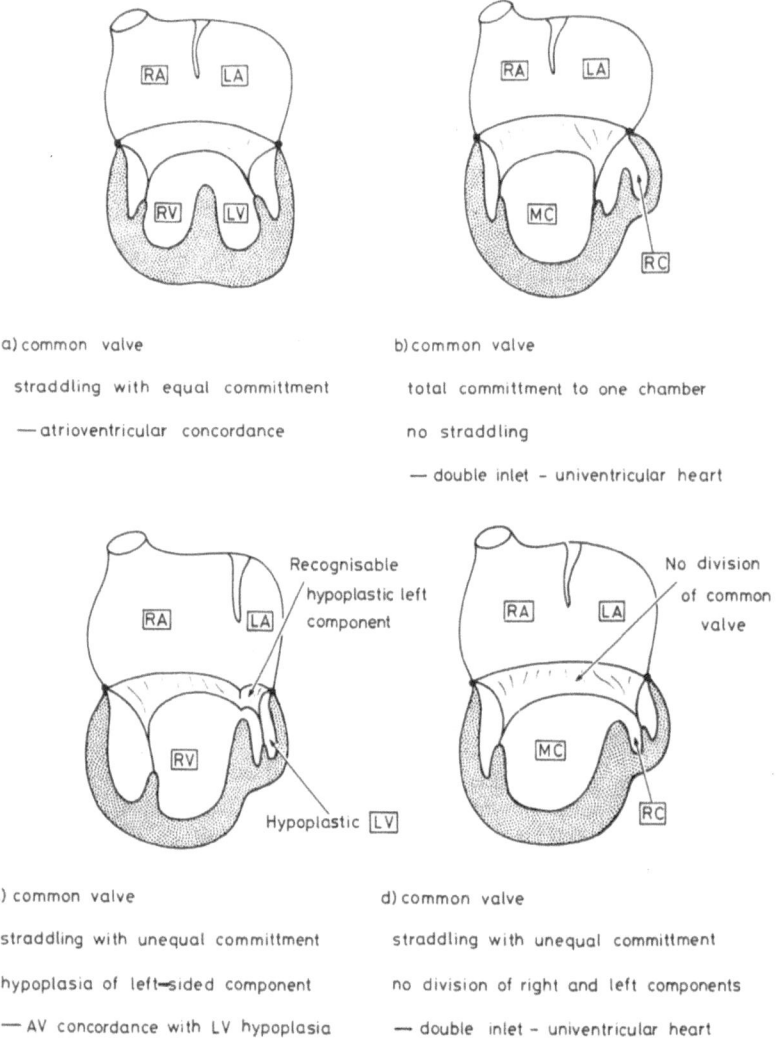

a) common valve

straddling with equal committment

— atrioventricular concordance

b) common valve

total committment to one chamber

no straddling

— double inlet – univentricular heart

Recognisable
hypoplastic left
component

Hypoplastic [LV]

No division
of common
valve

c) common valve

straddling with unequal committment

hypoplasia of left-sided component

— AV concordance with LV hypoplasia

d) common valve

straddling with unequal committment

no division of right and left components

— double inlet – univentricular heart

Fig. 4. Diagrams illustrating the problems of categorizing the atrioventricular connexion with different degrees of overriding of a common atrioventricular valve. Reproduced from reference 5 by kind permission of the *American Journal of Cardiology.*

balanced or "normal" situation with common orifice the common annulus is already shared 50–50 between the ventricular chambers. The degree of cutoff for determination of the type of atrioventricular connexion with a common valve is therefore 75% to the main ventricular chamber and 25% to the rudimentary ventricular chamber [5]. But it must then be recognised that not all hearts with the dominant right or dominant left form of atrioventricular defect are necessarily univentricular. This is because the left or right side of a common atrioventricular annulus may be properly apportioned between the chambers but yet hypoplastic, the chamber containing it being equally hypoplastic. In these instances a degree of judgement must be made as to whether there is an unequal commitment of a free-floating atrioventricular annulus in the setting of a univentricular heart or hypoplasia of the left or right side of a common atrioventricular orifice and valve in the setting of a dominant right or left type of atrioventricular defect (Fig. 4).

Common valve versus straddling right or left valve

Further problems can arise when considering straddling and overriding of a valve because it is also known that the valve connecting the right or left atrial chambers to the ventricular mass can straddle and override the septum in the absence of the other atrioventricular connexion (valve atresia with straddling atrioventricular valve [13, 15, 16]). When either the right or left valve connects the atrial chamber to two chambers in the ventricular mass, the overriding valve can have many of the features of a common atrioventricular valve. Indeed, it has been described as such by Van Mierop [17]. We believe it is preferable to define valves in such a way as to make it always possible to distinguish a common valve from an overriding single right valve or single left valve in the setting of absent atrioventricular connexion. We do this by defining a right atrioventricular valve as a valve which drains the right-sided atrial chamber. The left atrioventricular valve is defined as a valve which drains the left-sided atrial chamber. The morphologies of the right- and left-sided chambers will themselves depend upon atrial situs. In situs solitus the right-sided chamber will be a morphologically right atrium and the left-sided chamber a morphologically left atrium. In situs inversus the reverse will be the case. In atrial isomerism of right type both chambers will have characteristics of a morphologically right atrium and in left isomerism both chambers will have characteristics of a morphologically left atrium. But irrespective of atrial situs the right or left atrioventricular valves are always defined as the valves draining the right- or left-sided atrial chambers, respectively (Fig. 5a). A common valve is then defined as a valve which drains *both* atrial chambers. Thus, both atrial chambers are connected by a common atrioventricular connexion to the ventricular mass, the connexion being guarded by a sole valve (Fig. 5b). It is then an easy matter to distinguish a common valve from a single left or single right valve where there is absence of an atrioventricular connexion (Fig. 5c and d). When there is an absent atrioventricular connexion, the atrial septum will separate one of the atrial chambers from the single left or right valve. If this single left or right valve then connects to two ventricular chambers, it is readily diagnosed as a single valve because it connects only a single atrial chamber to two ventricular chambers (Fig. 6).

164

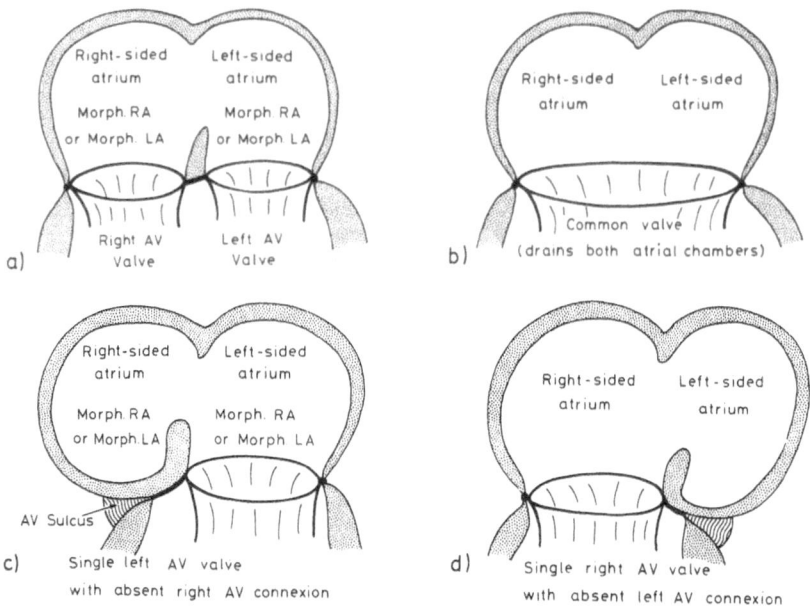

Fig. 5. Diagrams illustrating the difference between two valves, a common valve and a sole valve with absent connexion.

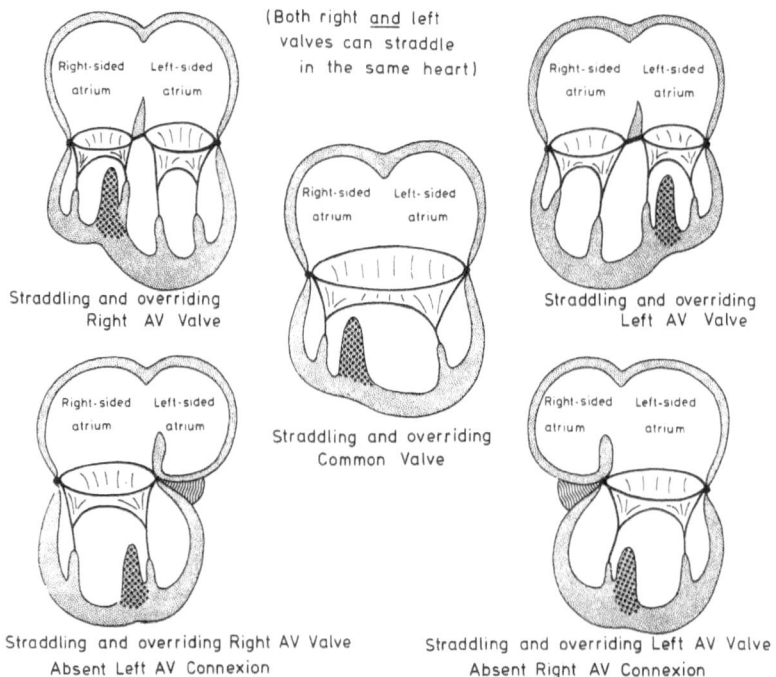

Fig. 6. Diagram illustrating how the right valve, the left valve, or a common valve can all straddle, but how additionally a right or left valve can straddle when one connexion is absent.

Straddling or overriding valves can connect the right- or left-sided atria to the ventricular mass in hearts with either situs solitus, situs inversus or isomeric atrial chambers. In basic terms the ventricular mass in hearts with these different atrial arrangements is comparable when there are straddling or overriding atrioventricular valves. In this section, therefore, we will describe only the arrangement in hearts with situs solitus, but it must be remembered that straddling and overriding can and does occur with situs inversus or when there is atrial isomerism. Equally, although we will describe only overriding of the right and left valves, the right or left side of a common valve can straddle or override in similar hearts with comparable morphology. We will describe three basic patterns: overriding of the left or the right valve, overriding of both valves, and overriding of a sole valve when one atrioventricular connexion is absent.

Straddling and overriding of the right valve

The right atrioventricular valve can itself override or straddle in two discrete patterns depending upon the pattern of ventricular morphology (Fig. 7). When there is right-hand pattern (right ventricle basically to the right [18, 19]), then the right valve is a morphologically tricuspid valve. A series of malformations is then found between primary commitment of this valve to the right ventricle (atrioventricular concordance with straddling tricuspid valve) to primary commitment of the valve to the left ventricular chamber (univentricular heart of left ventricular type with double inlet, straddling right atrioventricular valve and right-sided rudimentary chamber). Irrespective of the degree of override, the right valve overrides the posterior part of a septum which hardly ever extends to the crux (Fig. 8). Because of this, be there concordant or double inlet atrioventricular connexion, the conduction tissues arises from an anomalously located atrioventricular node (Fig. 9). It is possible that overriding of the right valve with right-hand pattern of ventricular architecture could occur when the septum extends to the crux and then it is anticipated that the connecting atrioventricular node would be regularly positioned. Such an arrangement would account for the grossly abnormal location of the atrioventricular bundle in one "Holmes heart" with double inlet which we studied [20].

A straddling right valve may also be found when there is left-hand pattern of ventricular architecture. Then the valve is a morphologically mitral valve and a series of hearts extends between atrioventricular discordance with straddling mitral valve (Fig. 10) and univentricular heart of right ventricular type with double inlet, straddling right valve and right-sided rudimentary

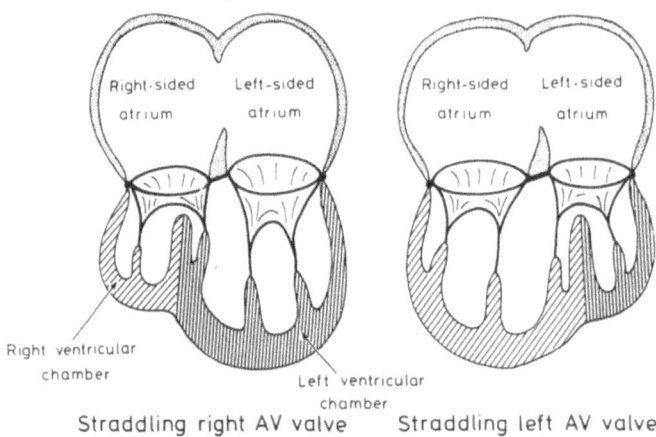

Straddling right AV valve   Straddling left AV valve
with right-hand pattern ventricular morphology

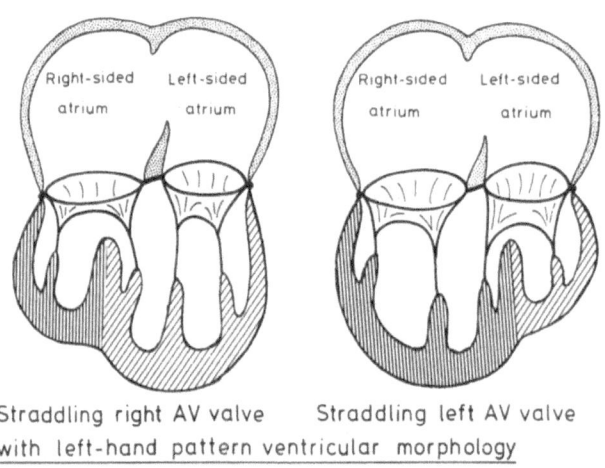

Straddling right AV valve   Straddling left AV valve
with left-hand pattern ventricular morphology

Fig. 7. Diagrams illustrating the effect of the pattern of ventricular morphology on straddling valves.

chamber. In these hearts, the valves straddle the anterior part of a septum which almost always extends to the crux. Despite this, the conduction tissue arises from an anterior node or else a sling of conduction tissue is formed [5, 21], the dominant force being the left-hand pattern of ventricular architecture (Fig. 11).

Straddling and overriding of the left valve

As with the right valve, the left valve can override or straddle in presence of either a right-hand or left-hand pattern of ventricular architecture. In a right-

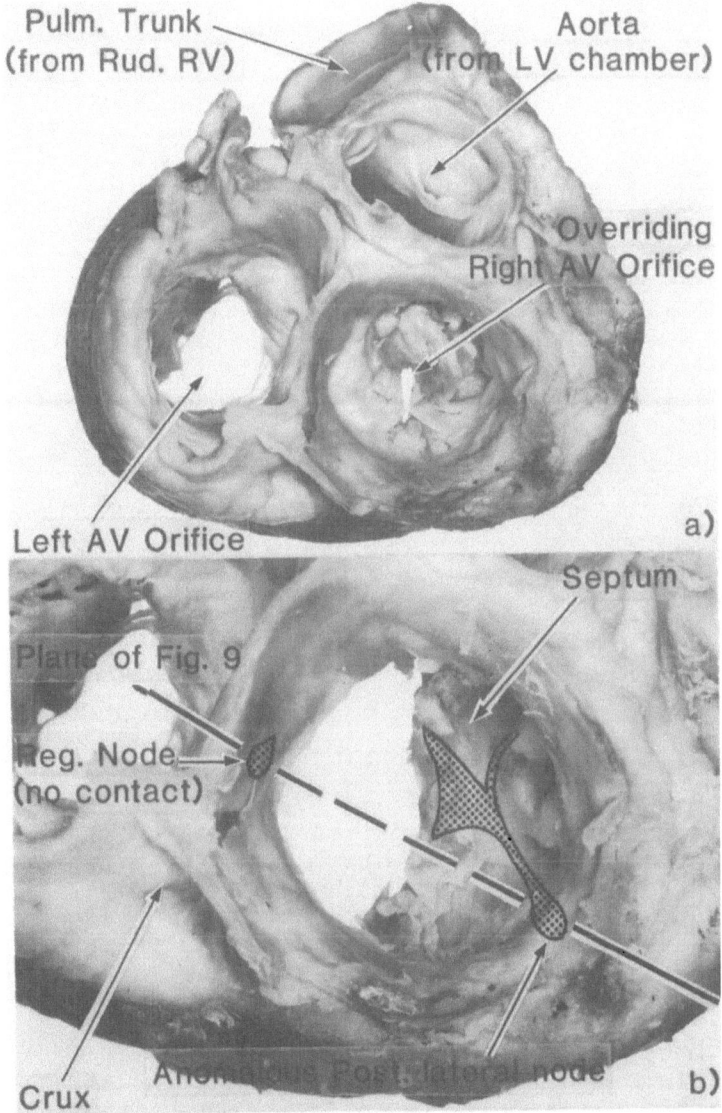

Fig. 8. View of the atrioventricular junction as seen from above in a case of univentricular heart of left ventricular type with right-sided rudimentary chamber and straddling right valve. Panel *a* shows the entire junction. Panel *b* is a detail of the overriding right orifice after removal of the valve leaflets. Note that the septum does not extend to the crux. The conduction tissue disposition has been marked on the photograph. The section in the plane indicated is shown in Figure 9.

168

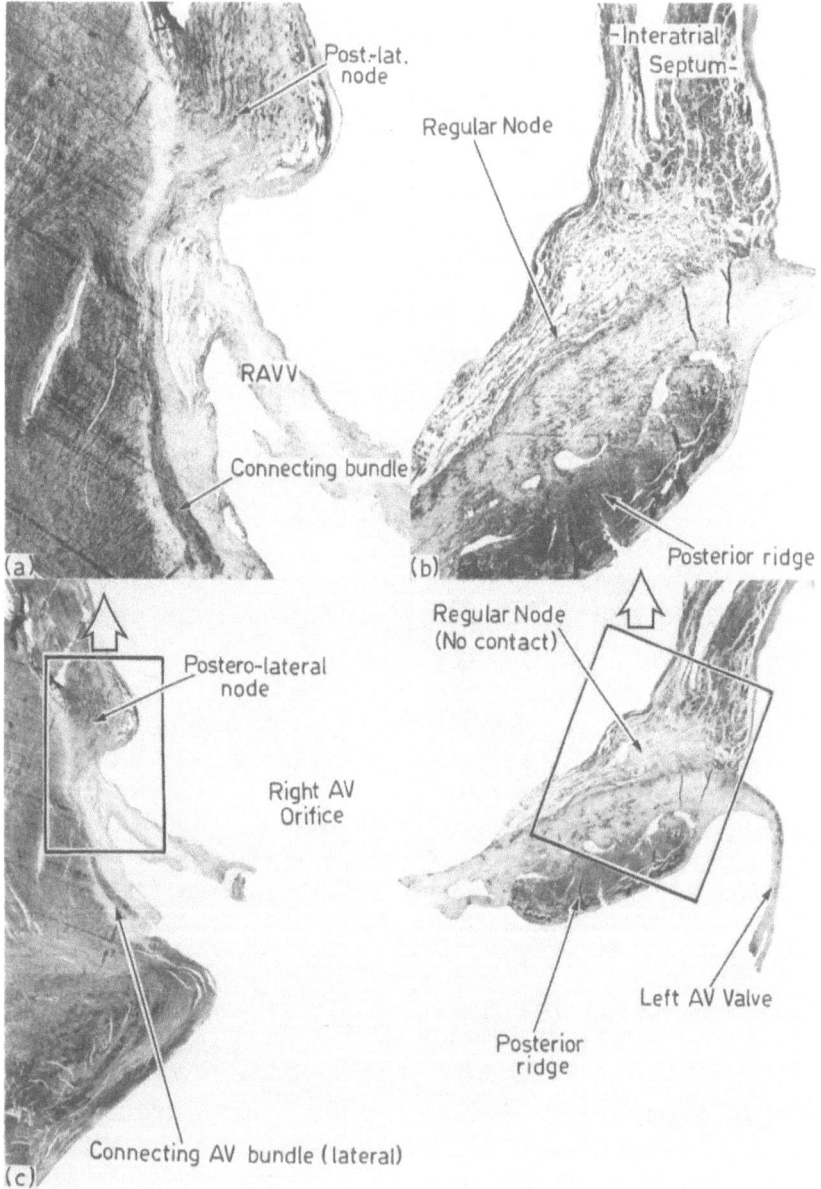

Fig. 9. The section in the plane shown in Figure 8. The lower panel (*c*) is an overall view of the right orifice and shows the regular node which does not give rise to a connecting bundle and the posterolateral node which does. The areas within the boxes are enlarged as Figure 9a and b, respectively. RAVV, right atrioventricular valve.

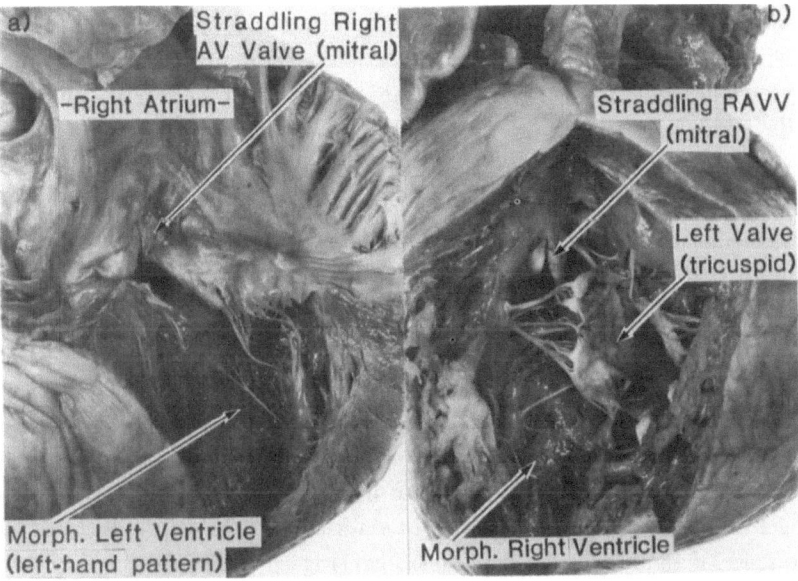

Fig. 10. Photographs of atrioventricular discordance with straddling mitral valve. (*a*) The view from the posterior aspect of the right-sided chambers (morphologically right atrium and left ventricle). (*b*) The view from the left-sided morphologically right ventricle. Specimen by permission of Dr. Marquis.

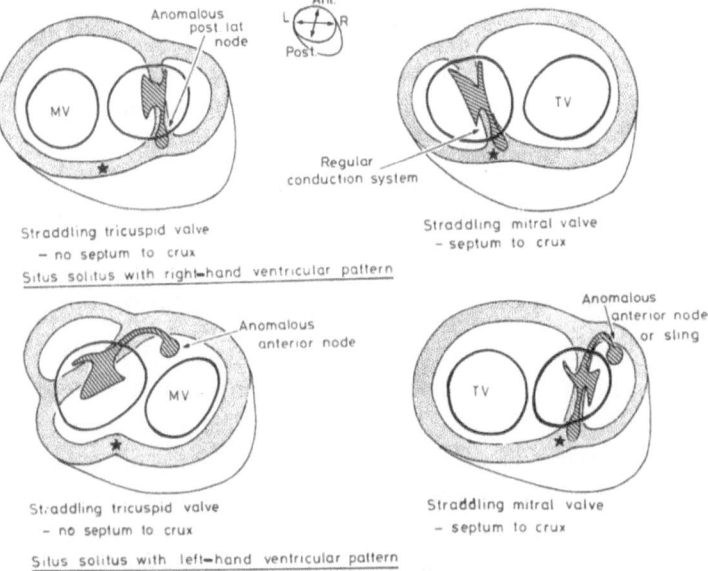

Fig. 11. Diagram illustrating the anticipated conduction tissue disposition with the basic patterns of straddling right and left valves.

hand pattern the valve is a morphologically mitral valve and depending on the degree of override a series is produced between atrioventricular concordance with straddling mitral valve and univentricular heart of right ventricular type with double inlet and straddling left valve. From the conduction tissue standpoint the significant feature is that the valve straddles the anterior part of a septum which almost always reaches the crux. Because of this the atrioventricular bundle originates from a regularly situated atrioventricular node (Fig. 11).

When there is a left-hand pattern of ventricular architecture with straddling left valve, the series of anomalous hearts extends between atrioventricular discordance with straddling tricuspid valve and univentricular heart of left ventricular type with double inlet, straddling left valve left-sided rudimentary chamber. Whatever the degree of override, the valve straddles the posterior part of a septum which hardly ever reaches the crux and this, together with the left-hand pattern of ventricular architecture, dictates the presence of an anterior conduction system (Fig. 11).

Straddling or overriding of both atrioventricular valves

This is a much rarer anomaly and thus far we have encountered three examples. In all there was a right-hand pattern of ventricular architecture with the right ventricle situated in anterior position. The ventricular septum was located more or less in the frontal plane and did not reach to the crux. The degree of commitment of the two overriding valves varied amongst the hearts, but when added together the valve orifices were more or less equally shared between the two ventricles. Although we have yet to study the conduction tissues in these hearts, we anticipate an anomalous lateral atrioventricular node in the right atrioventricular orifice. Straddling of both valves should also be anticipated when there is left-hand pattern ventricular architecture.

Overriding and straddling valves with absent atrioventricular connexion

This arrangement must be anticipated with the same variability of ventricular morphology (Fig. 12) as is found when one of two valves straddles or overrides (Fig. 7). Thus when the right atrioventricular connexion is absent, the left valve may straddle between a posterior left ventricular chamber and an anterior right ventricular chamber, or between a posterior right ventricular chamber and a right-sided left ventricular chamber. We have encountered examples of both these anomalies, studying the conduction systems in two of the latter and finding slings between an anterior node in the floor of the blind-ending right atrium and a posterior node in the wall of the left atrium [20]. When the left atrioventricular connexion is absent, the right valve may strad-

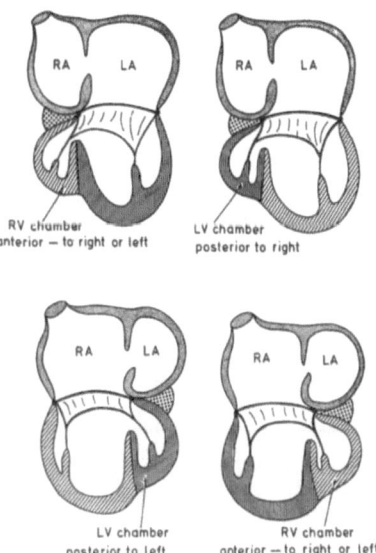

Fig. 12. Diagram illustrating the basic chamber arrangements in which straddling right and left valves can be found when there is absence of the other atrioventricular connexion: RA, morphologically right atrium; LA, morphologically left atrium.

dle between a posterior left ventricular chamber and an anterior right-sided right ventricular chamber. Alternatively it may straddle between a left-sided right ventricular chamber and a right-sided left ventricular chamber. Again we have encountered examples of both types, an important point being that in the heart with posterior left-sided left ventricular chamber the septum did not extend to the crux and an anomalous lateral right atrial node was present. It is a matter of choice as to whether these hearts are categorized as biventricular or univentricular. When the commitment of the sole valve is disproportionately in favour of one ventricular chamber, we would categorize the major chamber as a ventricle and consider the second chamber to be rudimentary. Contrariwise, when the sole valve is equally committed to both ventricular chambers, it seems reasonable to consider both as ventricles (Fig. 13).

VENTRICULO-ARTERIAL JUNCTION

The variability described in ventricular morphology is independent of ventriculo-arterial connexions. Any ventriculo-arterial connexion must be anticipated with any variety of straddling overriding valve. However, one significant association can be observed and that is the combination of double outlet right ventricle with sub-pulmonary ventricular septal defect and a straddling mitral valve, either in the basic setting of atrioventricular concordance [22] or discordance [21].

172

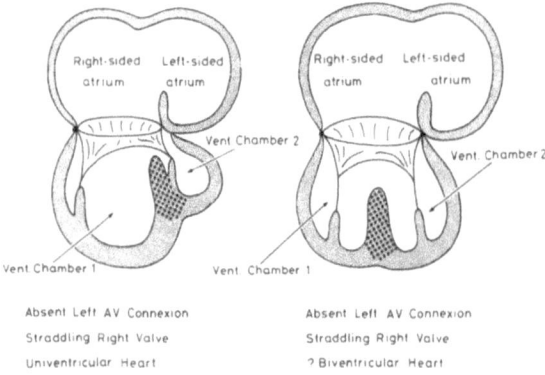

Fig. 13. Diagram illustrating the difficulties in nomenclature of ventricular chambers when one valve straddles and the other atrioventricular connexion is absent.

Acknowledgements. We are greatly indebted to all our friends and colleagues who have contributed to the concepts expressed herein, particularly Anton Becker, Arnold Wenink, Adri Gittenberger-de Groot, Simcha Milo, Jim Wilkinson, Audrey Smith, Fergus Macartney, Elliot Shinebourne and Mike Tynan. We thank Joan Otto and Christine Anderson for their help in preparing the manuscript. This work has been supported by grants from the British Heart Foundation.

REFERENCES

1. Seward JB, Tajik AJ, Ritter DG: Echocardiographic features of straddling tricuspid valve. Mayo Clin Proc 50:427–434, 1975.
2. Bargeron LM, Elliott LP, Soto R, Bream PR, Curry GC: Axial angiography in congenital heart disease. I. Technical and anatomical considerations. Circulation 56:1075–1083, 1977.
3. Tabry IF, McGoon DC, Danielson GK, Wallace RB, Tajik AJ, Seward JB: Surgical management of straddling valve. J Thorac Cardiovasc Surg 77:191–200, 1979.
4. Pacifico AD, Soto B, Bargeron LM Jr: Surgical treatment of straddling tricuspid valves. Circulation 60:655–664, 1979.
5. Milo S, Ho SY, Macartney FJ, Wilkinson JL, Becker AE, Wenink ACG, Gittenberger-de Groot A, Anderson RH: Straddling and overriding atrioventricular valves morphology and classification. Am J Cardiol 44:1122–1134, 1979.
6. Bharati S, McAllister HA, Lev M: Straddling and displaced atrioventricular orifices and valves. Am J Cardiol 43:364, 1979.
7. Bharati S, Lev M: The relationship between single ventricle and small outlet chamber and straddling and displaced tricuspid orifice and valve. Herz 4:176–183, 1979.
8. Van Praagh R, Plett JA, Van Praagh S: Single ventricle. Herz 4:113–150, 1979.
9. Ellis K: Angiography in complex congenital heart disease: single ventricle, double inlet, double outlet and transposition. In: Davila JC (ed) 2nd Henry Ford Hospital International Symposium on Cardiac Surgery, New York, Appleton-Century-Crofts, 1977, pp 222–234.
10. Edwards JE: Discussion. In: Davila JC (ed) 2nd Henry Ford Hospital International Symposium on Cardiac Surgery. New York, Appleton-Century-Crofts, 1977, pp 242.
11. Van Praagh R, Ongley PA, Swan HJC: Anatomic types of single or common ventricle in man: morphologic and geometric aspects of sixty necropsied cases. Am J Cardiol 13:367–386, 1964.

12. Kirklin JW, Pacifico AD, Bargeron LM, Soto B: Cardiac repair in anatomically corrected malposition of the great arteries. Circulation 48:153–159, 1973.
13. Liberthson RR, Paul MH, Munster AJ, Arcilla RA, Eckner FAO, Lev M: Straddling and displaced atrioventricular orifices and valves with primitive ventricles. Circulation 43:213–226, 1971.
14. Bharati S, Lev M: The spectrum of common atrioventricular orifice (canal). Am Heart J 86:553–561, 1973.
15. Rosenquist GC: Overriding right atrioventricular valve in association with mitral atresia. Am Heart J 87:26–32, 1974.
16. Navarro-Lopez F, Marin-Garcia J, Zomeno M, Lorian ARC: Mitral atresia and occlusive left atrial thrombus. A case with 11 years of survival. Br Heart J 31:649–652, 1969.
17. Van Mierop LHS: Pathology and pathogenesis of endocardial cushion defects. Surgical implications. In: Davila JC (ed) 2nd Henry Ford Hospital International Symposium on Cardiac Surgery. New York, Appleton-Century-Crofts, 1977, pp 201–207.
18. Van Praagh R, Weinberg PM, Van Praagh S: Malposition of the heart. In: Moss AJ, Adams FH, Emmanouilides GC (eds) Heart disease in infants, children and adolescents, 2nd edn. Baltimore, Williams and Wilkins, 1977, pp 394–416.
19. Anderson RH, Becker AE, Freedom RM, Macartney FJ, Quero-Jimenez M, Shinebourne EA, Wilkinson JL, Tynan M: Analysis of the atrioventricular junction – connexions, relations and ventricular morphology. In: Godman M (ed) Paediatric cardiology, vol 4. Edinburgh, Churchill Livingstone (in press).
20. Becker AE, Wilkinson JL, Anderson RH: Atrioventricular conduction tissues: a guide in understanding the morphogenesis of the univentricular heart. In: Van Praagh R, Takao A (eds) Etiology and morphogenesis of congenital heart disease. Mt. Kisco, New York, Futura, pp 489–514.
21. Becker AE, Ho SY, Caruso G, Milo S, Anderson RH: Straddling right atrioventricular valves in atrioventricular disordance. Circulation 61:1133–1141, 1980.
22. Kitamura N, Takao A, Ando M, Imai Y, Konno S: Taussig–Bing heart with mitral valve straddling: case reports and post-mortem study. Circulation 49:761–767, 1974.

13. THE VENTRICULAR SEPTUM IN HEARTS WITH A STRADDLING TRICUSPID VALVE

ADRIANA C. GITTENBERGER-DE GROOT AND ARNOLD C.G. WENINK

INTRODUCTION

Straddling of an atrioventricular valve is a condition in which the tension apparatus of that valve is related to both sides of a septum in the ventricular mass. In most cases this is accompanied by overriding of the orifice. Dependent on the degree of involvement of orifice and tension apparatus, there exists, at one extreme, overriding of the orifice without the tension apparatus contributing to the anomaly and, at the other, only the tension apparatus taking part in the straddling without overriding of the orifice [1].

The straddling valve may be either a left- or right-sided valve or a common valve. The common atrioventricular valve is not discussed here. The atrioventricular valve can be of tricuspid, mitral, or undetermined nature dependent on the anatomy of the underlying ventricular chambers. A mitral valve is normally related to a left ventricle whereas a tricuspid valve is seen in conjunction with a right ventricle.

Whether in the case of straddling the naturally related chambers are identical to the ventricles seen in cases with normally situated valves will be discussed in the paragraph on developmental aspects. Until then the chamber containing not only its own inlet orifice but also part of the straddling valve will be referred to as the primary chamber. The other chamber containing only part of the straddling valve is called the secondary chamber.

In this chapter we will highlight the characteristics of a straddling tricuspid valve in its relation to the septum and the septal defect. A similar approach is given in the next chapter with regard to the straddling mitral valve.

MORPHOLOGY

In normal hearts the ventricular septum is composed of an inlet component, a bulboventricular, and an infundibular component. The inlet septum is posterior in position and the tension apparatus of the septal tricuspid valve leaflet is attached to it. The borderline between inlet and bulboventricular septa is the trabecula septomarginalis seen in the right ventricle. No tension apparatus has been seen to cross the borderline between these two septal components.

A.C.G. Wenink et al. (eds.) The Ventricular Septum of the Heart, *175–183. All rights reserved.*
Copyright ©1981 by Martinus Nijhoff Publishers, The Hague/Boston/London.

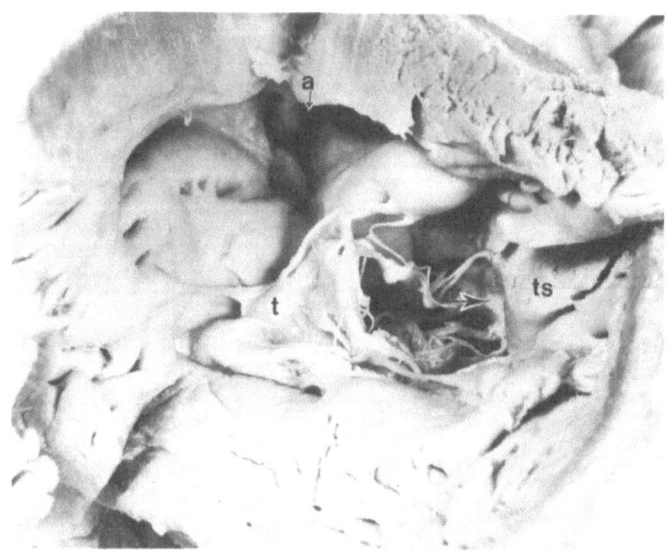

Fig. 1. View into the right-sided secondary chamber with right ventricular morphology of a heart with straddling tricuspid valve (t). The trabecula septomarginalis (ts) has the tension apparatus attached to its free rim. Part of the inlet septum is visible with valve tissue connected to it (large arrow); a, aortic orifice.

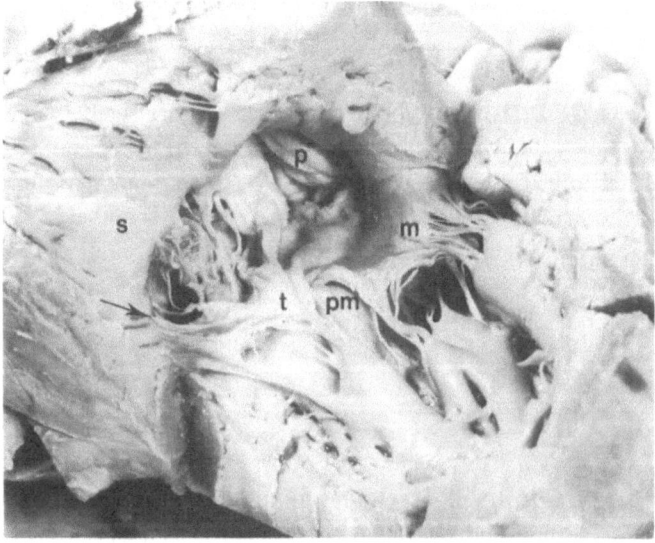

Fig. 2. View into the left-sided primary chamber with left ventricular morphology of a heart with a straddling tricuspid valve (t). The septum (s) is not directed to the crux, indicated by the position of the posteromedial muscle (pm) which separates the tricuspid valve and mitral valve (m). The tricuspid valve straddles over the posterior part of the septum and tension apparatus is seen to cross to the right into the secondary chamber (arrow); p, pulmonary orifice.

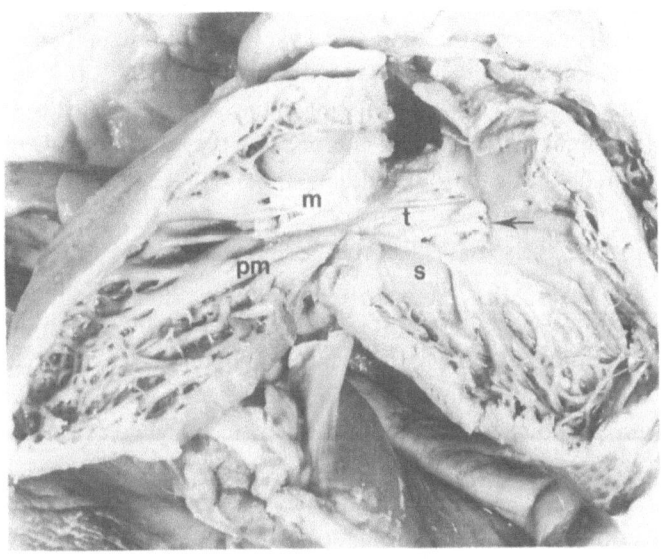

Fig. 3. View into the right-sided primary chamber with left ventricular morphology of a heart with minor straddling of the tricuspid valve (t). The secondary chamber with right ventricular morphology is left-sided. In this case the septum (s) is directed to the posteromedial muscle (pm) but is not in line with this part of the inlet septum. The septal defect is in posterior position. Part of the straddling tricuspid tension apparatus is attached to the left aspect of the inlet septal component of the septum as well as to the free rim of the defect (arrow) also constituted by inlet septum; m, mitral valve.

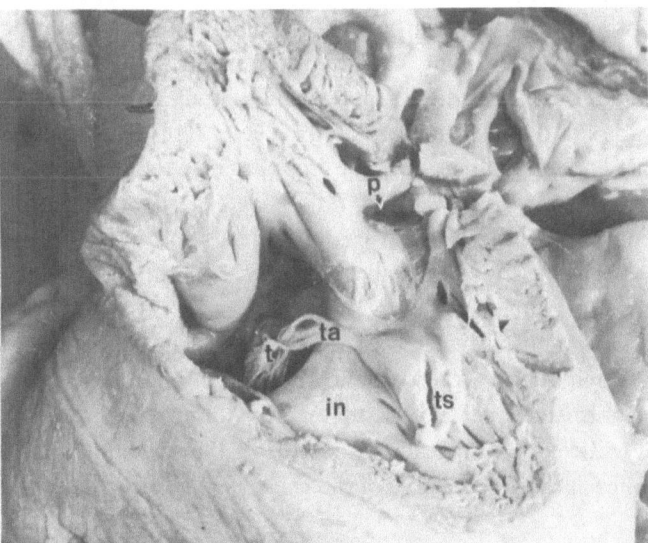

Fig. 4. View into the right-sided secondary chamber with right ventricular morphology of case with almost 100% straddling of the tricuspid valve (t). A small amount of tension apparatus (ta) is still attached to a papillary muscle which is continuous with the trabecula septomarginalis (ts). Clearly visible is the inlet septum (in) component posterior to the ts forming the free rim of the defect; p, pulmonary orifice.

In all of the 11 cases of straddling tricuspid valve studied, in the secondary chamber, most resembling a morphological right ventricle, a trabecula septomarginalis was distinguished; posterior to this structure a part of the inlet septum with papillary muscles and chordae was present (Fig. 1). Dependent to some extent on the degree of straddling, the size of the secondary chamber could vary from very small to normal.

The position of the septal defect was posterior in all cases with a variable degree of extension anteriorly. This implies that the inlet septum was in all cases involved in the septal defect. On the posterior wall of the ventricular chambers the septum reached to the tricuspid annulus in all but one case. The attachment of the valvular tissue could be to the side of the inlet septum or to the posterior part of the inferior rim of the defect also constituted of inlet septum.

The situation in the primary chamber, most resembling a morphological left ventricle, differed markedly from the normal situation. This chamber not only received the complete mitral valve but also the straddling part of the tricuspid valve. In all cases there was a muscle ridge present on the posterior wall of the chamber between tricuspid and mitral orifice. This muscle ridge is the posteromedial muscle (PMM) to which in most cases the tension apparatus of the straddling tricuspid valve was attached (Fig. 2).

The relation of the septum, which with its smooth surface most resembled the left ventricular side of the septum, to this PMM was peculiar. It could be directed to the PMM contacting it at the annular level at a certain angle (Fig. 3), or it could sway away along the posterior rim of the tricuspid orifice. In the most extreme form the posterior part of the septum deviated almost completely to one side of the orifice, resulting in nearly 100% overriding with only a very limited amount of tension apparatus present in the secondary chamber (Fig. 4).

It is remarkable that, in the 11 cases studied, minor straddling was rare (three cases) whereas in eight instances the valve straddled for more than 50% into the primary chamber.

A straddling tricuspid valve was found on the right or left side in atrioventricular concordance or discordance, dependent on the loop of the heart. Additional anomalies such as concomitant straddling mitral valve, atresia of the mitral orifice, septal defects not related to the straddling, and varying abnormalities at the arterial pole of the heart were also encountered.

NOMENCLATURE

Nomenclature of straddling tricuspid valve is in the literature at the moment very confusing. The simplest approach as given by Milo et al. [1] does not reflect developmental theories. A proportion of the cases with a straddling tricuspid valve are classified as biventricular; others dependent on the degree of straddling as univentricular. In biventricular hearts the ventricle containing only part of the atrioventricular valve is called the secondary chamber, whereas the other ventricular cavity containing the whole of the other atrioventricular valve and part of the straddling valve is called the primary chamber. As soon as straddling is more than 50%, these hearts are classified as univentricular hearts of left ventricular type with straddling. The secondary chamber can then also be referred to as rudimentary chamber, which can either be an outlet chamber or a trabeculated pouch; the primary chamber can then be called a ventricle or main chamber having a morphology of left ventricular type. It is essential to differentiate the univentricular hearts of left ventricular type with straddling from those cases without straddling, as will become evident from the paragraph on the developmental aspects, as they are not a natural entity from an embryological point of view.

Classification on basis of developmental concepts is more complicated. Bharati and Lev [2] describe a continuous spectrum between straddling atrioventricular valve and complete displacement into the main chamber. This latter category is differentiated from what they refer to as cases of single ventricle with small outlet chamber on basis of the morphology of this outlet chamber (in terminology of Anderson and co-workers [3] this is the rudimentary chamber of a univentricular heart). This outlet chamber morphology reflects, in Bharati and Lev's opinion, embryological components of the primary heart tube and enables a classification which is partly based on developmental theories that are not identical to ours.

We prefer to use the nomenclature as suggested by Milo et al. [1], although from the following paragraph on the development of straddling tricuspid valve, it will be evident that natural entities have not always been grouped together under the same name. This is, however, not as confusing as the introducing of again a new terminology based on our own developmental theories.

DEVELOPMENTAL ASPECTS

A study of the development of the ventricular septum during early embryogenesis, shows that the septum is formed by the fusion of the embryonic inlet septum with the bulboventricular fold (Chapter 3, Fig. 5c). The embryonic inlet septum, being a loose trabecular mass in midline position on the posterior wall of the embryonic ventricle, forms the posterior part of the septum. The anterior part is formed by the bulboventricular fold, which fuses with the embryonic inlet septum at an angle (Chapter 3, Fig. 5d). From above the infundibular septum completes the septation [4]. During normal septation the tricuspid annulus is led to the right without an actual shift of the atrioventricular canal region to the right. This latter mode of development has been erroneously postulated by several authors [5–7]. The lack of shift of the atrioventricular canal region is important for our further concepts concerning development of a straddling tricuspid valve. It also forms a solution to some hitherto unexplained phenomena in cases of straddling which will be referred to later.

In normal hearts the left and right ventricle are not simply the result of a midline septation of the embryonic ventricle. The left ventricle is derived from embryonic ventricle with a small part of bulbus in the left ventricular outflow tract, whereas the right ventricle is mainly derived from bulbus and that small part of the embryonic ventricle, present underneath the right half of the atrioventricular canal, which will be the inlet part of the future right ventricle. The inlet component of the right ventricle is initially very small, and so are the dimensions of the embryonic inlet septum. Hemodynamic influences are supposed to remodel this region, resulting in a normal position of the tricuspid orifice with an adequate size of the inflow tract of the right ventricle. In this situation the septum separating both atrioventricular orifices runs to the crux and the embryonic inlet septum cannot be detected separately. The loose trabeculations of the inlet septum have, however, contributed to the valvular and tension apparatus of the definitive atrioventricular valves [4].

Straddling tricuspid valve always associated with a defect in the posterior part of the septum is thought to be the result of an abnormal development of the embryonic inlet septum. It is assumed that an abnormal excavation of the embryonic inlet septum has taken place after fusion with the other septal components, resulting in the formation of two main inlet septum components joined by a thinned-out region on the posterior wall of the primary chamber (Fig. 5a and b). One part of the inlet septum is a muscle ridge running over the posterior wall of the primary chamber, and the other part contacts the tricuspid annulus as posterior part of a septum between the primary and secondary chambers (Fig. 5a and b). The separation of the two inlet septal components may be more or less marked, accounting for the variation in deviation of the septum from the crux. The muscle ridge on the posterior wall of the primary chamber is always interposed between both atrioventricular orifices and indicates the position of the crux. This muscle bundle has been described in the literature by several authors [8, 9] as the posteromedial muscle bundle (PMM). It is encountered in various heart anomalies and very rarely in "normal" hearts. As will be evident from the above embryonic concepts the presence of a separate PMM reflects in our opinion a disturbance of the modeling of the embryonic inlet septum.

The current views in the literature regarding the development of a straddl-

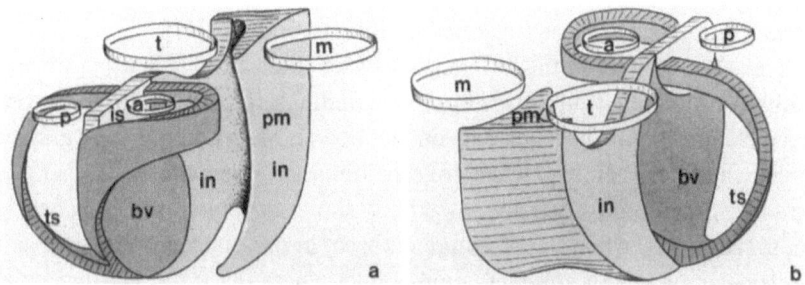

Fig. 5. (a) Schematic representation of the septal components in a left frontal view in case of straddling tricuspid valve. There has been a normal contact between the bulboventricular (bv), the inlet septum (in) component, and the infundibular septum (is). The tricuspid valve straddles over a posterior defect of the inlet septum (in) which is malformed and consists of two parts. One part is the posteromedial muscle (pm) while the other constitutes the posterior part of the septum; m, mitral orifice; a, aortic orifice; p, pulmonary orifice; ts, trabecula septomarginalis. (*b*) Right posterior view indicating the separation of inlet septum components with resultant straddling of the tricuspid valve (t).

ing tricuspid valve can be distinguished in two major concepts. According to one concept, there is a displacement of the ventricular septum as a whole by deviation of this structure to the right [10]. These authors do not accept the PMM as part of the embryonic septal components. The other explanation is based on the theory of shifting of the atrioventricular canal region [5–7], straddling, almost 100% overriding to complete overriding and straddling Both concepts allow for a sliding scale from cases with minor tricuspid straddling, almost 100% overriding to complete overriding and straddling also referred to as displacement of an atrioventricular orifice [11]. This implicates that, according to their views, the septum is identical in all these cases with a varying degree of embryonic ventricle being incorporated in the secondary chamber.

Bharati and Lev [2, 11] separately distinguish a group of hearts with single ventricle and small outlet chamber that they think belong to a different developmental complex. Here the septum is solely of bulboventricular origin and the small outlet chamber composed of bulbus only. This latter group and the cases of displacement of an atrioventricular orifice are identical to what Anderson and co-workers [3] have described as univentricular hearts of left ventricular type with complete double inlet. These authors do not classify according to embryological concepts but nevertheless have come to the conclusion that the septum in all these univentricular hearts is of bulboventricular origin. We agree with this view and are also of the opinion that the septum in univentricular hearts of left ventricular type with complete double inlet is in fact bulboventricular and lacks an inlet septum component, and then see no reason to distinguish a separate group with displacement of an atrioventricular orifice as suggested by Bharati and Lev [11].

That there is an essential difference between the septum in hearts with and without straddling is supported by several findings. Exploration of the secondary chamber (which dependent on the degree of straddling may also be called an outlet chamber) in case of straddling, independent of whether this straddling is minor or extreme, constantly shows the presence of a trabecula septomarginalis, while this structure is absent in univentricular hearts of left ventricular type with complete double inlet where the trabecula forms the inferior rim of the defect.

Part of the tension apparatus of the tricuspid valve is derived from the embryonic inlet component in the ultimate septum in a later stage of development [4]. If no tension apparatus is connected to the posterior part of the septum, this suggests that an embryonic inlet component is lacking. On the other hand, the constant relation between the tension apparatus of the tricuspid valve and the PMM supports the theory that this structure is derived from the embryonic inlet septum. In the case of straddling tricuspid valve, there is an additional component in the septum, while in univentricular hearts of left ventricular type with complete double inlet, the PMM is the only remnant of the embryonic inlet septum.

A final support for the above differentiation between univentricular hearts of left ventricular type with and without straddling is given by the difference in localization of the conducting system. In a univentricular heart of left ventricular type with complete double inlet, an anterior node is always to be expected [12], whereas those cases that present with straddling have a posterior though abnormally placed node at the site of junction of the inlet septum and the ring of the tricuspid annulus. This latter differentiation is valid only in the case of normally related chambers. In atrioventricular discordance there always is an anterior node [1].

Typical for a straddling tricuspid valve is its relation to the posterior aspect of the septum. In straddling mitral valve, there is a mode of development that is more nearly related to the anterior part of the septum (Chapter 14). The inlet septum is not involved and runs to the crux normally. This implies that a straddling mitral valve is not the mirror image of straddling tricuspid valve as is sometimes suggested on basis of the theory of shifting of the atrioventricular canal region to the right [8, 13].

REFERENCES

1. Milo S, Yen Ho S, Macartney FJ, Wilkinson JL, Becker AE, Wenink ACG, Gittenberger-de Groot AC, Anderson RH: Straddling and overriding atrioventricular valves: morphology and classification. Am J Cardiol 44:1122–1134, 1979.

2. Bharati S, Lev M: The relationship between single ventricle and small outlet chamber and straddling and displaced tricuspid orifice and valve. Herz 4:176–183, 1979.

3. Anderson RH, Tynan M, Freedom RM, Quero Jimenez M, Macartney FJ, Shinebourne EA, Wilkinson JL, Becker AE: Ventricular morphology in the univentricular heart. Herz 4:184–197, 1979.

4. Wenink ACG: Embryology of the ventricular septum. Separate origin of its components. Virchows Arch [Pathol Anat] 390:71–79, 1981.

5. De la Cruz MV: Double-outlet and double-inlet ventricular complexes. In: Davila JC (ed) 2nd Henry Ford Hospital International Symposium on Cardiac Surgery. New York, Appleton-Century–Crofts, 1977, pp 214–220.

6. Munoz-Castellanos L, De la Cruz MV, Cieslinski A: Double inlet right ventricle. Two pathological specimens with comments on embryology. Br Heart J 35:292–297, 1973.

7. Liberthson RR, Paul MH, Muster AJ, Archilla RA, Eckner FAO, Lev M: Straddling and displaced atrioventricular orifices and valves with primitive ventricles. Circulation 43:213–226, 1971.

8. Devloo-Blancquaert A, Ritter D: Muscle ridge between atrioventricular valves and mal-alignment of junction of these valves with ventricular septum. Br Heart J 40:1267–1274, 1978.

9. Wenink ACG: Considerations pertinent to the embryogenesis of transposition. In: Van Mierop LHS, Oppenheimer-Dekker A, Bruins CLDC (eds) Embryology and teratology of the heart and the great arteries. Leiden, Leiden University Press, 1978, pp 129–135.

10. Van Praagh R, Plett JA, Van Praagh S: Single ventricle. Pathology, embryology, termi-nology and classification. Herz 4:113–150, 1979.

11. Bharati S, McAllister HA, Lev M: Straddling and displaced atrioventricular orifices and valves. Circulation 60:673–684, 1979.

12. Becker AE, Wilkinson JL, Anderson RH: Atrioventricular conduction tissues in uni-ventricular hearts of left ventricular type. Herz 4:166–175, 1979.

13. Aziz KU, Paul MH, Muster AJ, Idriss FS: Positional anomalies of atrioventricular valves in transposition of the great arteries including double outlet right ventricle, atrioventricular valve straddling and malattachment. Am J Cardiol 44:1135–1145, 1979.

14. THE VENTRICULAR SEPTUM IN HEARTS WITH A STRADDLING MITRAL VALVE

ARNOLD C.G. WENINK

INTRODUCTION

The typical anatomy of a straddling mitral valve has not always been fully appreciated. The striking difference from a straddling tricuspid valve was recognized only recently [1]. To stress this difference, two separate chapters of this book are devoted to the two anomalies, respectively.

The description of hearts with a straddling mitral valve can be less complicated than that of cases with a straddling tricuspid valve. From the preceding chapter, it is clear that a straddling tricuspid valve has a tendency to override for more than 50%. This means that, according to the classification principles explained in Chapter 12, the secondary chamber (i.e., the chamber in which the straddling valve would actually belong) has to be called a rudimentary chamber and not a right ventricle in most of the cases. The situation is different in hearts with a straddling mitral valve. Here, overriding for more than 50% into the primary chamber is the exception rather than the rule. Therefore, in this chapter the terms of left and right ventricle are used as in the normal heart. Only additional pathology, such as absence of one atrio-ventricular connection, may demand the disuse of these terms.

MORPHOLOGY

The ventricular septal defect, a prerequisite for a valve to be able to straddle, is characteristic for the anatomical type of valve that is straddling. With a straddling mitral valve, the ventricular septal defect has an anterior position. It is always bordered by the infundibular septum. In typical cases, the infundibular septum is malaligned with the anterior (bulboventricular) septum and is freely visible in the right ventricle, producing the anatomy of double-outlet right ventricle. In the literature [2–6], the straddling mitral valve has often been described as associated with the Taussig–Bing anomaly. Figure 1 shows such a case.

If the defect is completely muscular, its posterior border is formed by the trabecula septomarginalis. However, the defect may be larger and reach more posteriorly. Then, it also has a perimembranous component and in some

186

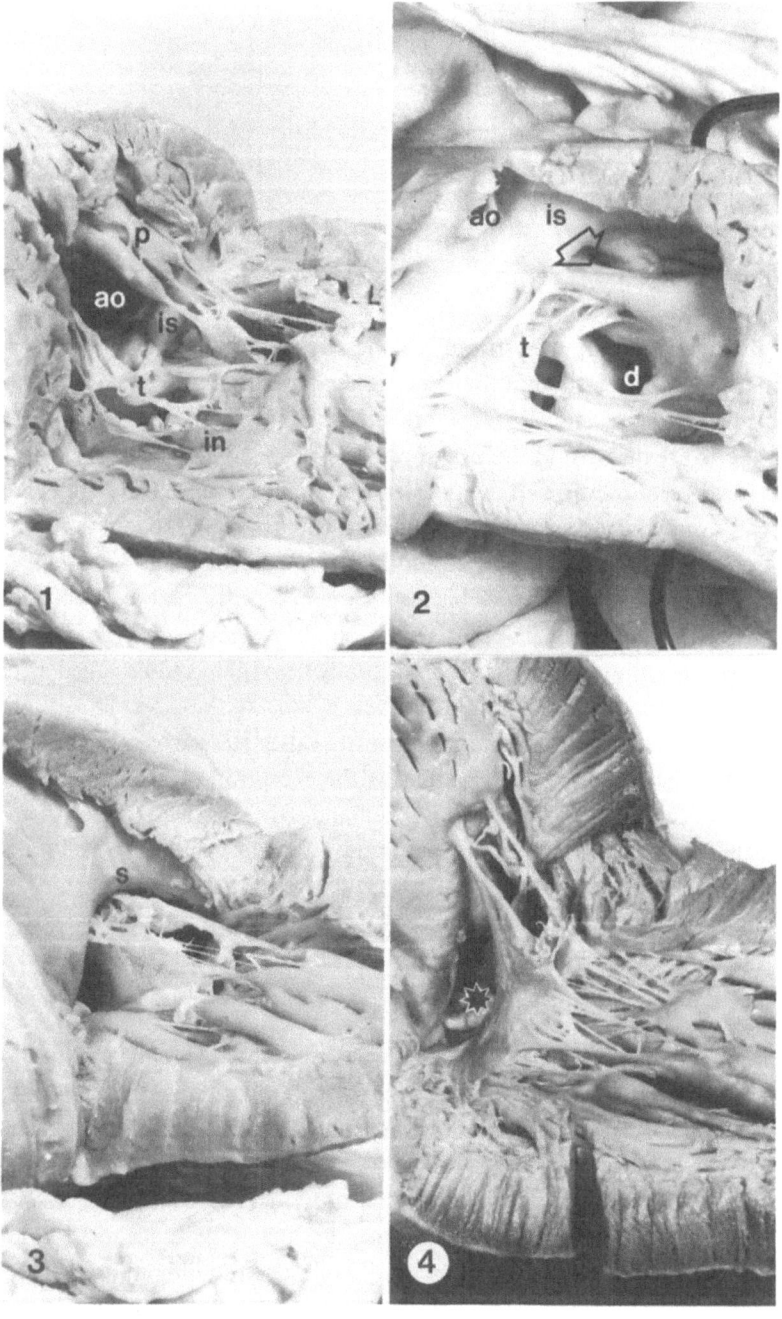

Figs. 1–4. (*1*) Right ventricular view of a heart with the Taussig–Bing anomaly and a straddling mitral valve. Papillary muscles (p) of the mitral valve are attached to the right ventricular anterior wall, to the right of the infundibular septum (is). The pulmonary orifice is hidden by mitral

hearts it may even reach into the inlet septum. The latter extension is not typical and, even in hearts with a large defect (Fig. 2), the mitral valve straddles across the anterior portion of the septum and the posterior part of the defect seems to be coincidence.

In the purest forms, there is malalignment of infundibular and bulboventricular septa only, and the inlet septum is not involved. It is not deficient and its position is normal. Thus, the ventricular septum extends to the crux of the heart, and abnormalities of the conducting tissues are not to be expected.

Usually, the percentage of overriding of a straddling mitral valve is minimal. The papillary muscles holding the straddling portion of the valve tend to maintain position high in the right ventricular outflow tract (Fig. 1). Commonly, they are related to the rim of the defect. The anatomy of the mitral valve, stenosing the left ventricular outflow tract (Fig. 3) and sometimes being partly attached to the rim of an infundibular defect, may be identical to the anatomy of a malattached mitral valve as occurs in hearts with complete transposition of the great arteries (Fig. 4). This malformation can even occur in the absence of a ventricular septal defect and represents neither overriding nor straddling.

A straddling mitral valve may occur together with other malformations. Different septal pathology may be added to the infundibular malalignment. This can be major pathology, as in hearts with an absent right atrioventricular connection (tricuspid atresia). The only septum present is constituted by the infundibular and bulboventricular septa, and the remnant of the inlet septum is visible in the main chamber of left ventricular morphology as the posteromedial muscle bundle. The main chamber, containing the mitral valve, communicates with the outlet chamber via the outlet foramen. This foramen is bordered by infundibular and bulboventricular septa. If in these hearts a straddling mitral valve is also present, the characteristic pathology does not differ from that seen in biventricular hearts. Again, there is malalignment of the infundibular and bulboventricular septa, causing a discontinuity in the borders of the outlet foramen. The malalignment tends to create a double-outlet outlet chamber and the infundibular septum runs freely to the anterior

---

valvular tissue. The inlet septum (in) is not involved in the anomaly; t, tricuspid valve; ao, aortic orifice.

(2) Right ventricular view of a heart with transposition and a large ventricular septal defect. Although the posterior part of the defect (d) lies in the inlet septum, the mitral valve straddles only anteriorly. The mitral valve itself is not seen, but a thick chorda (arrow) is attached in this right ventricle; ao, aortic orifice; t, tricuspid valve; is, infundibular septum.

(3) Left ventricle of a heart with straddling mitral valve. The arterial orifice is not visible, because the mitral valve straddles across the anterior portion of the septum (s).

(4) Left ventricle of a heart with transposition of the great arteries and malattached mitral valve. A direct view of the arterial orifice (asterisk) is impossible because of the anterior position of the mitral valve. Compare with Figure 3.

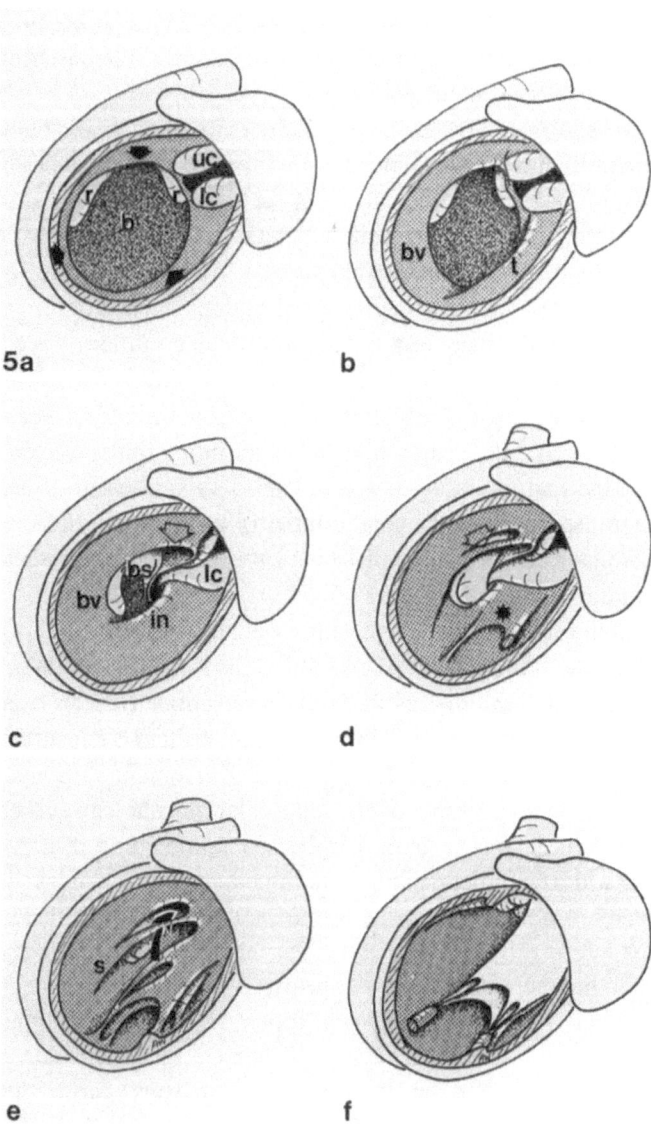

Fig. 5. Diagram to show ventricular septation. Left lateral view. The left parietal wall of the embryonic ventricle has been removed. Compare whith Figure 5 in Chapter 3, p. 26.

(*a*) Preseptation stage. The bulboventricular orifice is bordered by the bulboventricular fold (arrows). Through the orifice, the bulbar cavity (b) is seen, with two endocardial bulbar ridges (r). The atrioventricular orifice, which opens into the embryonic ventricle, is guarded by the upper (uc) and lower (lc) atrioventricular endocardial cushions.

(*b*) Outgrowth of the bulbar and ventricular cavities leads to accentuation of the bulbo-ventricular fold (bv). From individual trabeculations, a ridge (t) is formed on the posterior ventricular wall.

(*c*) The posterior ventricular ridge has grown out to form the inlet septum (in), and the anterior wall of this chamber. Between the infundibular septum and the basal protion of the bulboventricular septum, papillary muscles are found to hold the straddling portion of the mitral valve.

The typical anatomy of hearts with a straddling mitral valve has often been overlooked. Some authors [6–8] appreciated the anatomy, but others stressed a supposed analogy with hearts with a straddling tricuspid valve [9–11]. This analogy has been described particularly in relation to the univentricular heart. A spectrum should exist with, on one side, the double-inlet left ventricle and, on the other, the double-inlet right ventricle [10, 12–14]. This spectrum was further illustrated by the description of malalignment of atrial and ventricular septa [11, 12, 15]. According to this concept, the straddling mitral valve is described as part of a malformation of the inlet portion of the heart, for it is the inlet septum that has to be aligned with the atrial septum. As stated above, such an inlet malformation is not a feature of hearts with a straddling mitral valve.

There is a completely different spectrum of malformations to which straddling of the mitral valve belongs. Actual straddling is the most serious form. From there, the spectrum goes via malattached or cleft mitral valves [16–21] (Fig. 4) toward an abnormally short distance between the papillary muscles and the septum [19]. The existence of this spectrum, together with the fundamental difference from the straddling tricuspid valve, may be understood from normal development.

DEVELOPMENTAL CONSIDERATIONS

During the sixth week of embryonic development, closure of the interventricular communication is effected mainly by downward growth of the bulbar septum (i.e., the adult infundibular septum). This septation process causes part of the bulboventricular fold to end up in the left ventricle (Fig. 5).

---

portion of the bulboventricular fold has formed the bulboventricular septum (bv). The cranial portion of the bulboventricular fold (arrow) encircles the future left ventricular outflow tract. This outflow tract is further bordered by the bulbar septum (bs), resulting from fusion of the bulbar ridges. The upper (uc) and lower (lc) atrioventricular cushions have fused to separate the left and right atrioventricular orifices. Note that the right atrioventricular orifice is partly bordered by the bulboventricular fold.

(*d*) The interventricular communication is closed. Part of the bulboventricular myocardium (arrow) is moved away from the site of final clusure, to contribute to the anterior leaflet of the mitral valve. At the same time, the posterior ventricular wall and the inlet septum are undermined to contribute to the posterior leaflet (asterisk).

(*e*) Loosening of myocardium has proceeded, but part of the future mitral valve is still attached to the septum (s). The arrow points at the entrance of the aortic vestibulum.

(*f*) Mature left ventricle. The mitral valve has no septal papillary muscles. Distinction between the different septal components cannot be made.

It is continuous with the anterior (bulboventricular) septum and encircles the aortic orifice. In these early stages, there are no definitive valve leaflets and the "mitral" orifice is temporarily guarded by endocardial cushions. Formation of the valve takes place by invagination of sulcus tissue and undermining of ventricular myocardium [22]. The actual topography causes some differences in the development of the anterior and posterior mitral valve leaflets. The posterior leaflet has to be elaborated from ventricular myocardium. The anterior leaflet, however, is already present in a primitive form in relatively early stages (Fig. 6). It is the left ventricular portion of the bulboventricular fold (Fig. 5). During subsequent development, this fold or flap is attenuated and by an undermining process loosened from the bulboventricular septum. Thus, in an embryo of 23-m CR length, there is a muscular anterior mitral leaflet that only apically has contact with the ventricular septum (Figs. 5 and 7). In later stages, part of the flap becomes fibrous to form the valve leaflet and its chordae, and the papillary muscles are quite separated from the ventricular septum.

From the earliest stages on, the anlage of the anterior leaflet surrounds the aortic orifice and this condition persists to form the mitral-aortic fibrous continuity. Part of the fibrous mitral ring is incorporated into the aortic wall [23]. Development in this region is not quantitatively uniform since the distance between aortic and mitral valves has appeared to be variable [24].

Development of the papillary muscles implies that the bulboventricular

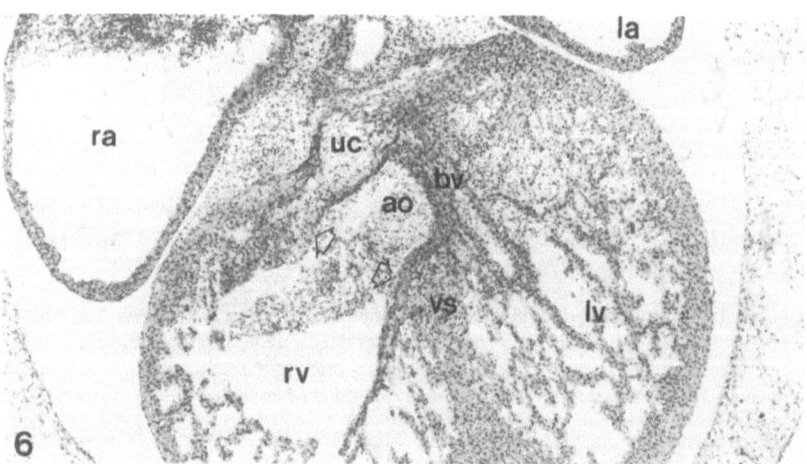

Fig. 6. Transverse section of the heart of a human embryo of 11-m CR length. The cranial portion of the bulboventricular fold (bv) forms the left-hand boundary of the aortic vestibulum (ao). Note its trabeculations coursing apically on the left side of the ventricular septum (vs); ra, right atrium; la, left atrium; rv, right ventricle; lv, left ventricle; uc, upper atrioventricular cushion; arrows, bulbar ridges.

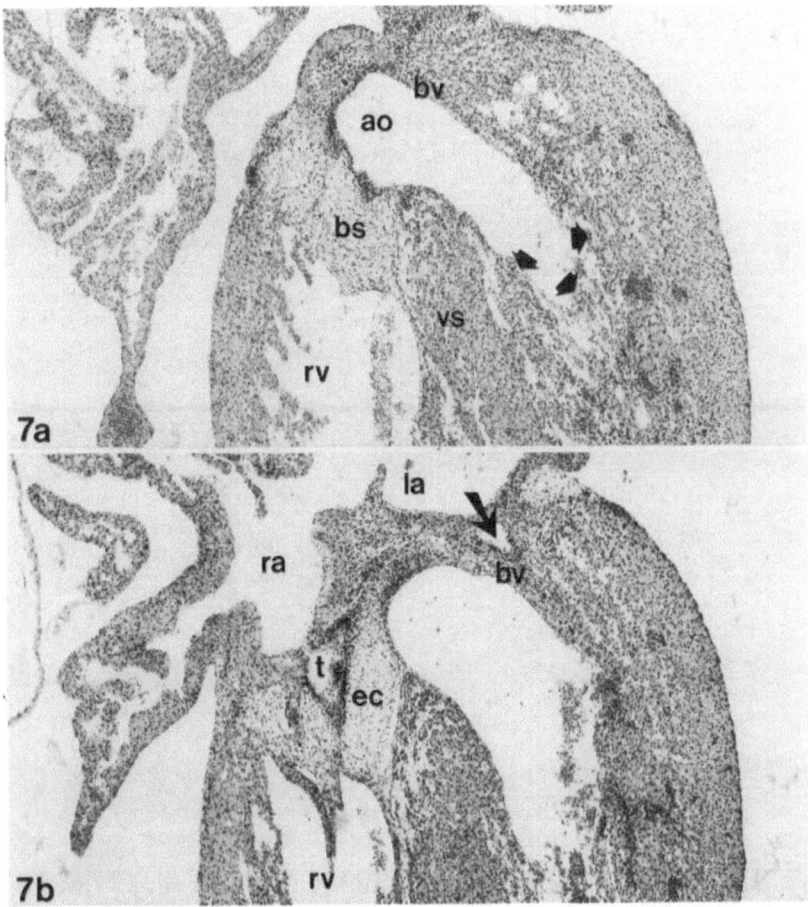

Fig. 7. Transverse sections of the heart of a human embryo of 22-mm CR length. (*a*) At the level of the bulbar septum (bs). The cranial portion of the bulboventricular fold (bv) still borders the aortic vestibulum (ao), but its attachment to the septum (vs) has a more apical position (arrows); rv, right ventricle. (*b*) More caudal section to show the contribution of the bulboventricular fold (bv) to the mitral valve. The arrow points to the mitral orifice; ra, right atrium; la, left atrium; t, tricuspid orifice; ec, atrioventricular endocardial cushion; rv, right ventricle.

myocardium in the direct proximity of the bulbar (adult infundibular) septum is undermined and "moved away" toward the apex and, finally, toward the ventricular free wall (Fig. 8). This description of migration of papillary muscles ignores the probable differential growth of the ventricular wall and the fact that much of these dimensional changes is only relative.

Probably, the anatomy of the normal mitral valve illustrates the somewhat different mechanisms by which the anterior and posterior leaflets develop. The anterior leaflet has an early predecessor in the bulboventricular fold,

192

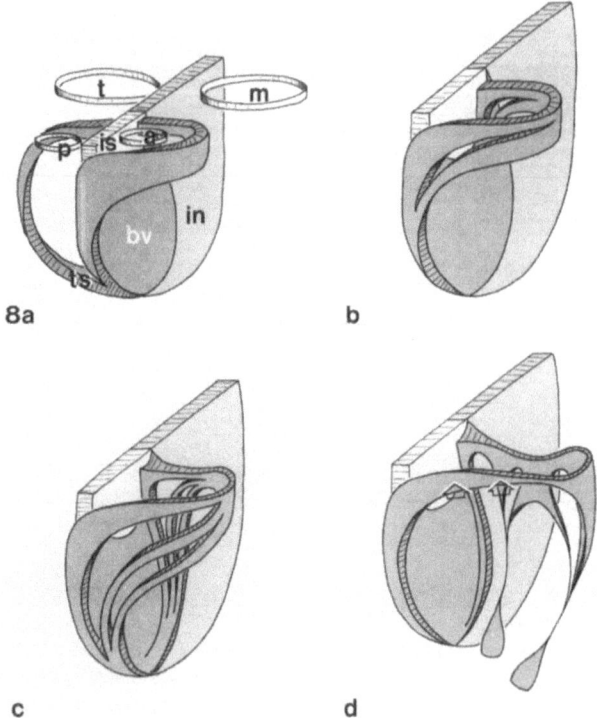

8a   b

c   d

Fig 8. Diagrams to show schematically the elaboration of the aortic leaflet of the mitral valve. Left anterior view.

(*a*) Septal components after complete septation; in, inlet septum; bv, bulboventricular septum; is, infundibular septum; ts, trabecula septomarginalis. Note that part of the bulboventricular fold, still in continuity with the septum, encircles the aortic orifice (a). It also forms the anterior boundary of the mitral orifice (m); p, pulmonary annulus; t, tricuspid annulus.

(*b–d*) Consecutive stages of elaboration of the aortic leaflet of the mitral valve from bulbo-ventricular myocardium. The trabecula septomarginalis and the valve annuli have been left out. Note that in *d* the papillary muscles of the mitral valve have lost their attachment to the septum. The arrowed portion of the bulboventricular fold is no longer traceable in normal hearts.

whereas the posterior leaflet has to be elaborated from the left ventricular free wall. This might explain the uniform anatomy of the anterior leaflet and the variable morphology, with two or more scallops, of the posterior leaflet [25].

Normal development of the anterior mitral leaflet explains the anatomy of a straddling mitral valve. The characteristic ventricular septal defect lies at the very site at which elaboration of bulboventricular myocardium is initiated (Fig. –). In the case of the typical malalignment, the undermining process is not localized by the bulbar septum, but can freely extend into the right

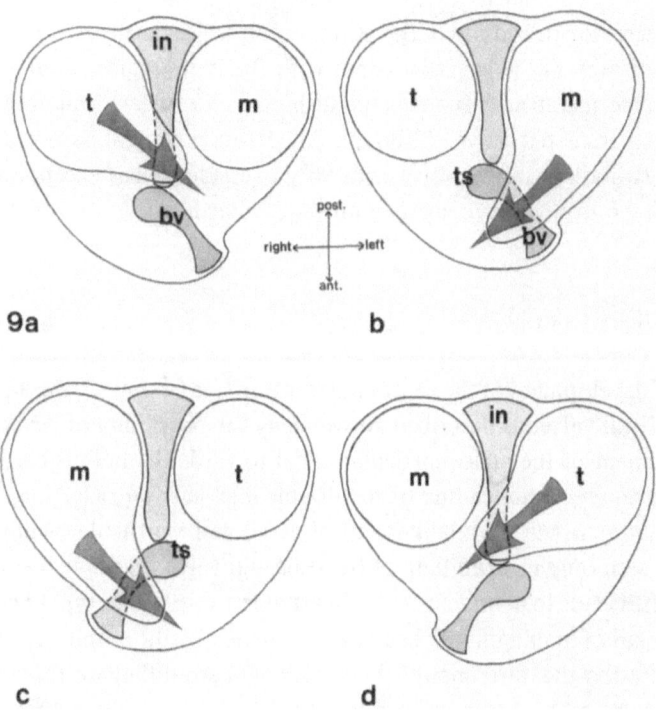

Fig. 9. Diagrams to illustrate the result of extreme overriding of straddling valves.

(*a*) Straddling tricuspid (t) valve, posterior to the bulboventricular septum (bv). More than 50% overriding would create a univentricular heart of left ventricular type. Musculature between tricuspid (t) and mitral (m) valves is inlet septum (in).

(*b*) Straddling mitral valve (m), across the bulboventricular septum (bv). More than 50% overriding would create a univentricular heart of right ventricular type. Musculature between tricuspid (t) and mitral (m) valves is trabecula septomarginalis (ts).

(*c*) Ventricular inversion with straddling mitral valve. With more than 50% overriding, the leftsided main chamber of right ventricular type would show trabecula septomarginalis (ts) between tricuspid (t) and mitral (m) valves.

(*d*) Ventricular inversion with straddling tricuspid valve. With more than 50% overriding, the right-sided main chamber of left ventricular type would show inlet septum (in) between tricuspid (t) and mitral (m) valves.

ventricular outflow tract. Once papillary muscles have been elaborated in that position, the subsequent process of migration toward the apex and the free wall becomes impossible. Straddling is present. Two different explanations may still be given for the malattached anterior mitral leaflet (Fig. 4). In developmental stages, there may have been straddling, with subsequent closure of the ventricular septal defect. Alternatively, the migration process of the papillary muscles might have stopped halfway, which could explain the spectrum of anomalies proposed above.

From these developmental considerations, it becomes clear that the mitral annulus is not primarily involved. Thus, normal development provides an explanation for straddling of the mitral valve, while the necessity of overriding is not present. This is consistent with the pathological findings. For a mitral valve, it is an additional distinguishing feature when compared with the straddling tricuspid valve. Although Anderson et al. [26] have described a case of straddling mitral valve with 90% overriding, it is exceptional for a straddling mitral valve to create a univentricular heart.

UNIVENTRICULAR HEARTS

Normal development of the ventricular septum (see Chapter 3, this book) and of the mitral valve, as described above, deny the possibility of "exaggerated displacement of the atrioventricular canal towards the bulbus cordis" [10]. There is no spectrum leading from "double inlet left ventricle" into "double inlet right ventricle". Malalignment of atrial and ventricular septa [11, 12] may be seen only in straddling of the tricuspid valve. Extreme overriding in these cases leads to a univentricular heart of left ventricular type. The reverse of this kind of malalignment has never been seen by the author. Kitamura et al. [6] stressed the difference of their cases with straddling mitral valve from those described by Muñoz-Castellanos et al. [12] and Quero Jiménez et al. [10]. In univentricular hearts, it is not always easy to distinguish between morphologically tricuspid and mitral valves. Often other anatomical details have to be considered. Thus, the diagram produced by Tandon et al. [27] to illustrate the anatomy of a straddling mitral valve has more features of a straddling tricuspid valve with ventricular inversion, since the posteromedial muscle is depicted in the right-sided ventricular chamber (see Gittenberger-de Groot and Wenink, this book, Chapter 13).

Some cases of univentricular heart of right ventricular type have been described as having a common atrioventricular valve [10, 28]. Such hearts are probably closely related to atrioventricular defects with right ventricular dominance [29]. Although this latter anomaly was suggested as comparable to the straddling mitral valve [30], the present data do not support this suggestion.

Since the mitral valve always straddles the anterior portion of the septum, the musculature between the tricuspid valve and the straddling mitral valve is trabecula septomarginalis (Fig. 9). It is not a remnant of the inlet septum as was described by Devloo-Blancquaert and Ritter [14]. Thus, while a univentricular heart of right ventricular type with a straddling atrioventricular valve has to have trabecula septomarginalis separating the two valves, in a univentricular heart of left ventricular type with a straddling atrioventricular valve a remnant of the inlet septum is found to separate the valves.

Further investigations are needed to show whether or not the uni-ventricular heart of right ventricular type is a uniform entity. A thorough study of ventricular morphology, topography of ventricular septal defects, and anatomy of the valve or valves and the papillary muscles must solve the problem.

REFERENCES

1. Dickinson DF, Wilkinson JL, Smith A, Becker AE, Anderson RH: Atrioventricular con-duction tissues in univentricular hearts of left ventricular type with absent right atrio-ventricular connection ("tricuspid atresia"). Br Heart J 42:1–8, 1979.
2. Lev M, Bharati S, Meng CCL, Liberthson RR, Paul MH, Idriss F: A concept of double outlet right ventricle. J. Thorac Cardiovasc Surg 64:271–281, 1972.
3. Sondheimer HM, Freedom RM, Olley PM: Double outlet right ventricle: clinical spectrum and prognosis. Am J Cardiol 39:709–914, 1977.
4. Bharati S, McAllister HA, Lev M: Straddling and displaced atrioventricular orifices and valves. Circulation 60:673–684, 1979.
5. Muster AJ, Bharati S, Azis KU, Idriss FS, Paul MH, Lev M, Carr I, De Boer A, Anagnos-topoulos C: Taussig–Bing anomaly with straddling mitral valve. J Thorac Cardiovasc Surg 77:832–842, 1979.
6. Anderson RH, Shinebourne EA, Becker AE, Macartney FJ, Wilkinson JL, Tynan MJ: Letter to the Editor: tricuspid atresia and univentricular heart. Pediatr Cardiol 1:165, 1979/1980.
7. Danielson GK, Tabry JF, Fulton RE, Hagler DJ, Ritter DC: Successful repair of straddling atrioventricular valve by technique used for septation of univentricular heart. Ann Thorac Surg 28:554–560, 1979.
8. Milo S, Stark J, Macartney FJ, Anderson RH: Parachute deformity of the tricuspid valve. Thorax 34:543–546, 1979.
9. Liberthson RR, Paul MH, Muster AJ, Arcilla RA, Eckner FAO, Lev M: Straddling and displaced atrioventricular orifices and valves with primitive ventricles. Circulation 43:213–226, 1971.
10. Quero Jinénez M, Pérez Martínez VM, Maitre Azcárate MJ, Merino Batres G, Moreno Granados F: Exaggerated displacement of the atrioventricular canal towards the bulbus cordis (rightward displacement of the mitral valve). Br Heart J 35:65–74, 1973.
11. Aziz KU, Paul MH, Muster AJ, Idriss FS: Positional anomalies of atrioventricular valves in transposition of the great arteries including double outlet right ventricle, atrioventricular valve straddling and malattachment. Am J Cardiol 44:1135–1145, 1979.
12. Muñoz-Castellanos L, De la Cruz MV, Cieslinski A: Double inlet right ventricle. Two pathological specimens with comments on embryology. Br Heart J 35:292–297, 1973.
13. De la Cruz MV: Double-outlet and double-inlet ventricular complexes. In: Davila JC (ed) 2nd Henry Ford Hospital International Symposium on Cardiac Surgery. New York, Ap-pleton-Century-Crofts, 1977, pp 214–220.
14. Devloo-Blancquaert A, Ritter D: Muscle ridge between atrioventricular valves and mal-alignment of junction of these valves with ventricular septum. Br Heart J 40:1267–1274, 1978.
15. Tabry IF, McGoon DC, Danielson GK, Wallace RB, Tajik AJ, Seward JB: Surgical management of straddling atrioventricular valve. J Thorac Cardiovasc Surg 77:191–201, 1979.
16. Layman TE, Edwards JE: Anomalies of the cardiac valves associated with complete trans-position of the great vessels. Am J Cardiol 19:247–255, 1967.

17. Rosenquist CC, Stark J, Taylor JFN: Congenital mitral valve disease in transposition of the great arteries. Circulation 51:731–737, 1975.
18. Shrivastava S, Tadavarthy SM, Fukuda T, Edwards JE: Anatomic causes of pulmonary stenosis in complete transposition. Circulation 54:154–159, 1976.
19. Rosenquist GC, Stark J, Taylor JFN: Mitral valve abnormalities associated with transposition of the great arteries. Am J Cardiol 35:166, 1975.
20. Van Gils FAW: Left ventricular outflow tract obstruction in transposition with interventricular communication: anatomical aspects. In: Van Mierop LHS, Oppenheimer-Dekker A, Bruins CLDC (eds) Embryology and teratology of the heart and the great arteries. Leiden, Leiden University Press, 1978, pp 160–171.
21. Van Gils FAW, Moulaert AJ, Oppenheimer-Dekker A, Wenink ACG: Transposition of the great arteries with ventricular septal defect and pulmonary stenosis. Br Heart J 40:494–499, 1978.
22. Van Gils FAW: The development of the human atrioventricular valves. J Anat 128:427, 1979.
23. Walmsley R: Anatomy of human mitral valve in adult cadaver and comparative anatomy of the valve. Br Heart J 40:351–366, 1978.
24. Rosenquist GC, Clark EB, Sweeney LJ, McAllister HA: The normal spectrum of mitral and aortic valve discontinuity. Circulation 54:298–301, 1976.
25. Ranganathan N, Lam JHC, Wigle ED, Silver MD: Morphology of the human mitral valve. II. The valve leaflets. Circulation 41:459–467, 1970.
26. Anderson RH, Tynan M, Freedom RM, Quero-Jiménez M, Macartney FJ, Shinebourne EA, Wilkinson JL, Becker AE: Ventricular morphology in the univentricular heart. Herz 4:184–197, 1979.
27. Tandon R, Moller JH, Edwards JE: Communication of mitral valve with both ventricles associated with double outlet right ventricle. Circulation 48:904–908, 1973.
28. Keeton BR, Macartney FJ, Hunter S, Mortera C, Rees P, Shinebourne EA, Tynan M, Wilkinson JL, Anderson RH: Univentricular heart of right ventricular type with double or common inlet. Circulation 59:403–411, 1979.
29. Bharati S, Lev M: The spectrum of common atrioventricular orifice (canal). Am Heart J 86:553–561, 1973.
30. Freedom RM, Bini M, Rowe RD: Endocardial cushion defect and significant hypoplasia of the left ventricle: a distinct clinical and pathological entity. Eur J Cardiol 7:263–281, 1978.

15. CLASSIFICATION VERSUS ANATOMY

ADRIANA C. GITTENBERGER-DE GROOT AND ARNOLD C.G. WENINK

INTRODUCTION

For many years the lack of an unambiguous stable nomenclature for the classification of congenital cardiac malformations has led and still leads to misunderstanding and confusion.

The creation of a system that classifies on the basis of a set of definitions dealing with anatomical features, not taking into consideration embryological aspects, is a possible solution. Such a system has been offered by a London group of investigators [1–5] and we will refer to it in short as the sequential chamber analysis (SCA). This system has two major disadvantages. The first disadvantage is that it names the ventricular chambers on the basis of their inlet and outlet connections and not on the basis of their intrinsic morphology. This intrinsic anatomy is needed, however, to differentiate between morphologically right and left sides of the heart. To achieve completeness, detailed morphological information should therefore always be added to the description of specimens when using this classification system. A second disadvantage is that anomalies that are closely related from an embryological aspect are not always grouped together under the same name, whereas anomalies of various developmental origins may be classified within a single category.

Another way to solve nomenclature problems would be to group together malformations that are developmentally linked. The advantage of such a classification, based on embryology, would be that it provides a better basis for the understanding of groups of malformations and their characteristic features. A disadvantage is the lack of unity with regard to developmental concepts on normal and abnormal development of the heart and the use of these concepts by cardiac morphologists [6–17]. This leads to a confusing variety of almost identical terms.

Recently one of us [15] has introduced a new developmental concept concerning ventricular septation (Chapter 3) which, of course, influences our views on normal and abnormal development. We can now either choose for a classification adjusted to this new developmental concept, with resultant introduction of new terms and perhaps redefinition of old ones, or choose the already mentioned SCA, which has no embryological background. We tend

A.C.G. Wenink et al. (eds.) The Ventricular Septum of the Heart, *197–202. All rights reserved.*
Copyright ©1981 by Martinus Nijhoff Publishers, The Hague/Boston/London.

to opt for the SCA system since investigations of development continue to be carried out, which might imply an instability of nomenclature. We are, however, also very well aware of the hazards of the SCA system.

To illustrate this and to exemplify in more detail the problems of a classification with an embryological background, we will discuss in more detail a group of cardiac malformations that are classified according to the SCA as univentricular heart of left ventricular type (UVH of LV type).

While talking about UVH, we have to distinguish between left ventricular, right ventricular, and indeterminate types (Chapter 16). Essential for the definition of a univentricular heart is the general agreement as to what has to be called a ventricle and what not. In SCA, a chamber in the ventricular mass is called a ventricle on basis of its inlet orifice. When it receives more than 50% of an inlet, it should be called a ventricle [3]. In univentricular hearts, therefore, only one chamber deserves the name of ventricle, although there may be more than one cavity within the ventricular mass. Under the heading of univentricular heart, several malformations are grouped together that are not developmentally related. This will be evident from the following examples of UVH of LV type.

UVH OF LV TYPE WITH COMPLETE DOUBLE INLET

These hearts with two separate atrioventricular valves, which are solely and completely committed to one ventricular chamber with a trabeculation pattern of the left ventricular type, have more features in common than merely a double-inlet ventricle. Nearly always there is a rudimentary chamber below one of the great arteries, and there is a septum that does not run to the crux cordis. On the posterior wall of the ventricle a muscle ridge is seen that separates the two inlet orifices. The connecting atrioventricular node is invariably anterior [18].

First we will refer to the developmental aspects of this group of hearts which, according to our views, should be considered as a single natural entity. The septum separating the rudimentary chamber from the ventricle and running to the acute margin of the heart is of crucial importance. We think this septum to be solely constituted by bulboventricular and infundibular components. The septal defect is in fact the bulboventricular foramen, i.e., the ostium between embryonic ventricle and bulbus, which is now relatively restricted by excessive outgrowth of the bulboventricular fold. We consider the posterior muscular ridge identical to the "posteromedial muscle" [19, 20] and the remnant of the embryonic inlet septum. The actual septum of these hearts has no embryonic inlet component and therefore is not directed toward the crux. For the same reason the posterior atrioventricular node does not connect. In this concept the chamber receiving both inlet orifices is not identical to a normal left ventricle, as it also contains part of the normal right ventricle.

Van Praagh et al. [11] refer to the UVH of LV type with complete double inlet as single left ventricle. Our disagreement with the latter term does not concern the adjective "single", since the prefix "uni" does not mean anything different. It is the term "left ventricle" that we think unadvisable. Although the trabecular pattern may be morphologically that of a left ventricle, this does not make this cavity a normal left ventricle. As has been mentioned already, we are of the opinion that the "left ventricle" (main chamber) in these UVH hearts contains the inlet portion of the right ventricle. This does not lead, however, to such changes in this chamber that the essential morphological characteristics of a normal left ventricle [11] have disappeared.

Van Praagh et al. [11], however, have a different developmental explanation for cases of single left ventricle that supports a terminology using the terms "left ventricle" in these hearts. They claim that, in embryonic stages, the "future left ventricle" receives the entire atrioventricular canal.

This short discussion on developmental concepts and the interpretation thereof may illustrate how difficult it is to use terms as right and left ventricle in these malformed hearts as a generally accepted definition of these terms, either morphologically or embryologically.

A similar reasoning may be pertinent with respect to some descriptions by Bharati et al. [12]. Apart from their "single ventricle with small outlet chamber", which is Van Praagh's "single left ventricle" and what we call here "univentricular heart of left ventricular type with complete double inlet", they distinguish hearts with "displaced tricuspid valve". These hearts would contain within their rudimentary chambers more of a "sinus portion". The only way in which we are able to understand their description is by assuming that they base their arguments on the embryological views of the Heidelberger School [8–10]. These authors have described a shift of the atrioventricular canal toward the right, and, apart from that, they distinguish between three separate cavities in the embryonic heart, which finally form the two adult ventricles. Since Bharati et al. [12] distinguish between a proampulla, a metampulla, and a bulbus, they have created a basis for understanding the different stages of incomplete rightward shift of the atrioventricular canal. Only therefore, we believe, do they distinguish between "single ventricle with small outlet chamber", "displaced tricuspid valve", and "straddling tricuspid valve". On purely morphological grounds, we see no reason for distinction between the last two categories. Their illustrations of displaced tricuspid valve [12] show at least septal attachments of the right atrioventricular valve, which we consider to be an indication of straddling.

UVH OF LV TYPE WITH STRADDLING

As has been explained in the chapter on straddling tricuspid valve (p. 179), there is in our opinion a sliding scale from cases with minor straddling, which for reasons of nomenclature are referred to as biventricular hearts (straddling less than 50%), to cases with more than 50% straddling, which are called univentricular. Thus, the nomenclature dictated by the SCA here classifies hearts with an identical developmental background into two different groups. It would be tempting to classify all hearts with a straddling tricuspid valve in a single group that would form a natural entity from an embryological point of view. Here again rises the problem that not all investigators have identical embryological concepts. For instance, a group of authors [11–13] have, on the basis of their embryological views, not only grouped together all straddlers, but also included within this category the UVH of LV type with complete double inlet. This again illustrates that it is not advisable to use developmental concepts to create a stable nomenclature.

We believe that the cases with and without straddling do not belong to one natural entity. In cases of straddling tricuspid valve, the septum is indeed almost never directed to the crux, but its position and morphology are not directly comparable to the anatomy in hearts without straddling. In straddling tricuspid valve, the atrioventricular node may not be in its regular position but is posterior. In complete double inlet, there is an anterior connecting node (N.B. these differences only hold good for the normal bulboventricular loop).

Here, oversimplification has occurred in the work by Milo et al. [5], who using the SCA classification suggest in their summary that all univentricular hearts of left ventricular type, i.e., those with and without straddling, have an abnormal position of the septum which position would have consequences for the conducting tissues. We believe that this simplification is caused by grouping together all univentricular hearts of left ventricular type. Erroneously it might be supposed that such a group constitutes a natural entity, with more characteristics in common than those demanded by the definitions.

There are, however, more problems to be expected from a nomenclature that deliberately does not depend on developmental views. The following case of straddling tricuspid valve from the Leiden collection may illustrate this. The heart possessed a left-sided chamber of left ventricular morphology in which all of the mitral valve and more than 50% of the tricuspid valve were found. Thus, any additional chamber cannot contain more than 50% of the tricuspid orifice and the heart is classified as a univentricular heart of left ventricular type. If we add "with straddling tricuspid", the diagnosis is still not complete. As has to be expected in these hearts, there was an outlet chamber. However, this outlet chamber did not contain any inlet at all. Instead, there was a second rudimentary chamber that contained part of the straddling tricuspid valve. The two rudimentary chambers were almost completely separated by a septum, a very small muscular defect forming the only communication. Thus, the tricuspid valve straddled from a trabeculated pouch, and in addition there was a separate outlet chamber.

This malformation clearly illustrates that the terms used in the rigid system of the SCA have been very closely defined. Additional information is required to distinguish between different entities. Essential is the definition of a ventricle on basis of its inlet. Without this definition, an alternative option would be to term this malformation "two-chambered right ventricle with straddling tricuspid valve".

So far we have explained that important developmental and anatomical differences may exist between individual cases that are all classified under the term univentricular heart of left ventricular type. Evidently, it is always necessary to add a description of the status of the atrioventricular valves. The SCA provides for subgroups based on the presence of a complete double inlet, straddling, absent atrioventricular connection, or a common valve. These differentiations allow the embryologist or the cardiac morphologist using embryological concepts to classify the anomalies according to specific points of view. For instance, if he is studying straddling tricuspid valves as a natural entity, there is no doubt that this entity is dispersed throughout the groups of univentricular as well as biventricular hearts.

Sometimes there is a very wide dispersion of a developmental entity throughout the classification system. This is illustrated by the anatomy of hearts with concomitant straddling of both the tricuspid and the mitral valve. Obviously, such hearts, combining two circumscript developmental entities, form a new entity. What happens to this entity if these hearts are classified according to the SCA? If both valves override for less than 50%, a biventricular heart is present. A univentricular heart of left ventricular type exists if mitral overriding is less than 50% and tricuspid overriding is more than 50%. A univentricular heart of right ventricular type would have tricuspid overriding of less than 50%, but more than 50% overriding of the mitral orifice. Such a case is not purely theoretical and has been described by Bharati et al [21]. If both orifices override for more than 50%, then again the heart would be biventricular but very different from the first biventricular form within this category. The atrioventricular bloodstreams would cross each other, although not in the way described in hearts with a horizontal septum [21].

Summarizing the above considerations, we believe that the ideal classification system does not exist. However, as long as unambiguous definitions as used in the SCA system are our guide and as long as we keep filling in the classifying system with actual morphology, we are able to communicate in a common tongue.

REFERENCES

1. Shinebourne EA, Macartney FJ, Anderson RH: Sequential chamber localization. Logical approach to diagnosis in congenital heart disease. Br Heart J 38:327–340, 1976.
2. Tynan MJ, Becker AE, Macartney FJ, Quero Jimenez M, Shinebourne EA, Anderson RH: Nomenclature and classification of congenital heart disease. Br Heart J 41:544–553, 1979.
3. Anderson RH, Becker AE, Freedom RM, Quero Jimenez M, Macartney FJ, Shinebourne EA, Wilkinson JL, Tyan M: Problems in the nomenclature of the univentricular heart. Herz 4:97–106, 1979.
4. Keeton BR, Macartney FJ, Hunter S, Mortera G, Rees P, Shinebourne EA, Tynan M, Wilkinson JL, Anderson RH: Univentricular heart of right ventricular type with double or common inlet. Circulation 59:403–411, 1979.
5. Milo S, Yen Ho S, Macartney FJ, Wilkinson JL, Becker AE, Wenink ACG, Gittenberger-de Groot AC, Anderson RH: Straddling and overriding atrioventricular valves: morphology and classification. Am J Cardiol 44:1122–1134, 1979.
6. Davis CL: Development of the human heart from its first appearance to the stage found in embryos of twenty paired somites. Contrib Embryol 19:247–293, 1927.
7. Streeter GL: Developmental horizons in human embryos. Descriptions of age groups XV, XVI, XVII and XVIII. Contrib Embryol 32:133–204, 1948.
8. Pernkopf E, Wirtinger W: Die Transposition der Herzostien – Ein Versuch der Erklärung dieser Erscheinung. Z. Anat Entwicklungsgesch 100:563, 1933.
9. Asami I: Beitrag zur Entwicklung des Kammerseptums im menschlichen Herzen mit besonderer Berücksichtigung der sogenannten Bulbusdrehung. Z Anat Entwicklungsgesch 128:1–17, 1969.
10. Chuaqui B: Doerr's theory of morphogenesis of arterial transposition in light of recent research. Br Heart J 41: 481–485, 1979.
11. Van Praagh R, Plett JA, Van Praagh S: Single ventricle. Pathology, embryology, terminology and classification. Herz 4:113-150, 1979.
12. Bharati S, Lev M: The relationship between single ventricle and small outlet chamber and straddling and displaced tricuspid orifice and valve. Herz 4:176–183, 1979.
13. Van Mierop LHS: Embryology of the univentricular heart. Herz 4:78–85, 1979.
14. Dor X, Corone P: Experimental creation of univentricular heart in the chick embryo. Herz 4:91–96, 1979.
15. Wenink ACG: Embryology of the ventricular septum. Separate origin of its components. Virchows Arch [Pathol Anat] 370:71–79, 1981.
16. Lev M, Liberthson RR, Kirkpatrick JR, Eckner FAO, Arcilla RA: Single (primitive) ventricle. Circulation 39:577–591, 1969.
17. Van Gils FAW: The development of the human atrioventricular heart valves. J Anat 128:427, 1979.
18. Becker AE, Wilkinson JL, Anderson RH: Atrioventricular conduction tissues in univentricular hearts of left ventricular type. Herz 4:166–175, 1979.
19. Devloo-Blancquaert A, Ritter D: Muscle ridge between atrioventricular valves and malalignment of junction of these valves with ventricular septum. Br Heart J 40:1267–1274, 1978.
20. Wenink ACG: Considerations pertinent to the embryogenesis of transposition. In: Van Mierop LHS, Oppenheimer-Dekker A, Bruins CLDC (eds) Embryology and teratology of the heart and the great arteries. Leiden, Leiden University Press, 1978, pp 129–135.
21. Bharati S, McAllister HA, Lev M: Straddling and displaced atrioventricular orifices and valves. Circulation 60:673–684, 1979.

16. THE MORPHOLOGY OF SEPTAL STRUCTURES IN UNIVENTRICULAR HEARTS

ROBERT H. ANDERSON, SIEW YEN HO, AND ANTON E. BECKER

INTRODUCTION

Of necessity we must first address ourselves to the conundrum of the very existence of septal structures in univentricular hearts. It would be simpler if a univentricular heart were defined as having a sole chamber within the ventricular mass. Such hearts could then possess a septum dividing the ventricular outflow tracts, which on occasion could produce a discrete sub-arterial chamber, but this would be the only possible septal structure, namely an infundibular septum. From our knowledge of congenital malformations we know that such anomalies are exceedingly rare. Perhaps unfortunately they are not the only hearts referred to as "single ventricles". Far more common, although infrequent when considered in the whole range of congenital heart disease, are the hearts most usually described as "single ventricle" which paradoxically possess a second chamber within the ventricular mass [1, 2]. By general consensus [3, 4] the criterion for inclusion of a heart as a "single ventricle" is the presence of double inlet atrioventricular connexion. The itself controversial, since those authorities who initially accepted and for- acceptance of double inlet ventricle as the essence of single ventricle is now in itself controversial, since those authorities who initially accepted and for- mulated this approach [1] now argue that the approach is non-morphological [5]. Yet, despite their adoption of a "morphological approach", the same authorities continue to describe as "single ventricle" hearts with two discrete chambers in the ventricular mass when the major chamber is of left ventricular morphology while arguing that comparable hearts with two ventricular chambers but with the major chamber of right ventricular morphology are not univentricular [5].

Thus while there is general acceptance that hearts *can* be single ventricles and still possess two ventricular chambers, there is no agreement on precisely which hearts deserve to be considered univentricular [6–8]. In this chapter we present our own approach [9, 10], taking as our point of departure the general agreement that the anomaly most frequently termed "single ventricle with outlet chamber" or "single ventricle complex" [6] is indeed univentricular. We reiterate at this opening point that if there was general acceptance that hearts with two chambers in the ventricular mass should not be considered

A.C.G. Wenink et al. (eds.) The Ventricular Septum of the Heart, *203–224. All rights reserved.*
Copyright ©1981 by Martinus Nijhoff Publishers, The Hague/Boston/London.

"single ventricles", then the logic for our use of "univentricular heart" would vanish. Equally, having said that, it would be necessary to find another collective term for the hearts we group together as univentricular and which we will describe here. They have in common the feature that they possess one ventricular chamber connected to the atria and one chamber in the ventricular mass which lacks an atrioventricular connexion [10].

Since we have taken the malformation usually termed "single ventricle with outlet chamber" as our paradigm, and since it is unlikely that the world at large will stop calling this heart "single ventricle" [3, 4], it seems eminently reasonable to group the hearts as *univentricular*. To justify this use it is our convention [10, 11] to describe the chamber without a connexion to the atria as a rudimentary chamber; a rudimentary ventricular chamber but not a ventricle. By definition we demand that a chamber in the ventricular mass possess an atrioventricular connexion before we describe it as a *ventricle*.

OUTLET CHAMBER MORPHOLOGY IN "SINGLE VENTRICLE WITH OUTLET CHAMBER"

Since this anomaly is the cornerstone of our approach to univentricular hearts, it is appropriate to analyse the morphology and components of its second ventricular chamber which, if logic is to prevail, cannot be considered a ventricle. Others who categorize this anomaly as a "single ventricle" do so because they argue that the second chamber is an infundibular chamber and lacks a "sinus" [1, 2]. But definitions of a ventricular "sinus" are disappointingly vague [2, 8]. It is perhaps more fruitful to concentrate on the definition of an infundibulum. Most would agree that an infundibulum is that part of a ventricular chamber supporting an arterial valve, exemplified by the right ventricular infundibulum. Implicit in this use is that the infundibulum is a complete muscular structure, and on occasions it is well recognized that there may be bilateral infundibula, as for example frequently seen in double outlet right ventricle. It is also well known that in anomalies such as tetralogy of Fallot the infundibulum may become sequestrated as a discrete and smooth-walled *infundibular chamber*. If the second chamber in "single ventricle" is an infundibular chamber, it should therefore be comparable with the infundibular chamber to be found in tetralogy of Fallot. As may be expected, in tetralogy this chamber is separated from the rest of the ventricular mass by the infundibular septum (Fig. 1a). But the "outlet chamber" in single ventricle is of totally different morphology. It possesses an apical trabecular component (Fig. 1b). Its sub-arterial part is indeed infundibulum, and is separated from the main ventricular chamber by the infundibular septum. In contrast, an apical septal structure separates the trabecular part of the chamber from the

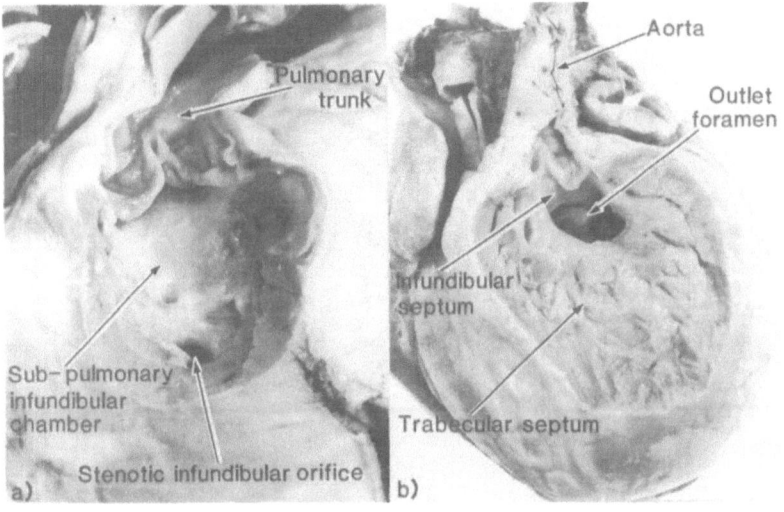

Fig. 1. Photographs illustrating the difference between an infundibular chamber in tetralogy of Fallot (*a*) and an outlet chamber in a univentricular heart (*b*). The infundibular chamber has only an outlet portion (i.e. is simply an infundibulum) while the outlet chamber has an infundibulum together with the trabecular component of right ventricular type. The trabecular component is separated by the trabecular septum from the main ventricular chamber. Figure *a* is reproduced by kind permission of Dr S.P. Allwork.

main chamber, and the foramen between main and outlet chambers is sandwiched between the infundibular and trabecular components of the septum (Fig. 2). Thus the justification for the second chamber not being a ventricle cannot be that it is simply an infundibulum. For us the justification of its rudimentary ventricular status is that it lacks an atrioventricular connexion, or in other words it lacks an inlet portion. This brings us to an important point which simplifies description of the hearts under discussion, however we categorize them. That is to consider the normal ventricular mass as possessing three components [12] rather than "sinus" and "conus".

THE TRIPARTITE VENTRICULAR SUB-DIVISION

If we open a normal heart and simply observe its ventricular endocardial surfaces, then from a descriptive standpoint it is inescapable that each ventricle possesses three parts (Fig. 3). The inlet portion extends from the atrioventricular annulus to the attachment of the papillary muscles. The trabecular component extends from the papillary muscles towards the apex while the outlet component supports the arterial valve, being in fibrous continuity

206

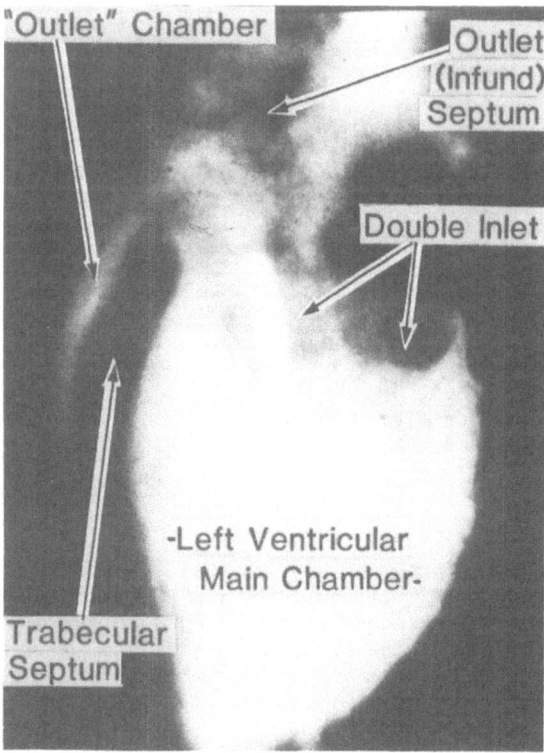

Fig. 2. Angiogram of a univentricular heart of left ventricular type with double inlet taken in a plane so as to profile the septum between the main and outlet chambers. If the outlet chamber were simply an infundibulum it would be separated from the main chamber by the infundibular septum. As can be seen, this is not the case, the chamber being separated from the main chamber by the extensive trabecular septum. Angiogram taken and provided by kind permission of Drs L.M. Bargeron, Jr., and B. Soto.

with the inlet component in the normal left ventricle (Fig. 3b). In the normal heart there are no discrete lines of demarcation between these ventricular components, nor is there any need to demand such demarcations. However, as we will see, the separate components are easily recognized and described in rudimentary ventricular chambers of malformed hearts since each of the components can exist in isolation.

Having divided the ventricles into three parts, it is then a logical extension to consider the ventricular septum as possessing three muscular components; inlet, trabecular and outlet septa, respectively. The right-sided trabecula septomarginalis, often accentuated by a leftward septal bend, overlies the boundaries of the inlet and trabecular septum and extends upwards to overlie the junction of the trabecular and outlet septa. The normal ventricular septum is completed by a fourth component, the membranous septum.

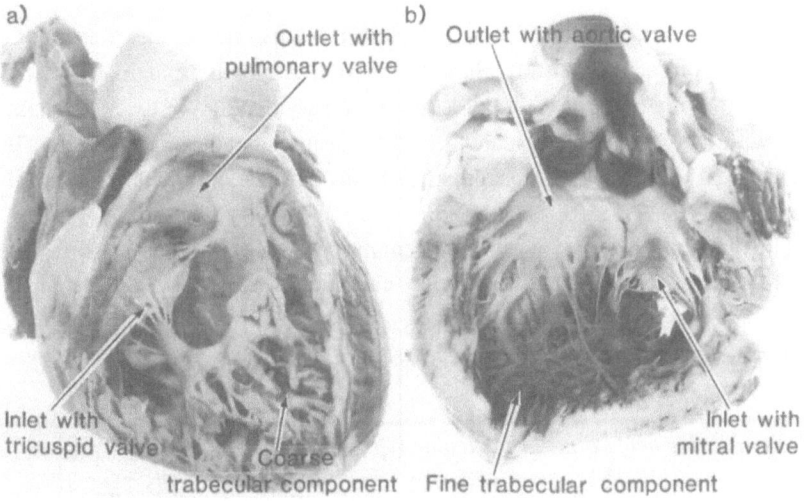

a)

Outlet with
pulmonary valve

b)

Outlet with aortic valve

Inlet with
tricuspid valve

Coarse
trabecular component

Fine trabecular component

Inlet with
mitral valve

Fig. 3. Photographs illustrating the tripartite nature of the normal right (*a*) and left (*b*) ventricles. Note the difference in trabecular pattern between the chambers.

When considering univentricular hearts we must also take account of septal orientation. To do this, the crux of the heart is distinguished as the point where the line of the atrial septum crosses the atrioventricular junction posteriorly. The acute and obtuse points of the junction are then 1 o'clock and 11 o'clock on the right and left atrioventricular orifices, respectively (Fig. 4).

SEPTAL MORPHOLOGY IN UNIVENTRICULAR HEARTS OF LEFT VENTRICULAR TYPE

A univentricular heart of left ventricular type exists when the main chamber connected to the atria has left ventricular trabecular pattern and the rudimentary chamber has the hypoplastic trabecular component of right ventricular

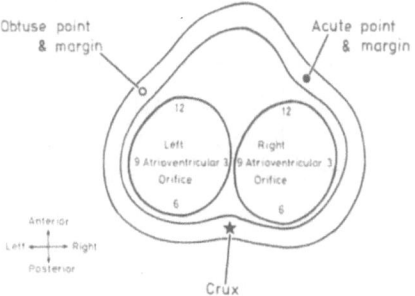

Obtuse point
& margin

Acute point
& margin

12

12

Left
9 Atrioventricular 3
Orifice

Right
9 Atrioventricular 3
Orifice

6

6

Anterior

Left ← → Right

Posterior

Crux

Fig. 4. Diagram illustrating the landmarks of the atrioventricular junction.

type. Within our definitions, size in itself is not a distinguishing criterion of a ventricle from a rudimentary chamber. A ventricle with an atrioventricular connexion may be large or small: similarly a rudimentary ventricular chamber without an atrioventricular connexion may be large or small. The anatomical components determine the status of a ventricular chamber, not its size.

Univentricular hearts of left ventricular type can exist when the atria are connected only to the left ventricular chamber because of double inlet or because either the right of left atrioventricular connexion is absent. These different connexions will be described separately.

Univentricular heart of left ventricular type with double inlet

This heart as we have seen is the paradigm of "single ventricle". Of necessity, the inlet ventricular septum is lacking. The trabecular septum separates the trabecular component of the rudimentary right ventricular chamber from the main chamber (Fig. 5). When both inlets have been exclusively committed to the main chamber, we have never seen an example of this anomaly in which the trabecular septum extended to the crux. In general terms, therefore, it can be stated that the hallmark of this heart is presence of a trabecular septum which does not extend to the crux. But this is not an inviolable criterion, since hearts can be imagined in which there could be double inlet to a left ventricular chamber and in which the trabecular septum might extend to the crux. We have seen one such heart in presence of overriding right atrioventricular valve (see below). It must be emphasized that our teminology has no embryological implications. From a developmental point of view, however, only the inlet septum can extend to the crux. This means that any septum extending to the crux must have an "embryonic" inlet component within it. In our terminology the inlet septum is used descriptively since it separates the two ventricular inlets. We therefore have to term the septum in hearts with overriding of the right atrioventricular valve just the trabecular septum. In our concept, as a general rule the trabecular septum in univentricular hearts of left ventricular type is an antero-superior structure. Its precise orientation varies with the relationship between main and rudimentary chambers. When the rudimentary chamber is right-sided, the septum usually extends posteriorly to the acute point of the atrioventricular junction. When the rudimentary chamber is left-sided, the trabecular septum extends to the obtuse point. When the chamber is directly anterior, then the septum is more or less in the frontal plane (Fig. 6).

The morphology of the rudimentary chamber, and hence its septal structure, is also related to the ventriculo-arterial connexion. In presence of double inlet atrioventricular connexion there is most usually a discordant ventriculo-

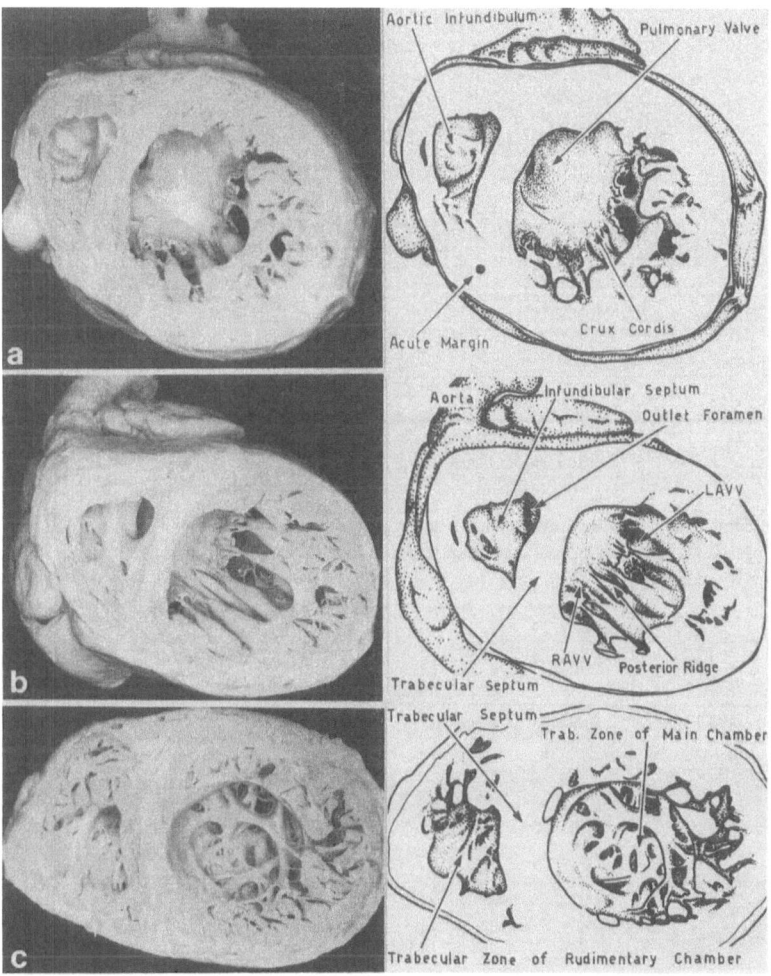

Fig. 5. Photographs illustrating the morphology of univentricular heart of left ventricular type with double inlet. The top two panels show the main chamber from different views and the septum between the chambers which does not extend to the crux. The lowest panel shows the removed apex of the heart and illustrates how each chamber has its own trabecular component. Reproduced by kind permission of Dr L.H.S. Van Mierop and the editors of *Herz*.

arterial connexion. Then, whatever the position of the rudimentary chamber, it is usual for the trabecular septum to be more extensive than the infundibular septum (the extent depending on the size of the trabecular component) and for the outlet foramen to be adjacent to the aortic valve (Fig. 7a). In contrast, in the rarer situation where there is ventriculo-arterial concordance, the infundibular septum is more extensive and the outlet foramen is positioned relatively centrally within the rudimentary chamber (Fig. 7b). When

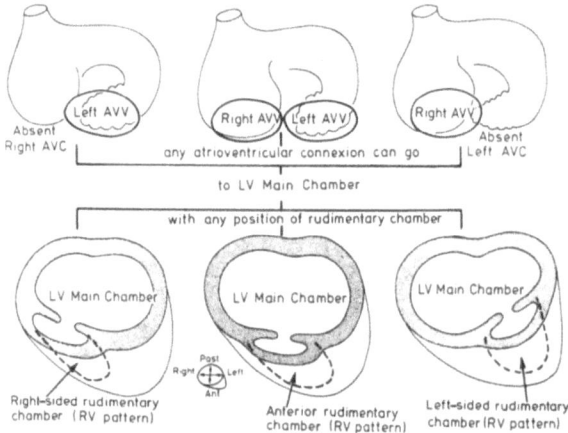

Fig. 6. Diagram illustrating how any atrioventricular connexion possible in a univentricular heart can co-exist with any position of the rudimentary ventricular chamber in a univentricular heart of left ventricular type.

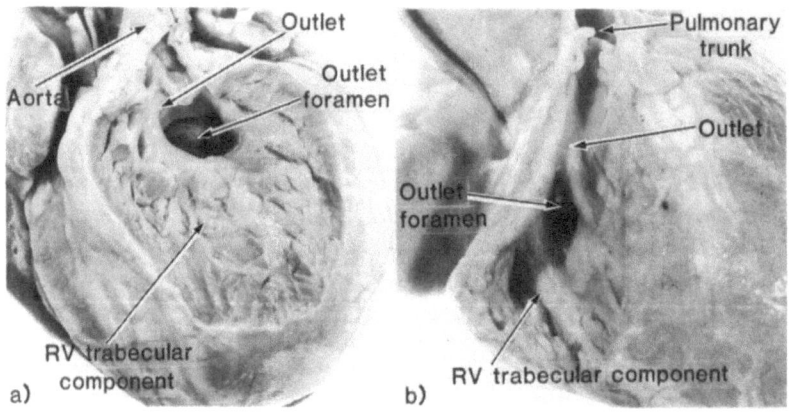

Fig. 7. Photographs illustrating the variable morphology of a rudimentary chamber of right ventricular type when there is ventriculo-arterial discordance (*a*) and ventriculo-arterial concordance (*b*).

there is double outlet from the main left ventricular chamber, then of necessity the rudimentary chamber lacks an outlet. It comprises solely the trabecular component of right ventricular type (Fig. 8). Exceedingly rarely both great arteries may arise from the rudimentary right ventricular chamber, and then each in our experience has had a well-formed infundibular component.

When univentricular hearts of left ventricular type with double inlet have

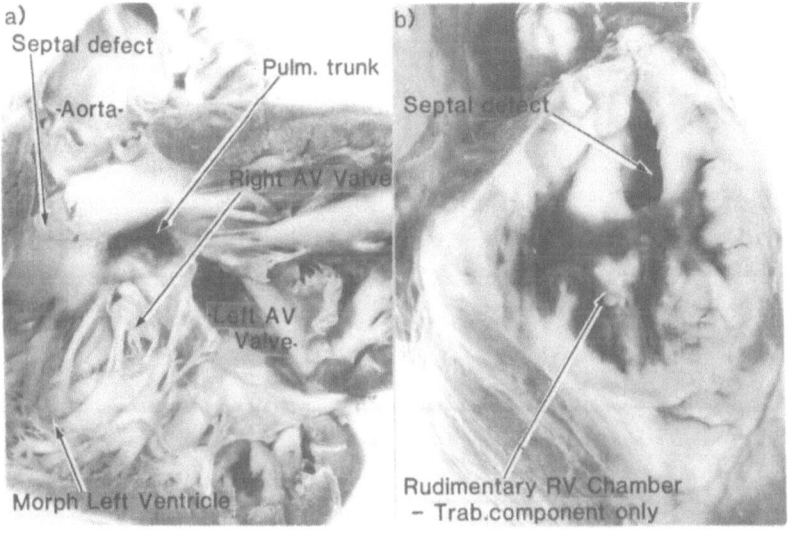

Fig. 8. Photographs showing how the trabecular component of the right ventricle can exist as a rudimentary chamber in its own right (*b*) when there is double inlet and double outlet to and from the left ventricular chamber.

an overriding atrioventricular valve, then the trabecular septum extends further towards the crux, but rarely reaches to the crux. These hearts were described in greater detail in the chapter devoted to septal morphology in hearts with straddling or overriding atrioventricular valves (see pp. 157–173).

Univentricular heart of LV type with absent right atrioventricular connexion

Assuming the presence of situs solitus, then univentricular hearts of left ventricular type with absent right atrioventricular connexion make up by far the greater majority of examples of "tricuspid atresia". This is not to say that all examples of tricuspid atresia are univentricular hearts. In a few cases an imperforate atrioventricular valve separates the right atrium from the right ventricle (Fig. 9). In these biventricular examples of tricuspid atresia the right ventricle has an inlet (albeit imperforate) and an inlet septum is present which extends to the crux. Usually there is a co-existing Ebstein's malformation (Fig. 9). But this type of tricuspid atresia is rare. In the classic type of tricuspid atresia the right ventricular chamber is rudimentary because it lacks an inlet (Fig. 10b), the right atrioventricular connexion being absent (Fig. 10a). By the token which makes "single ventricle with outlet chamber" a univentricular heart, then so is the classic type of tricuspid atresia [7]. As in "single ventricle with outlet chamber", the trabecular septum extends to the acute point of the

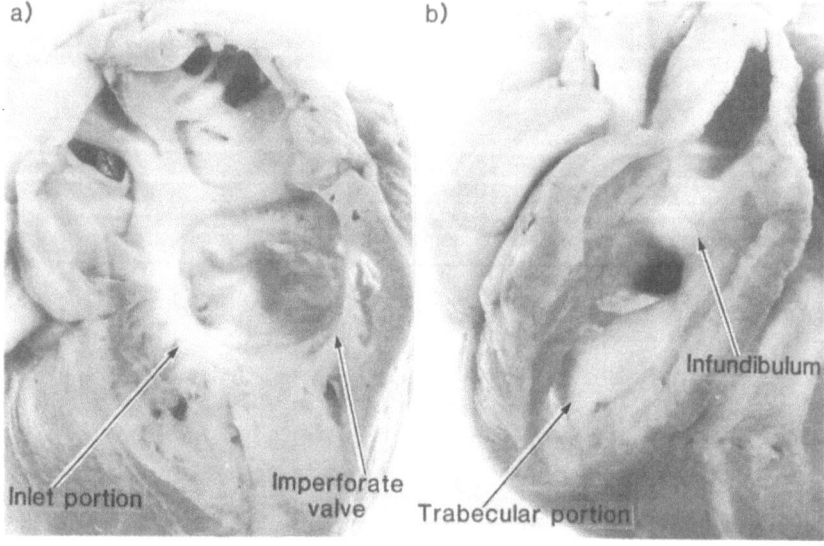

Fig. 9. Photographs illustrating the morphology of a biventricular heart with Ebstein's malformation and an imperforate tricuspid valve. (a) The imperforate valve membrane as viewed from the right atrium. The inlet component of the right ventricle is effectively part of the right atrium. (b) The trabecular and outlet components of the right ventricle which are separated by the imperforate valve from the right ventricular inlet portion. They are reached via a ventricular septal defect from the left ventricle.

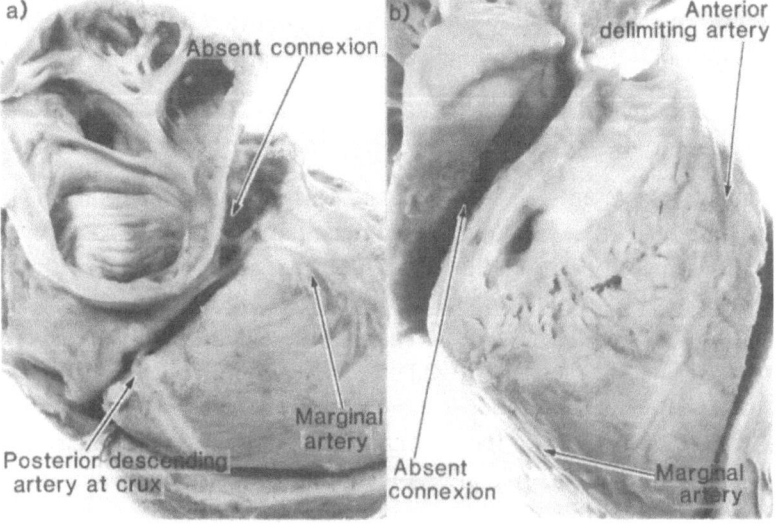

Fig. 10. Photographs illustrating the morphology of a univentricular heart of left ventricular type with absent right atrioventricular connexion (tricuspid atresia). (a) The absent right connexion is shown. (b) The rudimentary right ventricular chamber which possesses only trabecular and outlet components is shown.

atrioventricular junction and *not* to the crux, which means that it does not contain an embryonic inlet septal component. In both malformations the site of the septum is marked by delimiting arteries, the posterior extent being marked by a delimiting marginal artery (Fig. 10a).

A possible source of confusion when comparing right ventricular morphology in the two anomalies is that most frequently "single ventricle with outlet chamber" is found with ventriculo-arterial discordance, whereas "tricuspid atresia" exists usually with ventriculo-arterial concordance. But when the two anomalies are compared in presence of the same ventriculo-arterial connexion, then the morphology of the rudimentary right ventricular chamber is more or less identical (compare Figs. 7b and 10b). Furthermore, while the rudimentary chamber in classic tricuspid atresia is usually right-sided, it may be directly anterior or even on occasions *left-sided* [13] without altering its basic morphology. It is perhaps paradoxical that those authorities who proclaim the "morphological method" [5] would presumably be obliged to call a univentricular heart of left ventricular type with absent right atrioventricular connexion and left-sided rudimentary chamber an example of mitral atresia, since the left-sided rudimentary chamber would surely indicate an "l-loop".

What when the rudimentary chamber is directly anterior? Here presumably, because there is no intermediate "loop", the chamber will be judged to be left-sided or right-sided and the heart become mitral atresia or tricuspid atresia accordingly. This smacks of a 50% rule. This would surely be an uncharacteristic approach for one who criticizes us for our use of a similar rule in determining the connexion in hearts with overriding valves [5].

Univentricular hearts of LV type with absent left atrioventricular connexion

Exactly the same variability in rudimentary chamber position and septal orientation is to be found in hearts with main chamber of left ventricular pattern when the left atrioventricular connexion is absent. Here, however, it is more usual to find a left-sided rudimentary right ventricular chamber which lacks an inlet (Fig. 11b). Right-sided rudimentary right ventricular chambers (Fig. 11) are by no means uncommon. Again the trabecular septum is an anterior structure and rarely if ever extends to the crux. There is more general agreement that such hearts with right-sided rudimentary chambers should be considered univentricular [14, 15]. In this instance, then, any logic which permits a univentricular heart of left ventricular type with absent left atrioventricular connexion and right-sided rudimentary chamber to be a single ventricle [14, 15] cannot deny status to a similar heart just because the rudimentary chamber happens to be left-sided (compare Fig. 11a and b). Similarly it seems procrustean to call one of these hearts "mitral atresia" [14] and the other "tricuspid atresia" [16] simply because of the position of the

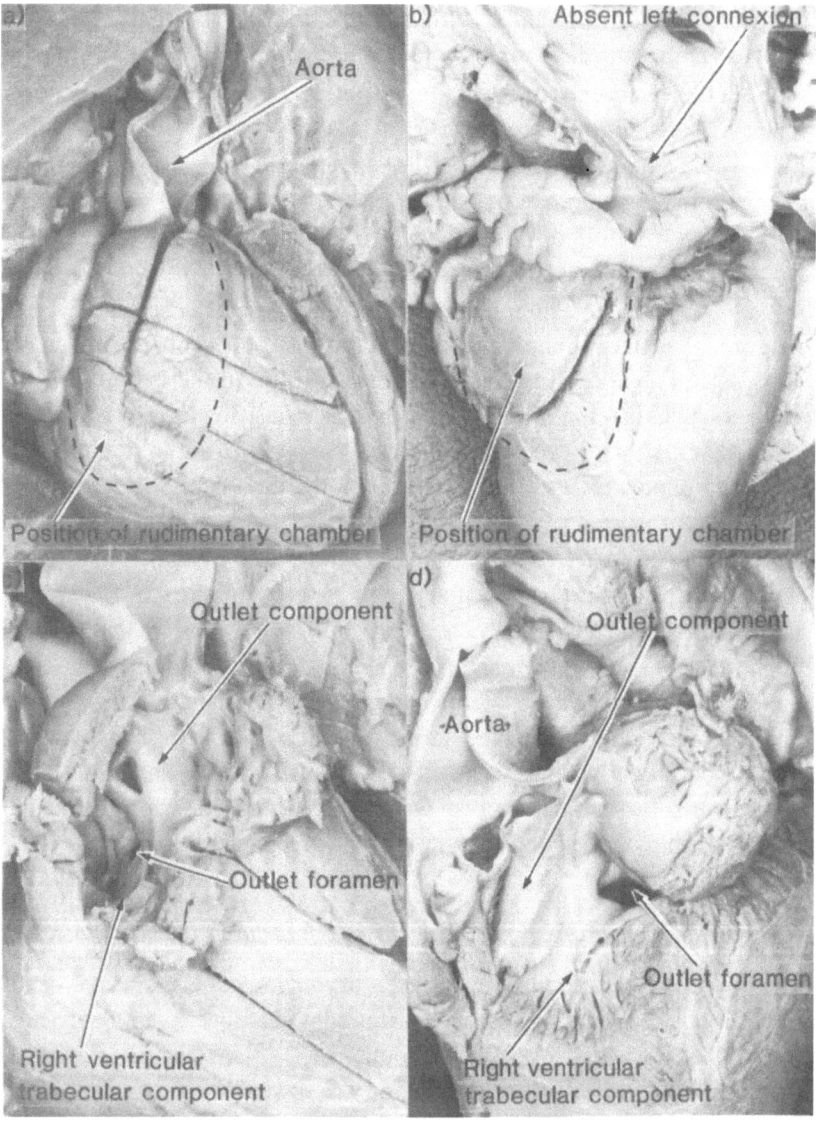

Fig. 11. Photographs illustrating the variability in position of the rudimentary chamber of right ventricular type in univentricular hearts of left ventricular type with absent left atrioventricular connexion. (*a* and *c*) The position and morphology of a right-sided rudimentary chamber. (*b* and *d*) A left-sided rudimentary chamber. The morphology of the hearts is the same apart from the position of the rudimentary chambers. Figures 11a and c are taken from the front, while 11b and d are taken from the left side. Hearts phonographed and reproduced by the kind permission of Dr. J.R. Zuberbuhler.

rudimentary chamber. It is less ambiguous to describe both as univentricular hearts of left ventricular type with absent left atrioventricular connexion and then describe the position of the rudimentary right ventricular chamber.

SEPTAL MORPHOLOGY IN UNIVENTRICULAR HEARTS OF RIGHT VENTRICULAR TYPE

When adjudicating the candidacy of hearts with main chamber of right ventricular type for univentricular status, a distinction must be drawn between, on the one hand, morphological features and, on the other hand, considerations of either embryology or homology. There can be little doubt that, during its development, a heart with double inlet to a main right ventricular chamber went through a stage in which the left ventricular chamber was connected to the atria [17]. This embryological history is discussed more fully elsewhere in this book (see Chapter 3). Equally, there is little doubt that the definitive left ventricular chamber in a heart with double inlet to a right ventricular chamber is remarkably similar to a left ventricle. This is hardly surprising since both possess the trabecular component of left ventricular pattern. But in this chapter we are concerned with neither embryological nor comparative considerations, but with morphology as it is observed in the definitive heart. As we have discussed above, the feature which for us denies a ventricular chamber the status of a ventricle is its lack of an inlet. Again, as with univentricular hearts of left ventricular type, the *size* of the chamber, be it ventricle or rudimentary, is of no definitive concern. This does not mean that the size of the chamber is unimportant, but simply that it does not influence our decision as to whether the chamber is to be considered a ventricle. Within the criteria we have established for distinction of univentricular hearts, it would be artificial if we were to exclude from the univentricular category hearts those with a main ventricular chamber of right ventricular trabecular pattern which possessed a second ventricular chamber of left ventricular pattern but in which the second chamber lacked an inlet portion [18–20]. Morphological and angiographic findings then show that such univentricular hearts of right ventricular type can, as with univentricular hearts of left ventricular type, be found with either double inlet [18, 19] or with absence of the right or left atrioventricular connexion [11, 20] (Fig. 12).

Univentricular hearts of right ventricular type with double inlet

These hearts have a main chamber of right ventricular type receiving both atrioventricular connexions through either two separate atrioventricular valves or a common valve, and possess a rudimentary left ventricular cham-

216

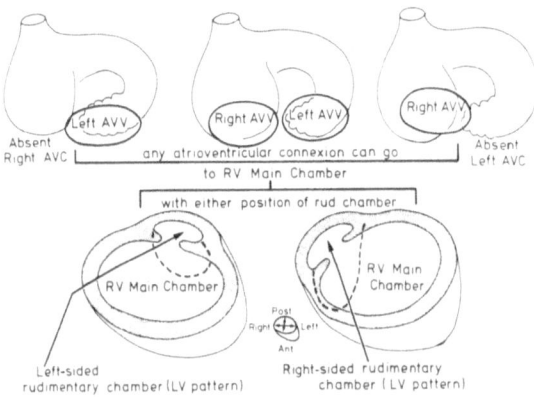

Fig 12. Diagram illustrating how atrioventricular connexions of double inlet or absent connexion can be found with different position of the rudimentary chamber in univentricular hearts of right ventricular type.

ber which of necessity lacks an inlet. The left ventricular chamber most frequently also lacks an outlet, there being either double outlet or single outlet from the main right ventricular chamber [18, 19]. Then the rudimentary chamber is made up solely of the left ventricular trabecular component, which may be large in the presence of a straddling or overriding valve (Fig. 13a) but which more frequently is tiny (Fig. 13b). In a minority of hearts the rudimentary chamber may give rise to a great artery, and then is a left ventricular outlet chamber (Fig. 14), usually of reasonable size. When the left ventricular chamber is only a pouch, then the septum between it and the main chamber is exclusively a trabecular septum (albeit that embryologically the septum may contain an inlet portion). When an outlet chamber is present, the outlet foramen will be the space between trabecular and outlet septa. The feature of the trabecular septum in univentricular hearts of right ventricular type with double inlet is that almost exclusively it extends to the crux (Fig. 12), witnessing the fact that it contains an embryonic inlet septal component. However, its orientation varies depending on the position of the rudimentary chamber which, although always posterior, may be left-sided (Fig. 13a) or less frequently right-sided (Fig. 13b). We have never encountered a univentricular heart of right ventricular type with double inlet in which the septum did *not* extend to the crux, but the possibility must exist.

Fig. 13. Photographs illustrating the varying size of rudimentary chambers in univentricular hearts of right ventricular type. (*a*) A good size rudimentary chamber when there is minimal straddling of the left atrioventricular valve. (*b*) The right-sided rudimentary chamber is tiny. However, each chamber has the same basic component, namely the trabecular component of left ventricular type. It is the lack of an inlet which determines that each chamber is rudimentary.

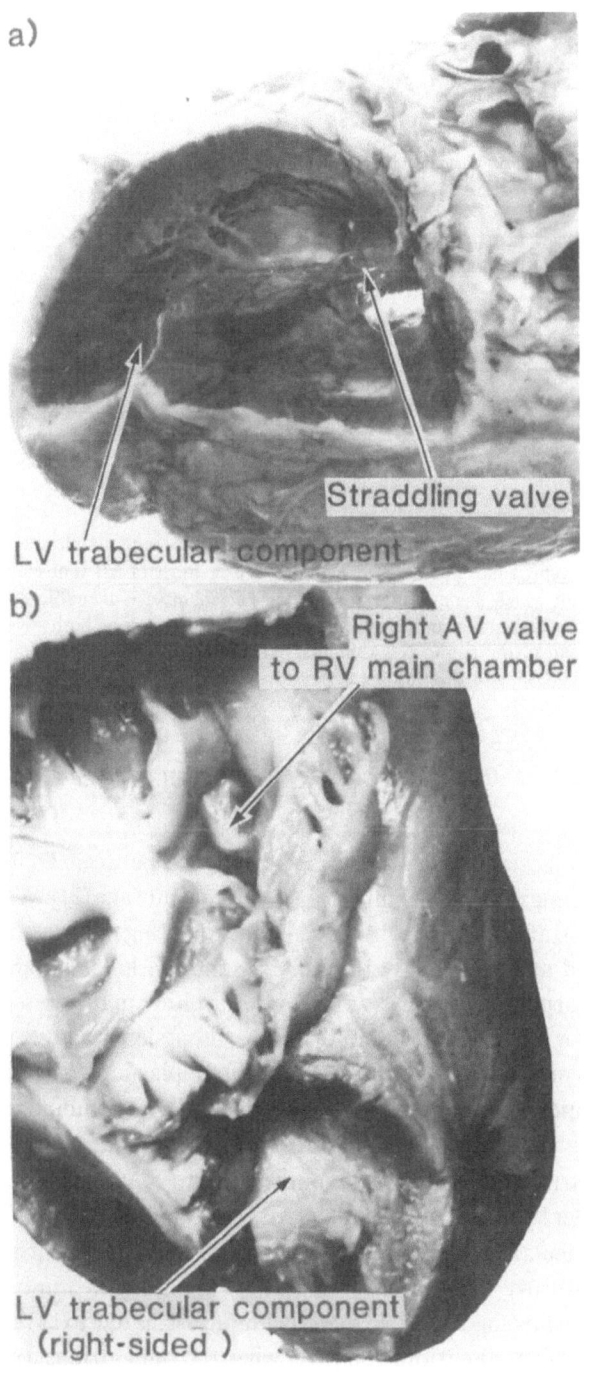

a)

Straddling valve

LV trabecular component

b)

Right AV valve
to RV main chamber

LV trabecular component
(right-sided)

218

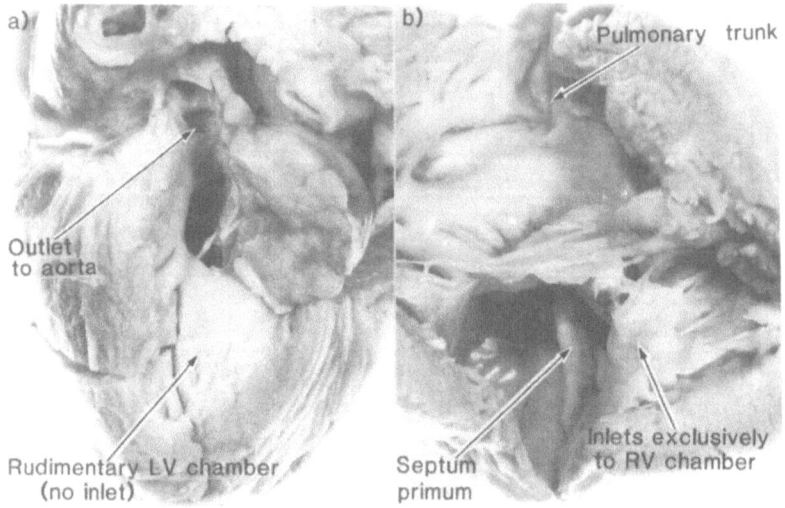

Fig. 14. Photographs of a univentricular heart of right ventricular type with double inlet and an outlet chamber of left ventricular type. (*a*) The rudimentary chamber of left ventricular type which lacks an inlet but which has an outlet, the aorta. The chamber is therefore an outlet chamber. (*b*) The main ventricular chamber of right ventricular type receiving both atrial inlets via a common valve and giving rise to the pulmonary trunk (i.e. there is ventriculo-arterial concordance).

Univentricular hearts of right ventricular type with absent left atrioventricular connexion

It is not generally accepted that there is a difference between an absent atrioventricular connexion and an imperforate valve membrane [21]. We have discussed the importance of this distinction in understanding the morphology of classic tricuspid atresia. Exactly the same distinction holds good when considering the morphology of classic mitral atresia, either in the presence of aortic atresia [22] or a patent aortic root [23]. This discussion is admittedly of more academic significance in the presence of "hypoplastic left heart syndrome", but of importance nonetheless. In some hearts with combined aortic and mitral atresia there is an unequivocal valve membrane to be found between the left atrium and a severely hypoplastic left ventricle. This can be demonstrated either by histology [24] or by gross examination (Fig. 15). Such hearts are biventricular hearts with severely hypoplastic left ventricles and imperforate mitral valves. In our experience, they make up the minority of examples of "mitral atresia". More frequently, the atresia is due to absence of the left atrioventricular connexion, and then, when the right atrium connects to a right ventricular chamber, the left ventricular chamber must perforce lack an inlet and hence be rudimentary (Fig. 16). As with double inlet to a

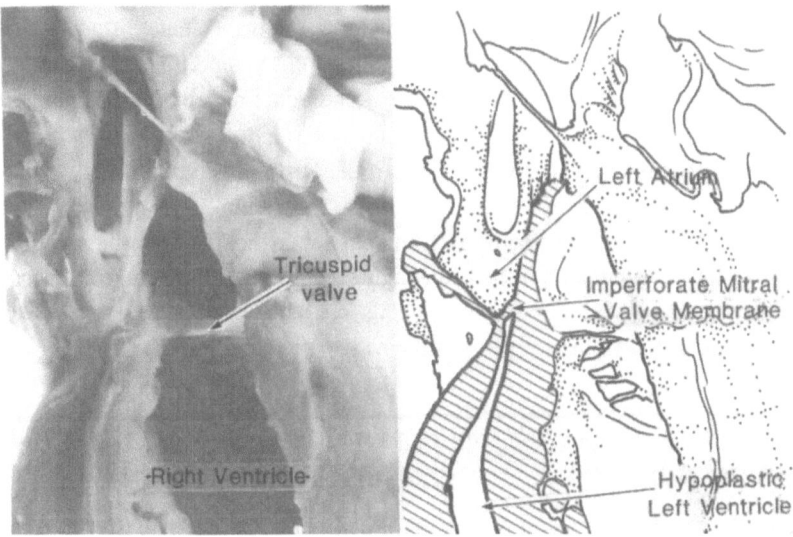

Fig. 15. A section through the left atrium and the hypoplastic left ventricle in a heart with atrioventricular concordance and an imperforate left atrioventricular valve (mitral atresia). The chambers are viewed from behind. The drawing shows the salient features.

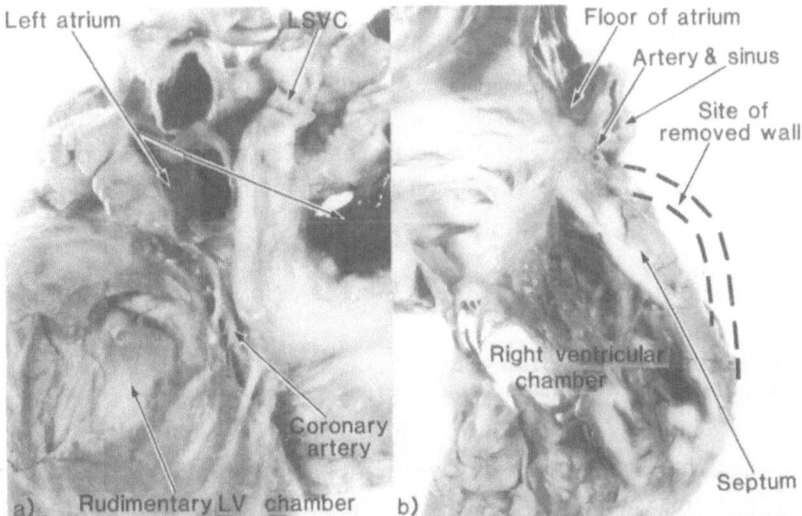

Fig. 16. Photographs illustrating the morphology of a univentricular heart of right ventricular type with absent left atrioventricular connexion (mitral atresia). (*a*) The left atrioventricular junction with the atrioventricular sulcus separating the floor of the left atrium from the rudimentary left ventricular chamber which comprises solely the trabecular component of left ventricular type. (*b*) A section through the junction viewed from the front. The part of the left ventricular parietal wall removed in the preparation of *a* has been inked in to show its position. Note how the coronary artery and coronary sinus (draining a persistent left superior vena cava – LSVC) interpose between left atrial floor and the rudimentary left ventricular chamber.

univentricular heart of right ventricular type, the trabecular septum almost always extends to the crux and the rudimentary chamber is posterior (Fig. 12). The rudimentary chamber, while usually left-sided, may on occasion be right-sided. It is usually a trabecular pouch but may be an outlet chamber. When it is an outlet chamber it usually gives rise to the aorta but in one heart we have studied it gave rise to the pulmonary trunk (ventriculo-arterial discordance) [22]. In one of the few examples of univentricular heart of right ventricular type we have seen in which the trabecular septum did not extend to the crux, there was an absent left atrioventricular connexion with straddling and overriding of the right atrioventricular valve (see Chapter 12).

Univentricular hearts of right ventricular type with absent right atrioventricular connexion

These hearts are uncommon, but perhaps their apparent paucity reflects a general unawareness of their existence. In our initial paper concerning tricuspid atresia [13], we described examples with sole ventricular chambers. While such hearts undoubtedly do exist, on re-examination of one of these hearts we found the main chamber to be of right ventricular pattern and discovered a small posterior right-sided left ventricular rudimentary pouch. Since then we have encountered similar hearts during angiographic examination [20] and found several examples with straddling and overriding left atrioventricular valves. Generally speaking, the trabecular septum extends to the crux, although this is not the case when the left valve overrides to any great extent. The rudimentary left ventricular chamber has always been right-sided and posterior, but there is no reason why it should not be left-sided (Fig. 12).

INFLUENCE OF SEPTAL MORPHOLOGY ON CONDUCTION TISSUE DISPOSITION

From our knowledge of development of conduction tissue [25–27] and its disposition in malformed hearts [20–31] we can deduce that two features are paramount in determining its morphology. They are firstly the presence or absence of a trabecular septum extending to the crux and secondly the pattern of ventricular architecture. When the trabecular septum, which carries the ventricular conduction tissues, does *not* extend to the crux, i.e. when it has not connected with the embryonic inlet septum carrying the proximal portion of the atrioventricular bundle, then the anomalous connecting atrioventricular node is found irrespective of the ventricular architecture. In univentricular hearts of left ventricular type the node is formed at the point where the trabecular septum reaches closest to the morphologically right atrioventricular junction. So, in presence of double inlet atrioventricular connexion, the node is formed anteriorly in the morphologically right atrioventricular orifice [28], be the rudimentary chamber right-sided or left-sided. The side of the rudimentary chamber affects only the relationship of the non-branching bundle to the outflow tract of the main chamber [32, 33]. In univentricular hearts of left ventricular type with absent left atrioventricular connexion, the connecting node is again anomalously located, being found anteriorly in the right atrioventricular orifice [30]. In contrast, when the right atrioventricular connexions absent in univentricular hearts of left ventricular type (classic tricuspid atresia), the septum approximates the crux but does not reach it. Because there is no right atrioventricular orifice to separate regular and anomalous nodes, a large node is formed in the floor of the blind-ending right atrium. Penetration into the ventricle and the course of the conduction tissue within the ventricle is directly comparable to that found in hearts of left ventricular type with double inlet [34].

The orientation of the septum in also an important feature in univentricular hearts of right ventricular type. When it does not extend to the crux, as in some examples with absent atrioventricular connexions and straddling valves, then grossly abnormal conduction systems are found with anomalous nodes at the junction of the trabecular septum with the atrioventricular junction [30]. However, when the septum does extend to the crux, then its influence is subordinate to the ventricular architecture. Thus in univentricular heart of right ventricular type with right-hand pattern ventricular architecture, there is a regular conduction system [35]. In contrast, when there is a left-hand pattern of ventricular architecture ("l-loop"), then an anomalous conduction system is formed despite the fact that the trabecular septum extends to the crux [36]. The basic rules are therefore – septum *not* to crux – anomalous conduction system; septum to crux – conduction system disposition subordinate to the pattern of ventricular architecture.

CONCLUSIONS

We have described septal morphology in a group of hearts unified by one feature, namely that only one of the two chambers present within the ventricular mass possesses an atrioventricular connexion. Whatever we choose to call these hearts, they warrant corporate consideration. It is our preference to consider them under the title of *univentricular hearts*. Univentricular hearts can then be divided into two sub-groups on the basis of ventricular trabecular pattern. The first group has main chambers of left ventricular pattern and rudimentary chambers of right ventricular pattern. The second group has main chambers of right ventricular pattern and rudimentary chambers of left ventricular pattern. Either sub-group can be found with double inlet atrioventricular connexion or with absence of the right or absence of the left atrioventricular connexion. Of necessity no heart in the overall group can possess an inlet septum in a descriptive anatomical sense, although remants of the embryonic inlet septum may be distinguished. Generally the disposition of the trabecular septum goes along with the sub-grouping. It is positioned in antero-superior position and rarely extends to the crux in univentricular hearts of left ventricular type. In contrast it is postero-inferior and almost always extends to the crux in univentricular hearts of right ventricular type. The presence or absence of a trabecular septum which extends to the crux is paramount in determining conduction tissue disposition. When *not* to the crux, there is always an anomalously positioned connecting atrioventricular node. When the septum does extend to the crux, then the pattern of ventricular architecture is the dominant feature.

Acknowledgements. We are indebted to our many friends and colleagues who contributed so much to the formulation of the concepts expressed herein; notably, Mike Tynan, Fergus Macartney, Elliot Shinebourne, Manuel Quero-Jiminez, Jim Wilkinson, David Dickinson, Audrey Smith, Bob Freedom, Bob Van Mierop, Arnold Wenink, Adriana Gittenberger-de Groot, Nienke Essed, Gaetano Thiene, Bob Zuberbuhler and John Mickell. We thank Joan Otto and Christine Anderson for their help in the preparation of the manuscript. This work has been supported by grants from the British Heart Foundation.

REFERENCES

1. Van Praagh R, Ongley PA, Swan HJC: Anatomic types of single or common ventricle in man: morphologic and geometric aspects of sixty necropsied cases. Am J Cardiol 13:367–386, 1964.
2. Lev M, Liberthson RR, Kirkpatrick JR, Eckner FAO, Arcilla RA: Single (primitive) ventricle. Circulation 39:577–591, 1969.
3. Ellis K: Angiography in complex congenital heart disease: single ventricle, double inlet, double outlet and transposition. In: Davila JC (ed) 2nd Henry Ford Hospital International Symposium on Cardiac Surgery. New York, Appleton-Century-Crofts, 1977, pp 223–224.
4. Edwards JE: Discussion. In: Davila JC (ed) 2nd Henry Ford Hospital International Symposium on Cardiac Surgery. New York, Appleton-Century-Crofts, 1977, p 242.
5. Van Praagh R, Plett JA, Van Praagh S: Single ventricle. Herz 4:113–150, 1979.
6. Bharati S, Lev M: The relationship between single ventricle and small outlet chamber and straddling and displaced tricuspid orifice and valve. Herz 4:176–183, 1979.
7. Anderson RH, Becker AE, Macartney FJ, Shinebourne EA, Wilkinson JL, Tynan MJ: Is "tricuspid atresia" a univentricular heart? Pediatr Cardiol 1:51–56, 1979.
8. Bharati S, Lev M: The concept of tricuspid atresia complex as distinct from that of the single ventricle complex. Pediatr Cardiol 1:57–62, 1979.
9. Wilkinson JL, Becker AE, Tynan MJ, Freedom R, Macartney FJ, Shinebourne EA, Quero-Jimenez M, Anderson RH: The nomenclature of the univentricular heart. Herz 4:107–112, 1979.
10. Anderson RH, Tynan MJ, Freedom RM, Quero-Jimenez M, Macartney FJ, Shinebourne EA, Wilkinson JL, Becker AE: Ventricular morphology in the univentricular heart. Herz 4:184–197, 1979.

11. Tynan MJ, Becker AE, Macartney FJ, Quero-Jimenez M, Shinebourne EA, Anderson RH: Nomenclature and classification of congenital heart disease. Br Heart J 41:544–553, 1979.
12. Goor DA, Lillehei CW: Congenital malformations of the heart. New York, Grune and Stratton, 1975, pp 11–13.
13. Anderson RH, Wilkinson JL, Gerlis LM, Smith A, Becker AE: Atresia of the right atrio-ventricular orifice. Br. Heart J 39:414–428, 1977.
14. Quero M: Atresia of the left atrioventricular orifice associated with a Holmes heart. Circulation 42:739–744, 1970.
15. Quero M: Coexistence of single ventricle with atresia of one atrioventricular orifice. Circulation 46:794–798, 1972.
16. Tandon R, Edwards JE: Tricuspid atresia. A re-evaluation and classification. J Thorac Cardiovasc Surg 67:530–542, 1974.
17. Quero-Jimenez M, Perez Martinez VM, Maitre Azcarte MJ, Merino-Batres G, Moreno Granados F: Exaggerated displacement of the atrioventricular canal towards the bulbus cordis (rightward displacement of the mitral valve). Br Heart J 35:65–74, 1973.
18. Keeton BR, Macartney FJ, Hunter S, Mortera C, Rees P, Shinebourne EA, Tynan MJ, Wilkinson JL, Anderson RH: Univentricular heart of right ventricular type with double or common inlet. Circulation 59:403–411, 1979.
19. Soto B, Bertranou EG, Bream PR, Souza A Jr, Bargeron LM Jr: Angiographic study of univentricular heart of right ventricular type. Circulation 60:1325–1334, 1979.
20. Shinebourne EA, Lau KC, Calcaterra G, Anderson RH: Univentricular heart of right ventricular type – clinical, angiographic and electrocardiographic features. Am J Cardiol 46: 439–445, 1980.
21. Bharati S, Lev M: Reply to letter. Pediatr Cardiol 1:165–166, 1980.
22. Thiene G, Daliente L, De Tomasi M, Macartney F, Anderson RH: The anatomical substrates producing atresia of the morphologically left atrioventricular orifice. Br Heart J 45: 393–401, 1981.
23. Mickell JJ, Mathews RA, Zuberbuhler JR, Lenox CC, Neches WH, Park SC, Fricker FJ, Anderson RH: The morphology of "mitral atresia" with patent aortic outflow tract. Am J Cardiol (submitted for publication).
24. Gittenberger-de Groot AC: Het links hypoplastische hart als aangeboren afwijking. Thesis, University of Leiden, Luctor et Emergo, Leiden, 1972, p 22.
25. Anderson RH, Taylor IM: Development of atrioventricular specialised tissue in human heart. Br Heart J 34:1205–1214, 1972.
26. Wenink ACG: Development of the human cardiac conducting system. J Anat 121:617–631, 1976.
27. Anderson RH, Becker AE, Wenink ACG: The development of the conducting tissues. In: Roberts NK, Gelband H (ed) Arrythmias in the neonate, infant and child. New York, Appleton-Century-Crofts, 1977, pp 1–28.
28. Anderson RH, Arnold R, Thaper MK, Jones RS, Hamilton DI: Cardiac specialized tissues in hearts with an apparently single ventricular chamber. (Double inlet left ventricle.) Am J Cardiol 33:95–106, 1974.
29. Bharati S, Lev M: The course of the conduction system in single ventricle with inverted (L) loop and inverted (L) transposition. Circulation 51:723–730, 1975.
30. Becker AE, Wilkinson JL, Anderson RH: Atrioventricular conduction tissues: a guide in understanding the morphogenesis of the univentricular heart. In: Van Praagh R, Takao A (eds) Etiology and morphogenesis of congenital heart disease. Mt. Kisco, New York, Futura, pp 489–514.
31. Anderson RH, Wilkinson JL, Becker AE: Conducting tissues in the univentricular heart. In: Van Mierop LHS, Oppenheimer-Dekker A, Bruins CLDC (eds) Embryology and teratology of the heart and great arteries. The Hague, Martinus Nijhoff, 1978, pp 62–78.
32. Wenink ACG: The conduction tissues in primitive ventricle with outlet chamber: two different possibilities. J Thorac Cardiovasc Surg 75:747–753, 1978.
33. Essed CE, Ho SY, Shinebourne EA, Joseph MC, Anderson RH: Further observations on conduction tissues in univentricular hearts. Eur Heart J 2:87–96, 1981.
34. Dickinson DF, Wilkinson JL, Smith A, Becker AE, Anderson RH: Atrioventricular con-

duction tissues in univentricular hearts of left ventricular type with absent right atrio-ventricular connection ("tricuspid atresia"). Br Heart J 42:1–8, 1979.

35. Wilkinson JL, Dickinson DF, Smith A, Anderson RH: Conducting tissues in univentricular heart of right ventricular type with double or common inlet. J Thorac Cardiovasc Surg 77:691–698, 1979.

36. Essed CE, Ho SY, Hunter S, Anderson RH: Atrioventricular conduction system in uni-ventricular heart of right ventricular type with right-sided rudimentary chamber. Thorax 35:123–127, 1980.

17. CROSS-SECTIONAL ECHOCARDIOGRAPHIC RECOGNITION OF SEPTAL STRUCTURES IN UNIVENTRICULAR HEARTS

DAVID J. SAHN, JOYCE HARDER, ROBERT FREEDOM, WALTER DUNCAN, AND RICHARD ROWE

INTRODUCTION

While surgical septation operations for patients with univentricular hearts are no longer widely practised, newer surgical techniques involving "Fontan"-type atrial to pulmonary artery connections for palliation of these complex malformations continue to require detailed delineation of the atrioventricular (AV) valve structure and outflow chamber morphology in these patients. M-mode echocardiography enables to some extent the non-invasive diagnosis of forms of univentricular hearts [1, 2] especially when combined with echocontrast techniques [3, 4]. Recent reports have suggested that two-dimensional echocardiography [5] has even greater utility in the examination of patients with univentricular hearts for defining atrioventricular valve morphology, the absences of valves or the degree of valve straddling. There has been some suggestion that 2D echo provides this type of information with details superior to those obtained by angiography.

Improvements in the resolution of two-dimensional systems and development of new views [6] have provided new capabilities for examination of these patients with two-dimensional echocardiography. A systematic approach to the morphology of these hearts [7] has aided the echocardiographer in defining and describing these malformations.

PATIENTS AND METHODS

We have recently reviewed two-dimensional echocardiographic data from 44 patients studied with electronically or dynamically focussed phased array sector scanners who were subsequently shown to have an angiographic, surgical or post-mortem diagnosis of univentricular heart. Only ten of the patients in this series have to this point in time had their hearts examined directly either by surgery or at autopsy. The remainder of the anatomical data was confirmed by angiographic evaluation.

For the performance of the two-dimensional echocardiogram, all the standard views were obtained on each exam [6] and special emphasis was placed on attempting to resolve the chordal structures of the valves, image the

A.C.G. Wenink et al. (eds.) The Ventricular Septum of the Heart, *225–233. All rights reserved.*

trabecular pattern of the main and rudimentary chambers as well as the divisions between the rudimentary and main chambers bordering the outlet foramen.

Of the patients, 33 had univentricular hearts of the left ventricular type with an angiographically definable rudimentary chamber. In five patients the left-sided and in 12 the right-sided AV connection was absent. Five patients had univentricular heart of the right ventricular type with a definable rudimentary chamber. Two of these had a blind trabecular pouch and no outflow from the rudimentary chamber. Six patients had indeterminate-type univentricular heart, all without angiographic visualisation of an outflow chamber.

RESULTS – DIAGNOSIS AND AV VALVE MORPHOLOGY

The correct diagnosis of univentricular heart was achieved by using two-dimensional echocardiography in all but two patients. The two patients who were missed occurred early in the series and had double inlet univentricular heart of left ventricular type with prominent papillary muscle ridges, which were mistaken for septation. In the recent studies, no diagnoses of double

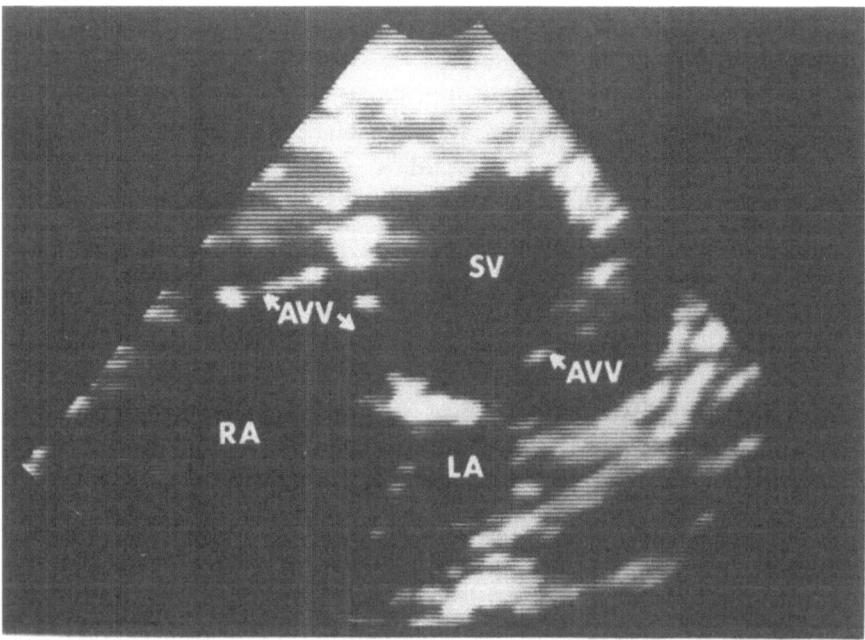

Fig. 1. An apical four chamber view shows two AV valves (AVV) with chordal-papillary muscle anchorings into the single ventricle (SV). The right AV valve was incompetent and therefore the right atrium (RA) was significantly larger than the left atrium (LA).

inlet type have been confused since with higher resolution the chordal attachments of the valves to the papillary muscle do not allow the confusion of these apical structures with septation. The 2D echoes correctly predicted 25 of the 27 patients with a double inlet main chamber and the five patients with absent left-sided and 12 with absent right-sided AV connection. This experience in the accuracy of defining the AV valve connection patterns (Fig. 1) agrees with the previous study by Picchio et al. [5]. In several instances (Fig. 2) overriding of an AV valve towards the rudimentary chamber could also be identified echocardiographically.

TRABECULAR AND SEPTAL STRUCTURES

More central to the main topic of this Boerhaave Conference on "the ventricular septum" have been our results with regard to the 2D echo imaging of septal structures partitioning the main from the rudimentary chamber, our imaging of the rudimentary chamber itself as well as our attempts to define

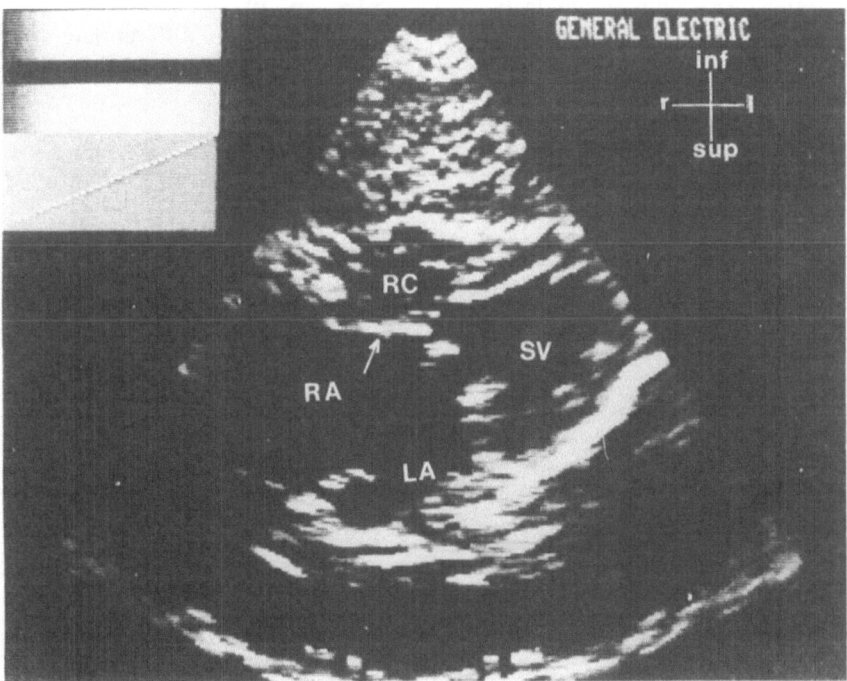

Fig. 2. A subcostal view shows a rim of interatrial septum and a single AV valve which overrides the partitioning between a single ventricle (SV) which was of right ventricular type and a small inferiorly placed blind rudimentary chamber (RC). The portion of the AV orifice opening towards the rudimentary chamber is denoted by a single arrow.

structures characteristic of left ventricular versus right ventricular morphology. The major advance in regard to echo imaging of rudimentary
chambers is the use of subcostal and apex echo views since the outflow or
rudimentary chambers often lie relatively high on the cardiac silhouette. With
these new views these chambers can be identified whether in right- or left-
sided position. Of the 33 rudimentary outlet chambers giving rise to a great
artery, 31 have been identified by using 2D echocardiography. In these
situations the lower division between the main chamber and the outlet chamber (inferior to the outlet foramen), the trabecular portion of the septum, can
be imaged (Fig. 3). The infundibular septum between the great arteries can
likewise be identified. Figure 4 shows a short-axis scan in a patient where this
identification has been achieved. The two outflow chambers which were
missed were both missed in patients with univentricular heart of the right
ventricular type in which the rudimentary chamber was posterior and somewhat inferior in position. Nonetheless one of the two blind trabecular pouches of left ventricular type was identified echocardiographically (Fig. 5) and
is shown as imaged inferiorly at the level of the AV groove and posteriorly.

When two-dimensional echos in the 44 patients were reviewed in coded
fashion, blinded as to patient's diagnosis in an attempt to differentiate uni-

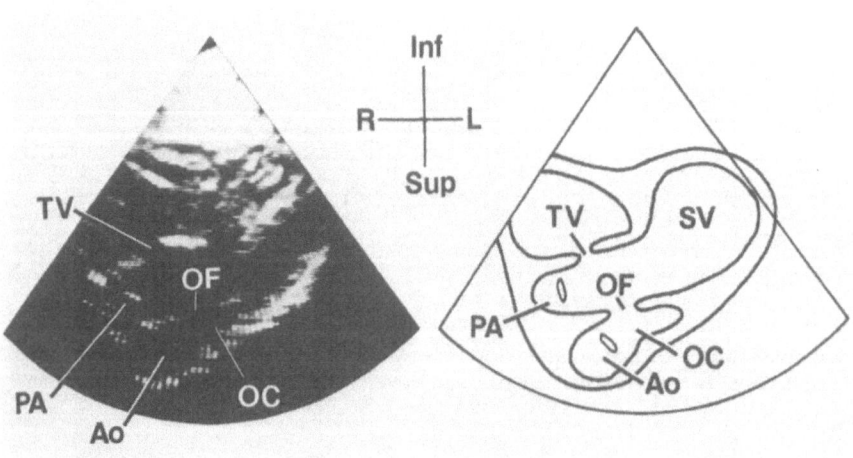

Fig. 3. A subcostal view shows a single ventricle (SV) and imaging of the outlet foramen (OF) and
the outlet chamber (OC). The portion of ventricular septum lying to the left of the outlet foramen
is trabecular septum, the portion separating the aorta (Ao) which arises from the outlet chamber
from the pulmonary artery (PA) is outlet or infundibular septum: Inf, inferior; Sup, superior;
R, right; L, left.

229

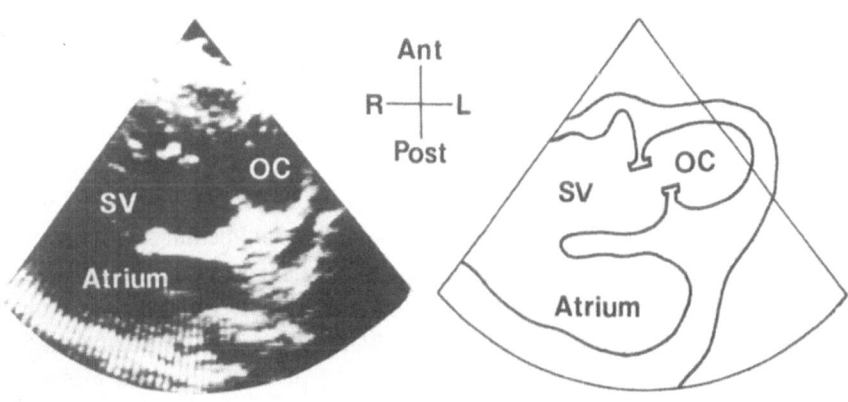

Fig. 4. A leftward anterior outlet chamber (OC) is visualised in short-axis section: Ant, anterior; Post, posterior; R, right; L, left.

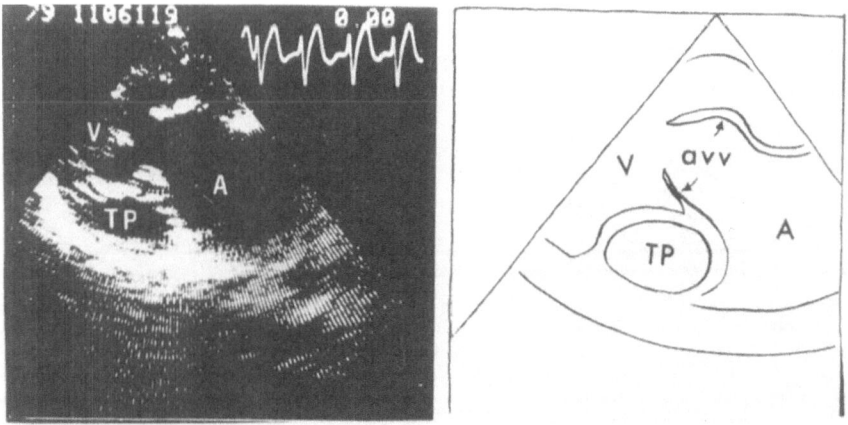

Fig. 5. A posteriorly inferiorly located blind trabecular pouch (TP) is seen at the level of the AV valve (avv) between the single ventricular cavity (V) and the atrial cavity (A). It lies on the AV ring at the crux of the heart and was a blind trabecular pouch of left ventricular type in a patient with univentricular heart of right ventricular type. The foramen providing communication into the blind trabecular pouch was visualised in another plane.

ventricular heart of the right ventricular type by assessing main chamber trabeculation, this distinction could be made in only one case. Nonetheless, in univentricular heart of the left ventricular type, the trabeculation of the outflow chamber as shown in Figure 6 was often so significantly more coarse than that in the main chamber that the correct diagnosis as to chamber type could also be achieved. Figure 6 shows an outlet chamber rotated somewhat posteriorly with the coarse trabecular pattern clearly identifying it as right ventricular type when compared with the smoother trabecular pattern in the main chamber which is not seen. The location of the outflow chamber as pointed out by Anderson et al. [7] is also useful in this regard. In univentricular heart of left ventricular type, the outlet or rudimentary chamber (a right ventricular outflow tract analog) is located high on the cardiac silhouette and does not come to the crux of the heart. In univentricular hearts of right ventricular type, the rudimentary chamber lies low on the cardiac silhouette at the level of the AV groove and the septum comes to the crux of the heart. We have found this distinction quite useful in evaluating patients with these malformations as shown in Figure 5.

Another anatomical structure which can be visualised in many of these patients with high resolution instruments as shown in Figure 7 is the posteromedial muscle bundle which comes down the posterior wall of univentricular hearts of the left ventricular type. It is indeed a remnant of the inlet septum

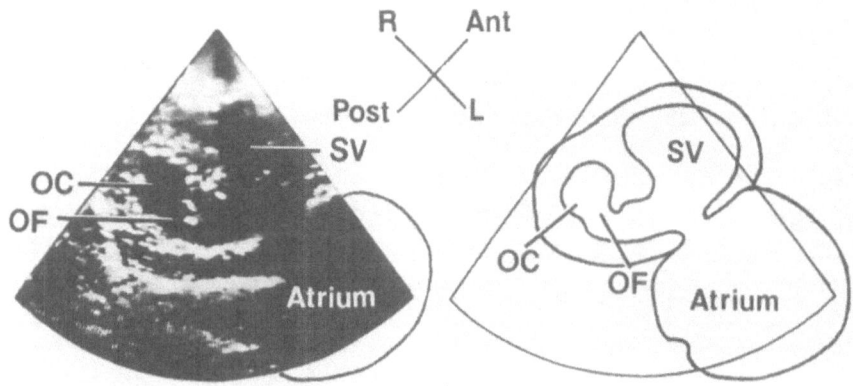

Fig. 6. In this patient whose heart was quite rotated, the outlet chamber (OC) communicating with the main chamber (SV) by the outlet foramen (OF) appears posteriorly located; but it is coarsely trabeculated and its superior location corresponded with an autopsy diagnosis of single ventricle of left ventricular type. The suggestion that the outlet chamber was of right ventricular morphology can be made by its coarse trabecular pattern on the echocardiogram.

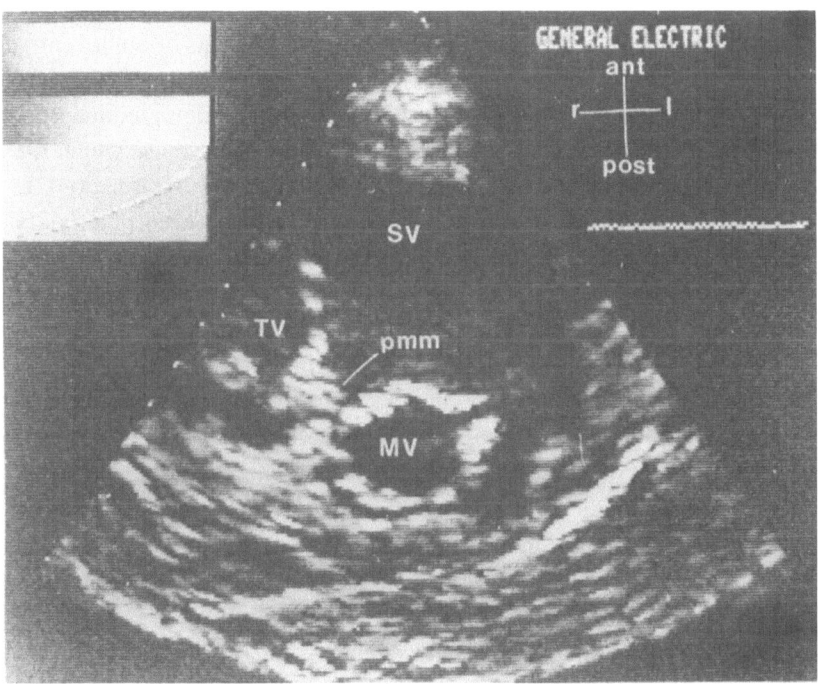

Fig. 7. In this patient, in short-axis section a single ventricle (SV) of left ventricular type with two AV valves is imaged. The left-sided mitral valve (MV) on the right side of the image has a fish-mouth-shaped orifice. Two leaflets of the right-sided tricuspid valve (TV) are visualised on the left side of the image. Between the two AV orifices the single arrow delineates the posterior medial muscle (pmm) which was quite prominent in this patient and is a remnant of the inlet septum.

posteriorly and it lies between the AV orifices. In short-axis scans it appears to be no more than an exaggerated posterior fold, an easily identified structure which should not be confused with ventricular septum.

A METHOD FOR TWO-DIMENSIONAL ECHO EVALUATION OF UNIVENTRICULAR HEARTS

Based on our observations and anatomical considerations, we recommend the following echo methodology:
1) The two-dimensional echocardiographic examination should consist of attempting to define with as many views as possible [6] the number of AV valves and the AV valve relationships, those connections which are absent or those valves which straddle and/or override the septum. The definition of chordal structures is helpful for distinguishing papillary muscle structures at the apex of the heart from true septation.

232

2) The rudimentary chambers and their separation in terms of bulboventri-cular or trabecular septation should be imaged by searching high on the cardiac silhouette as well as at the level of AV groove for those rudimentary outflow chambers which give rise to great arteries and those which are blind trabecular pouches. The great arteries may be distinguished on 2D echo by the characteristic bifurcation pattern of the imaged pulmonary artery which distinguishes the vast majority of these patients in whom the pulmonary artery arises posteriorly from the main chamber in the face of the transposed great artery orientation.

3) With regard to distinguishing the type of morphology, trabeculation may be useful, i.e. if the rudimentary chamber has a trabecular pattern which is significantly more coarse than that of the main chamber, univentricular heart of the LV type may be suggested. Also identification of the postero-medial muscle bundle is of assistance in finding univentricular heart of the LV type. Of additional assistance is the position of the posterior rudimentary chamber. With a septum coming to the crux of the heart and with a low outlet foramen, this suggests univentricular heart of right ventricular type. Superiorly located rudimentary chambers with high out-let foramen are almost routinely identified in the univentricular hearts of the left ventricular type.

THE ROLE OF TWO-DIMENSIONAL ECHOCARDIOGRAPHY

It is unlikely that two-dimensional echocardiography will replace angio-graphy in analysis of these malformations, especially with the new angled or hemiaxial angiographic views. Angiography is still quite superior for the imaging of the trabecular pattern of chambers, position of the outlet chamber and great vessel orientation. Two-dimensional echocardiography does, how-ever, have a significant role in this area for screening patients and providing definitive and accurate precatheterisation diagnosis. Two-dimensional echocardiography remains superior to angiography in defining AV con-nections [5] and anatomical relationship of those AV valves present to the septation of the main chamber and outlet chamber. Two-dimensional echo-cardiography appears to have an additional place in the definition of AV valve function where Doppler techniques can suggest which AV valve is insuf-ficient by specific interrogation of the area behind the AV valve by using two-dimensional range gating techniques.

Finally echo contrast injections performed with two-dimensional scanning aid in the evaluation of anatomy and function of the AV valves.

SUMMARY

The combined use of two-dimensional echocardiography with contrast injections or Doppler interrogation represents a unique way to define the inflow patterns, the structure and function of AV valves and the outflow patterns in the patient with univentricular heart. Combined with increased resolution for evaluating septation as described in this chapter, two-dimensional echocardiography appears to provide information which is highly complimentary to angiographic evaluation in these patients. Two-dimensional echocardiography therefore has significant utility for the evaluation of patients with univentricular heart.

REFERENCES

1. Bini BM, Bloom KR, Culham JAG, Freedom RM, William CM, Rowe RD: The reliability and practicality of single crystal echocardiography in the evaluation of single ventricle. Angiographic and pathological correlates. Circulation 57:269, 1978.
2. Felner JM, Brewer DB, Franch RH: Echocardiographic manifestations of single ventricle. Am J Cardiol 38:80, 1976.
3. Seward JB, Tajik AJ, Hagler DJ, Guilani ER, Gau GT, Ritter DG: Echocardiogram in common (single) ventricle: angiographic-anatomic correlation. Am J Cardiol 39:217, 1977.
4. Seward JB, Tajik AJ, Hagler DJ, Ritter DG: Contrast echocardiography in single or common ventricle. Circulation 53:513, 1977.
5. Picchio FM, Freedom RN, Harder JR, Moes CAF, Duncan WJ: Comprehensive assessment of atrio-ventricular valve morphology in single ventricle [abstr]. Am J Cardiol 45:428, 1980.
6. Goldberg SJ, Allen HD, Sahn DJ: Pediatric and adolescent echocardiography, 2nd edn. Chicago, Year Book Medical, 1980.
7. Anderson RH, Tynan M, Freedom RM, Quero-Jimenez M, McCartney FJ, Shinebourne EA, Wilkinson JL, Becker AE: Ventricular morphology in the univentricular heart. Herz 4:184, 1979.

INDEX

BOERHAAVE SERIES
FOR POSTGRADUATE
MEDICAL EDUCATION

1. Hemker HC, Loeliger EA, Veltkamp JJ, eds: Human blood coagulation. Biochemistry, clinical investigation, therapy. 1969 ISBN 90-6021-008-5
2. Goslings WRO, ed: Diseases of the gastro-intestinal tract. Some diagnostic, therapeutic and fundamental aspects. 1970. ISBN 90-6021-011-5
3. Haas JH de, Hemker HC, Snellen HA, eds: Ischaemic heart disease. 1970. ISBN 90-6021-012-3
4. Gevers RH, Ruys JH, eds: Physiology and pathology in the perinatal period. 1971. ISBN 90-6021-100-6
5. Elkerbout F, Thomas P, Zwaveling A, eds: Cancer chemotherapy. *Out of print*
6. Stoelinga GBA, Van der Werff ten Bosch JJ, eds: Normal and abnormal development of brain and behaviour. 1971. ISBN 90-6021-099-9
7. Spierdijk J, Feldman SA, eds: Anaesthesia and pharmaceutics. 1972. ISBN 90-6021-125-1
8. Snellen HA, Hemker HC, Hugenholtz PG, van Bemmel JH, eds: Quantitation in cardiology. 1972. ISBN 90-6021-139-1
9. Feldman SA, Leigh JM, Spierdijk J, eds: Measurement in anaesthesia. 1974. ISBN 90-6021-203-7
10. Hemker HC, Veltkamp JJ, eds: Prothrombin and related coagulation factors, 1975. ISBN 90-6021-236-3
11. Went LN, Vermeij-Keers C, van der Linden AGJM, eds: Early diagnosis and prevention of genetic diseases. 1975. ISBN 90-6021-237-1
12. Spierdijk J, Feldman SA, Mattie H, eds: Anaesthesia and pharmacology. With a special section on professional hazards. 1976. ISBN 90-6021-294-0
13. van Mierop LHS, Oppenheimer-Dekker A, Bruins CLDC, eds: Embryology and teratology of the heart and the great arteries. Conducting system; transposition of the great arteries; ductus arteriosus. 1978. ISBN 90-6021-424-2
14. de Wolff FA, Mattie H, Breimer DD, eds: Therapeutic relevance of drug assays. 1979. ISBN 90-6021-443-9
15. Keirse MJNC, Anderson ABM, Bennebroek Gravenhorst J, eds: Human parturition. 1979. ISBN 90-6021-445-5
16. van Oosterom AT, Muggia FM, Cleton FJ, eds: Therapeutic progress in ovarian cancer, testicular cancer and the sarcomas. 1980. ISBN 90-6021-452-8
17. van den Tweel JG, Taylor CR, Bosman FT, eds: Malignant lymphoproliferative diseases. 1980. ISBN 90-6021-451-X
18. Welvaart K, Blumgart LH, Kreuning J, eds: Colorectal Cancer. 1980. ISBN 90-6021-465-X
19. Daems WT, Burger EH, Afzelius BA, eds: Cell biological aspects of disease. The plasma membrane and lysosomes. 1981. ISBN 90-6021-466-8
20. Pauwels EK, Schütte HE, Taconis WK, Ell PJ, eds: Bone scintigraphy. 1981. ISBN 90-6021-476-5